DRUG DEVELOPMENT

MOLECULAR TARGETS FOR GI DISEASES

DRUG DEVELOPMENT

MOLECULAR TARGETS FOR *GI* DISEASES

Edited by

TIMOTHY S. GAGINELLA

School of Pharmacy, University of Wisconsin
Madison, WI

and

ANTONIO GUGLIETTA

Parke-Davis Pharmaceutical Research Division
Ann Arbor, MI

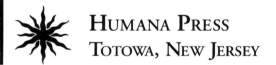

HUMANA PRESS
TOTOWA, NEW JERSEY

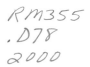

RM355
.D78
2000

Library of Congress Cataloging-in-Publication Data

Drug development : molecular targets for gastrointestinal diseases /
    edited by Timothy S. Gaginella and Antonio Guglietta.
        p.   cm.
    Includes bibliographical references and index.
    ISBN 0-89603-589-1 (alk. paper)
    1. Gastrointestinal agents. 2. Molecular pharmacology. 3. Drug
development. I. Gaginella, Timothy S. II . Guglietta, Antonio.
    RM355.D78   2000
    615'.73--dc21   99-35348
                                                        CIP

PREFACE

The application of molecular techniques to gastroenterology continues to yield important advances in the development of drugs to treat gastrointestinal disorders. Important new drugs have emerged through the collaborative and complementary efforts of basic scientists, clinicians, and clinical researchers in academia and the pharmaceutical industry. The challenge has been exciting, with a few surprises along the way. Consider peptic ulcer disease as an example. The discovery of H_2 receptors and the availability of potent and selective H_2-receptor antagonists signaled the beginning of a new era in the treatment of gastric hypersecretory states and peptic ulcers. Introduction of proton pump inhibitors offered another therapeutic option. Though H_2-receptor antagonists and proton pump inhibitors are important and useful drugs, the discovery of the link between *H. pylori* infection and peptic ulcer disease has led to even more effective pharmacotherapeutic regimens. Our intent in *Drug Development: Molecular Targets for GI Diseases* is to bring together hands-on experts to review promising areas of gastrointestinal pharmacology. The contemporary topics covered, from a mechanistic viewpoint, are relevant to gastrointestinal inflammation and motility disorders. Authoritative opinions are offered on both future research directions and potential applications for new therapies.

Although each chapter in *Drug Development: Molecular Targets for GI Diseases* stands alone, many of the experimental approaches and concepts that move drug development forward are interrelated. Just as the response of the gut at any instant depends upon the net effect of a multiplicity of mediators, so the reader may capture key ideas from several or all chapters and integrate them into his or her own research. The issues are complex, and at this time our understanding in many areas covered here remains incomplete.

For example, some arachidonic acid metabolites are clearly important for maintaining normal gastrointestinal functions, whereas others are deleterious and offer opportunities for therapeutic intervention. In this regard cyclooxygenase-2 inhibitors are currently promoted as "safer" nonsteroidal anti-inflammatory drugs, but as pointed out in Chapter 1, these drugs may worsen existing mucosal ulcers. Likewise, nitric oxide has both beneficial and injurious effects on the gut mucosa. The complexities of the nitric oxide pathway, with discussion of the roles of constitutive and inducible nitric oxide synthase, are presented in Chapter 2. The interplay among cytokines and other mediators of inflammation has a profound influence on the severity of inflammatory bowel disease. Chapter 3 provides an in-depth review of these pivotal regulators of immune function, in the context of new opportunities for pharmacotherapy. Maintenance and protection of the mucosa is influenced by a variety of peptide growth factors. The strengths and weaknesses of these agents as potential new gastrointestinal drugs is discussed in detail in Chapter 4. Peptides classified as tachykinins, particularly substance P and neurokinins, affect gut secretion, motility, and immune and vascular functions. Blocking or potentiating the effects of these mediators may be useful in disorders associated with altered gastrointestinal inflammation, secretion, and motility. Potential novel therapies involving tachykinins are presented in Chapter 5. The importance of cholecystokinin receptors as targets for new peptide and nonpeptide drugs is discussed in Chapter 6. Gut motility is greatly influenced by serotonin (5-hydroxytryptamine [5-HT]), and the existence of several subtypes of the 5-HT receptor offers the hope that subtype-selective 5-HT receptor agonists and antagonists might emerge as new anti-emetics and novel modulators of gut motility. Research in this area is discussed in Chapter 7.

Much of classical pharmacology was founded on the characterization of opiate actions on isolated strips of gut muscle. Subsequent research showed that opiates and opiate-like drugs could influence intestinal fluid secretion. The fact that multiple subtypes of opioid receptors reside in the gut supports the notion expressed in Chapter 8 that novel, selective drugs to act at such sites might be developed for treating diarrhea, certain motility disorders, and visceral pain. Finally, the discovery of H_3 receptors and the possibility that H_3-receptor agonists might find utility in treating gut inflammation or pain is reviewed in Chapter 9. Sadly, Giulio Bertaccini died before completion of the book. He was a pioneer in gastrointestinal pharmacology and a prolific contributor to the literature.

It is our hope that this book will stimulate further interest in bringing to light new, more effective drugs for treating gastrointestinal disorders.

This work would not have been possible without the efforts of the authors, and the support from our families, to whom we are grateful.

T. S. Gaginella
A. Guglietta

CONTENTS

CONTRIBUTORS

GIULIO BERTACCINI • *Institute of Pharmacology, School of Medicine, University of Parma, Parma, Italy (deceased)*

MICHEL R. BRIEJER • *Pharmacology Section, Yamanouchi Europe, The Netherlands*

GABRIELLA CORUZZI • *Institute of Pharmacology, School of Medicine, University of Parma, Parma, Italy*

MASSIMO D'AMATO • *Department of Clinical Pharmacology, Rotta Research Laboratorium SpA, Monza (MI), Italy*

CLAUDIO FIOCCHI • *Division of Gastroenterology, University Hospitals of Cleveland, Case Western Reserve University School of Medicine, Cleveland, OH*

ANTONIO GUGLIETTA • *Parke-Davis Pharmaceutical Research Division, Warner-Lambert Company, Ann Arbor, MI*

PETER HOLZER • *Department of Experimental and Clinical Pharmacology, University of Graz, Graz, Austria*

JEAN-LOUIS JUNIEN • *Ferring SA, Paris, France*

ALAN D. LEVINE • *Division of Gastroenterology, University Hospitals of Cleveland, Case Western Reserve University School of Medicine, Cleveland, OH*

FRANCESCO MAKOVEC • *Department of Preclinical Pharmacology, Rotta Research Laboratorium SpA, Monza (MI), Italy*

GIUSEPPINA MORINI • *Institute of Pharmacology, School of Medicine, University of Parma, Parma, Italy*

ENZO POLI • *Institute of Pharmacology, School of Medicine, University of Parma, Parma, Italy*

PIERRE J. M. RIVIÈRE • *Ferring Research Institute Inc., San Diego, CA*

LUCIO C. ROVATI, *Department of Clinical Pharmacology, Rotta Research Laboratorium SpA, Monza (MI), Italy*

SUSHIL K. SARNA • *Departments of Surgery and Physiology, Medical College of Wisconsin and Zablocki VA Medical Center, Milwaukee, WI*

JAN A. J. SCHUURKES • *Department of Gastrointestinal Pharmacology, Janssen Research Foundation, Beerse, Belgium*

B. L. TEPPERMAN • *Department of Physiology, University of Western Ontario, London, Ontario, Canada*

MARIJA VELJAČA • *PLIVA d.d. Research Institute, Zagreb, Croatia.*

JOHN L. WALLACE • *Department of Pharmacology and Therapeutics, University of Calgary, Calgary, Alberta, Canada*

B. J. R. WHITTLE • *The William Harvey Research Institute, St. Bartholomew's and the Royal London School of Medicine and Dentistry, London, UK*

1   The Arachidonic Acid Pathway

New Molecules and Enzymes

John L. Wallace

CONTENTS

1. INTRODUCTION

Arachidonic acid can be liberated from membrane phospholipids via the action of phospholipase A_2 or phospholipase C. The liberated arachidonic acid can then be metabolized via several enzymes to yield a vast array of vasoactive and immunomodulatory substances, termed "eicosanoids" (Fig. 1). Included in this group are the prostaglandins (PGs), leukotrienes (LTs) and thromboxanes (TXs). In general, eicosanoids have a short half-life (seconds to minutes), and act in a paracrine or autocrine manner. The enzymes that catalyze the formation of eicosanoids have been well characterized, and several new drugs have been

From: *Drug Development: Molecular Targets for GI Diseases*
Edited by: T. S. Gaginella and A. Guglietta © Humana Press Inc., Totowa, NJ

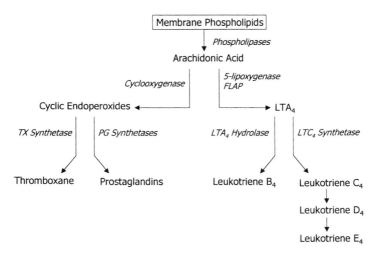

Fig. 1. Schematic diagram of the arachidonic acid cascade. Each of the enzymes shown represent potential targets for anti-inflammatory drugs, and selective inhibitors have been developed.

developed that inhibit their activity. In addition, the receptors for the eicosanoids have been identified and specific antagonists have been developed as potential therapies for a number of inflammatory conditions. This subject has been reviewed in detail by Halushka et al. (1989). In this chapter, the biological actions of the eicosanoids are reviewed, as are the enzymes through which they are formed, and the receptors through which they act. The potential of drugs that block the activity of these enzymes or the eicosanoid receptors is reviewed, particularly with respect to their potential utility in the treatment of inflammatory diseases of the gastrointestinal (GI) tract.

2. PROSTAGLANDINS

PGs are 20-carbon fatty acids produced from arachidonic acid through the actions of the enzyme. cyclo-oxygenase (COX) (Fig. 1). It is now clear that there are at least two isoforms of COX, and selective inhibitors of each have been developed. This is discussed in more detail below. The recognition of the ability of PGs to reduce or prevent GI injury induced by topical irritants, or cytoprotection (Robert et al., 1976), resulted in an explosion of research into the physiological roles of these substances in GI mucosal defense. It is now well established that suppression of PG synthesis, through inhibition of COX, is a key component of the mechanism underlying gastric ulceration caused by nonsteroidal anti-inflammatory drugs (NSAIDs) (Vane, 1971; Wallace, 1993), as well as the ability of these drugs to exacerbate mucosal injury (Kaufmann and Taubin, 1987; Wallace et al., 1992b). Although the mechanism through which PGs exert their cytoprotective actions has never been firmly established, it is known that these substances can stimulate mucus and bicarbonate secretion, maintain mucosal blood flow, and, through mechanisms that are not yet fully understood, enhance the resistance of epithelial cells to injury induced by cytotoxins (Wallace, 1997). PGs also exert a number of anti-inflammatory effects. This is exemplified by the fact that NSAIDs can greatly exacerbate mucosal inflammation in animal models of colitis (Woolverton et al., 1989; Wallace et al., 1992b; Reuter et al., 1996), and in human inflammatory bowel disease (IBD) (Kaufmann and Taubin, 1987).

The GI mucosa contains a substantial number of immunocytes, including mast cells, macrophages, neutrophils, and eosinophils. The number of these cells varies considerably along the length of the GI tract, to some extent reflecting the bacterial load in the lumen of each region. As in other external mucosae (e.g., skin, lungs, urogenital tract), some of these immunocytes play an important role in signaling the entry into the lamina propria of foreign material or antigens. These cells typically release soluble mediators (including eicosanoids) and cytokines which initiate an inflammatory response aimed at limiting the entry of the foreign matter into the systemic circulation. These mediators act on several targets. Some increase the permeability of the vascular endothelium, thereby permitting plasma exudation, and facilitating the movement of antibodies into the interstitium. Some inflammatory mediators also increase expression of adhesion molecules on the vascular endothelium and/or circulating leukocytes, thereby facilitating the recruitment of the white blood cells to a site of injury or infection. Many inflammatory mediators are chemotaxins; that is, after extravasating, the leukocytes will migrate up a concentration gradient of these chemicals, toward the source of their release. Some inflammatory mediators are also capable of priming or stimulating leukocytes, to release reactive oxygen metabolites, proteases, or other inflammatory mediators.

One of the mechanisms through which PGs downregulate inflammatory responses is through modulation of the activity of mucosal immunocytes. For example, effects of PGs or PG synthesis inhibitors on tumor necrosis factor (TNF-α) release from macrophages have been very well characterized. Prostaglandin E_2 (PGE$_2$) has been shown to be a potent suppressor of TNF-α release from macrophages (Kunkel et al., 1986b), and also reduces expression of the gene for TNF-α in these cells (Kunkel et al., 1988). NSAIDs, on the other hand, increase the release of TNF-α from macrophages and other cells (Martich et al., 1991; Spatafora et al., 1991; Santucci et al., 1994). For example, administration of indomethacin, at doses that caused gastric mucosal injury in rats, resulted in marked increases in serum TNF-α levels (Santucci et al., 1994; Appleyard et al., 1996). In humans given bacterial endotoxin, prior administration of an NSAID significantly increased the release of TNF-α into the systemic circulation (Martich et al., 1991). PGs also regulate the release of other cytokines, such as interleukin-1, from macrophages (Kunkel and Chensue, 1985; Kunkel et al., 1986a), and are able to suppress the release of other eicosanoids, such as leukotriene B_4 (LTB$_4$), from activated neutrophils (Ham et al., 1983; Haurand and Floh, 1989).

The anti-inflammatory effects of PGs may also be mediated via inhibition of mast cell degranulation. Raud et al. (1990) demonstrated that PGs could partially suppress acute mast cell-dependent inflammation; Hogaboam et al. (1993), using isolated mast cells from both the peritoneum and the intestinal mucosa, demonstrated that PGE$_2$ inhibited, in a dose-dependent manner, the release of platelet-activating factor (PAF), histamine, and TNF-α. These effects were observed at very low (i.e., picomolar) concentrations. For example, with the PGE$_1$ analog, misoprostol, PAF release from peritoneal mast cells was inhibited at concentrations as low as 10^{-10} molar, while PGE$_2$ suppressed TNF-α release from peritoneal mast cells at concentrations as low as 10^{-11} M.

In addition to acting on immunocytes that are resident within the lamina propria, and thereby decreasing the intensity of an inflammatory response, PGs can inhibit the recruitment of leukocytes from the vasculature (Fig. 2). Because infiltrating leukocytes can cause considerable mucosal injury in some circumstances, this effect of PGs may be

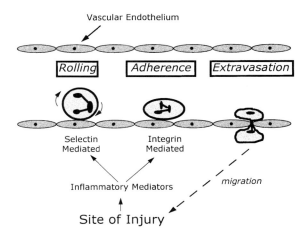

Fig. 2. Key events in the extravasation of leukocytes in response to tissue injury. Inflammatory mediators, including several of the eicosanoids, influence each step of the extravasation and migration process. PGs, particularly PGI_2 and PGE_2, are capable of suppressing most of the adhesive interactions that are depicted, as well as the activation of leukocytes to release free radicals and various enzymes.

one of the underlying mechanisms for the protective effects of these substances in experimental models of mucosal ulceration (e.g., ischemia-reperfusion [Hernandez et al., 1987], NSAID gastropathy [Wallace and Granger, 1992], colitis [Grisham and Granger, 1988; Wallace et al., 1992a]). As mentioned, neutrophils are recruited to a site of injury by the chemotaxins released from immunocytes within the lamina propria. The inflammatory response can also be amplified by the infiltrating neutrophils, because these cells have the capacity to release chemotaxins, such as LTB_4. Once again, PGs serve an important modulatory role by downregulating several neutrophil functions that contribute to inflammation and injury. For example, PGs can suppress the generation of reactive oxygen metabolites, which account for much of the tissue injury caused by neutrophils (Wong et al., 1981; Gryglewski et al., 1987), and the release of the chemotaxins, LTB_4 and interleukin-8 (Ham et al., 1983; Haurand and Floh, 1989; Wertheim et al., 1993). The observation that NSAIDs increase the numbers of neutrophils adhering to the vascular endothelium, and that this can be prevented by administering exogenous PGs (Asako et al., 1992a; 1992b), suggests that PGs are important physiological regulators of neutrophil adherence.

3. LEUKOTRIENES

The rate-limiting step in the synthesis of LTs from arachidonic acid is the enzyme 5-lipoxygenase (5-LO) (Fig. 1). This activity of this enzyme is in turn dependent on the activation of another protein, named 5-lipoxygenase-activating protein (FLAP), which appears to be involved in the translocation of 5-LO from the cytosol to the membranes from which arachidonic acid is liberated (Miller et al., 1990). The LTs can be conveniently subdivided into two main subclasses: LTB_4 and the peptido-leukotrienes (LTC_4, LTD_4, and LTE_4). As the name suggests, the peptido-LTs include amino acid moieties. LTs are produced chiefly by immunocytes, although there is some evidence for their production by epithelial and endothelial cells as well. In the mucosa, the mast cell appears to be the major source of peptido-LTs; the neutrophil appears to be the predominant source of LTB_4.

LTB_4 is a potent chemotaxin, particularly for neutrophils, and is able to prime a number of different types of immunocytes to secrete other vasoactive and immunomodulatory factors. LTB_4 exerts little, if any, effect on vascular permeability and mucosal blood flow, but can promote the recruitment of leukocytes from the vasculature (Gimbrone et al., 1984) by upregulating the expression on their surface of the β_2-integrins, CD11/CD18 (Lindstrom et al., 1990). LTB_4 can also stimulate neutrophils to release reactive oxygen metabolites, which contribute to tissue injury associated with mucosal inflammation (Schultz et al., 1991). Intra-arterial administration of LTB_4 does not alter the susceptibility of the rat stomach to damage induced by an irritant, but LTB_4 has been suggested to contribute to the pathogenesis of NSAID-induced gastric damage (Asako et al., 1992a; Hudson et al., 1993), probably through its ability to promote leukocyte adherence to the vascular endothelium. This process has been suggested to be an important event in the pathogenesis of NSAID-induced gastric damage (Wallace and Granger, 1992). Administration of LTB_4 receptor antagonists and inhibitors of 5-LO results in attenuation of NSAID-induced leukocyte adherence (Asako et al., 1992a), and a reduction in the severity of NSAID-induced mucosal damage (Vaananen et al., 1992). LTB_4 has also been suggested to play a role in promoting the leukocyte adherence to vascular endothelial cells that can be induced by water extracts of cultured *Helicobacter pylori* (Yoshida et al., 1993).

In contrast to LTB$_4$, the peptido-LTs exhibit little chemotactic activity, but they are potent stimulators of smooth muscle contraction, and are also capable of markedly increasing the permeability of the vascular endothelial lining of blood vessels (Ford-Hutchinson, 1990). Moreover, peptido-LTs have been shown to increase the expression of P-selectin on endothelial cells (Kanwar et al., 1995), thereby promoting the rolling (and subsequent extravasation) of leukocytes. Intra-arterial infusion of peptido-LTs can profoundly increase the susceptibility of the rat stomach to injury induced by topical irritants (Wallace et al., 1990), which is probably related to the vasoconstrictor properties of these substances, and could be blocked by pretreating the animals with a LTD$_4$ receptor antagonist.

One of the principal sources of peptido-LTs in the GI mucosa is the mast cell. Therefore, antigenic activation of mast cells leads to the release of peptido-LTs (Befus et al., 1988), and to effects on various target cells that are probably mediated by these substances. For example, the peptido-LTs have been implicated as mediators of the gastric damage associated with antigenic activation of mucosal mast cells (Rioux et al., 1994). Administration of an antigen to which rats had previously been sensitized resulted in a significant increase in the extent of damage induced by a topically applied irritant. Pretreatment of the rats with a LTD$_4$ receptor antagonist prevented this injury. Peptido-LTs have also been suggested to mediate the intestinal damage (Perdue et al., 1989) and the motor disturbances (Scott and Maric, 1991) associated with mucosal mast cell activation.

4. THROMBOXANE

TX is the major eicosanoid produced by platelet (via COX-1), which accounts for about 95% of serum TX levels. The neutrophil can also synthesize this substance, although in much smaller amounts (Higgs et al., 1985). In addition to being a potent stimulus for platelet aggregation, TX is a powerful vasoconstrictor. Because any reduction in mucosal blood flow can render the mucosa more susceptible to injury, it has been suggested that TX is an important contributor to the pathogenesis of ulceration in the GI tract. TX also has the capacity to stimulate LTB_4 release and the adherence of leukocytes to the vascular endothelium (Goldman et al., 1991), and therefore may contribute to mucosal injury throughout the GI tract via amplification of inflammatory responses.

The first evidence to support a role for TX in gastric mucosal defense was reported by Whittle et al. (1981), who showed that close-arterial administration of arachidonic acid into the dog gastric microcirculation resulted in a profound reduction of gastric blood flow. This effect was shown to be attributable to generation of TX from the arachidonic acid. Later, the same group (Whittle et al., 1985) demonstrated similar effects on gastric blood flow with a TX mimetic, and further demonstrated that the susceptibility of the gastric mucosa to injury could be profoundly increased by administration of this mimetic.

With the development of inhibitors of TX synthesis (blockers of TX synthetase), a number of studies were undertaken to determine the contribution of TX to mucosal injury in experimental models of gastric and colonic injury. For example, TX synthase inhibitors were shown to reduce the severity of gastric damage induced by bile salts (Konturek et al., 1983; Walt et al., 1987), ethanol, or indomethacin (Whittle, 1984). Given that indomethacin itself will block TX synthesis, however, it is difficult to implicate TX in the pathogenesis of that particular type of injury. This suggests that the TX synthase inhibitor used in that study may have reduced damage through a nonspecific effect. In support of this, Whittle (1984) showed that greatly reducing the capacity for TX synthesis, by rendering rats thrombocytopenic, did not alter the susceptibility of the stomach to damage induced by ethanol or indomethacin. Very few clinical studies have been performed to evaluate the role of TX in ulcer disease. Hawkey (1986) reported that there were no changes in TX levels in gastric tissue taken from ulcer patients vs controls, irrespective of where the biopsy was taken (at or distant to the ulcer site), or the presence or absence of inflammation at the biopsy site.

TX has also been implicated as a mediator of damage in the small intestine. Boughton-Smith et al. (1989) reported that endotoxin-induced damage in the jejunum was associated with markedly elevated TX and PAF synthesis. TX synthetase inhibitors were able to attenuate both the production of TX and the tissue injury, without affecting PAF synthesis. Bannerjee and Peters (1990) reported that selective inhibitors of TX synthetase were able to reduce the severity of indomethacin-induced small intestinal injury (epithelial permeability) and inflammation (granulocyte infiltration). However, the dose of indomethacin used to induce injury would itself cause a marked suppression of TX synthesis. It is surprising, given the availability of a number of selective TX receptor antagonists, that these agents have not been employed to further delineate the contribution of TX to the pathogenesis of GI mucosal injury.

5. GI-SPARING ANTI-INFLAMMATORY DRUGS

NSAIDs are among the most prescribed drugs in the world, and are also widely used in over-the-counter preparations. The first NSAID, aspirin, was first commercialized at the end of the nineteenth century. Since that time, dozens of more potent NSAIDs have been marketed. NSAIDs are used primarily for their anti-inflammatory, analgesic, and antipyretic effects, although, more recently, aspirin has been used increasingly for prevention of myocardial infarction and stroke. Although widely used, these drugs are not entirely safe, with well-documented toxicity in the GI tract and kidney.

The discovery, 5 yr ago, of a second isoform of the COX enzyme (Xie et al., 1991; Kujubu et al., 1991) confirmed a theory first suggested in 1972 that there is more than one form of COX (Flower and Vane, 1972). This discovery has led to a re-evaluation of the role of this enzyme in producing PGs in various circumstances. There is now a widely held belief that the PGs produced under normal circumstances, which play such an important role in modulating blood flow and such mucosal defense factors as mucus secretion, are derived from the constitutively expressed isoform, COX-1. PGs produced in the context of inflammation, on the other hand, are thought to be derived from the inducible isoform, COX-2 (Xie et al., 1992). This theory has been somewhat oversimplified to the following: COX-1 produces the PGs that perform beneficial functions, COX-2 produces PGs that exert pro-inflammatory effects. This hypothesis underlies the considerable resources being invested in the development of highly selective inhibitors of COX-2, which have been reported to exert anti-inflammatory and analgesic effects comparable to standard NSAIDs, but to lack ulcerogenic effects. However, there is considerable evidence emerging

Normal	Acute Injury or Inflammation	Ulcer
COX-1-derived PGs •mucus and bicarbonate secretion •mucosal blood flow	COX-1-derived PGs •mucus and bicarbonate secretion •mucosal blood flow	COX-1-derived PGs •unknown
COX-2-derived PGs •negligible (unknown)	COX-2-derived PGs •adaptive cytoprotection (resistance to damage induced by topical irritants)	COX-2-derived PGs •repair: cell proliferation, angiogenesis, maturation of granulation tissue

Fig. 3. Roles of PGs synthesized by COX-1 and COX-2 in gastric mucosal defense and repair in various circumstances. Note that COX-2 appears to become the more important isoform in conditions of mucosal injury.

for physiological roles for PGs produced from COX-2 (Shoda et al., 1995; Slater et al., 1995; Vinals et al., 1997; Gretzer et al., 1998), as well as some evidence that PGs produced from COX-1 contribute to inflammatory responses (Wallace et al., 1998).

Given the evidence that PGs play an important role in limiting inflammatory responses in the GI mucosa, it is perhaps not surprising that several groups have now demonstrated a crucial role for COX-2 in mucosal defense in various models of mucosal injury (Fig. 3). Studies performed recently in this laboratory provide evidence for marked upregulation of COX-2 (protein and mRNA) in the colon of the rat, following induction of colitis (Reuter et al., 1996). The vast majority of PGs produced by the inflamed colon were derived from COX-2. That these PGs were performing a vital function in terms of mucosal defense was confirmed by the finding that selective inhibitors of COX-2 exacerbated the colonic damage in this model of colitis.

There is also considerable evidence that the PGs derived from COX-2 are very important for promoting the healing of ulcers in the stomach. Administration of selective COX-2 inhibitors to rats with preexisting ulcers resulted in a marked retardation of healing (Mizuno et al., 1997; Schmassmann et al., 1998). These studies raise serious concerns about the widespread use of selective COX-2 inhibitors by patients at risk of ulcer disease (i.e., the elderly), particularly when one considers that the majority of these patients do not experience symptoms related to the ulcer, and therefore both the patient and their physician are unaware of its presence (Pounder, 1989).

6. TREATMENT OF IBD

6.1. LTs as a Target

In the past two decades, a significant body of evidence has suggested that LTB_4 makes an important contribution to the pathogenesis of IBD. Mucosal production of LTB_4 in human and experimental colitis was reported to be markedly increased over that in the normal colon (Sharon and Stenson, 1984; Sharon and 1985; Zipser et al., 1987; Wallace et al., 1989; Wallace and Keenan, 1990a). Moreover, LTB_4 accounted for the majority of the chemotactic activity that could be extracted from inflamed human colon (Lobos et al. 1987); intracolonic administration of LTB_4 exacerbated tissue injury in a rat model of colitis (Wallace and Keenan, 1990b). Treatment of rats with colitis with inhibitors of 5-LO resulted in a significant acceleration of healing in experimental colitis (Wallace et al., 1989; Wallace and Keenan, 1990a) (Table 1). A particularly important role for LTB_4 is supported by studies demonstrating significant anti-inflammatory effects of selective LTB_4 receptor antagonists in both the rat and the cotton-top tamarin (Fretland et al., 1989, 1995). Despite these data supporting a role for LTB_4 in IBD, clinical trials of inhibitors of LT synthesis (5-LO and FLAP inhibitors) have been disappointing. Inhibitors that produced a profound suppression of LT synthesis failed to significantly modify disease severity, or produced only modest effects (Stenson et al., 1991; Bukhave et al., 1991; Roberts et al., 1997). Despite this, it would be imprudent to completely dismiss the potential utility of LT synthesis inhibitors or receptor antagonists for treatment of IBD. IBD is a complex disease with many subsets of patients. It is entirely possible that there may be subsets of patients that would respond to modulators of LT synthesis or action.

A far less compelling case can be made for a role of peptido-LT in IBD. Elevated synthesis of peptido-LT has been demonstrated in the inflamed colon of rabbits (Zipser et al., 1987) and humans (Peskar et al., 1986). A small clinical trial suggested beneficial effects of a peptido-LT receptor

Table 1
Effects of Inhibitors of Eicosanoid Synthesis or Action in Experimental Colitis

Drug	Dose (mg/kg)	Route of Administration	Target	% Reduction of leukotriene synthesis	% Reduction of severity of colitis[a]	Ref.
5-ASA	100	ip	Multiple	0	0	Wallace et al., 1989
5-ASA	100	ip	Multiple	30	45	Wallace et al., 1989
L-651,392	10	ic	5-LO	67	60	Wallace et al., 1989
MK-886	3	po	FLAP	35	31	Wallace and Keenan, 1990a
MK-886	10	po	FLAP	90	64	Wallace and Keenan, 1990a
PF-5901	50	po	FLAP	41	10	Wallace et al., 1992b
PF-5901	100	po	FLAP	82	54	Wallace et al., 1992b
SC-41930	20	ic	LTB$_4$ receptor	N/A	50	Fretland et al., 1990
OKY-1581	10	po	TX synthetase	N/A	50	Vilaseca et al., 1990
R-70416	1	po	TX synthetase	N/A	61	Vilaseca et al., 1990
Prednisone	5	im	Multiple	73	57	Vilaseca et al., 1990

[a]Semiquantitative scoring of macroscopic ± histologic damage, or measurement of tissue granulocyte numbers. ip, intraperitoneal; ic, intracolonic; po, by mouth; im, intramuscular. 5-LO, 5-lipoxygenase; FLAP, 5-lipoxygenase-activating protein; LTB$_4$, leukotriene B$_4$; TX, thromboxane, NA, not assessed.

antagonist in the treatment of ulcerative colitis (Nielsen et al., 1991), but these results have not been confirmed or extended.

6.2. TX as a Target

There is considerable interest in the possibility that TX is an important mediator of mucosal injury in IBD (particularly Crohn's disease), because of the evidence for altered thrombogenesis in these patients (Hudson et al., 1996). Impaired mucosal perfusion, as could occur when a vasoconstrictor like TX is overproduced, has been suggested to be a precipitating event in the pathogenesis of Crohn's disease (Wakefield et al., 1995). In a rat model of colitis, mucosal TX synthesis was shown to be substantially elevated (Vilaseca et al., 1990). Treatment with 5-aminosalicylate or prednisone, both of which reduced the severity of colitis, also significantly reduced TX production. Moreover, treatment with either of two TX synthetase inhibitors reduced the severity of mucosal injury. The results of trials of a dual TX synthetase inhibitor/TX receptor antagonist, ridogrel, in the treatment of ulcerative colitis have been reported in abstract form (Van Outryve et al., 1996). Once-daily rectal treatment with ridogrel produced a reduction in the severity of colitis, comparable to what could be achieved with prednisolone. In another trial, ridogrel treatment for 8 wk was found to be effective in relieving the inflammation and symptoms of mild-to-moderate ulcerative colitis, with comparable efficacy to that seen with a standard dose of 5-aminosalicylic acid (Skandalis et al., 1996). These encouraging results need to be extended by larger trials. Moreover, studies are warranted to determine the mechanism through which the TX synthetase inhibitors and TX receptor antagonists produce their beneficial effects.

7. SUMMARY

Over the past decade, knowledge of the enzymes responsible for production of a number of vasoactive and immunomodulatory factors that share arachidonic acid as a common precursor has increased considerably. The identification of these enzymes has led to the development of selective inhibitors of their activity. Given the considerable evidence of a role for various eicosanoids in both mucosal protection and injury, the emerging enzyme inhibitors are being evaluated for their potential clinical utility. Extensive characterization of the receptors for the various eicosanoids is also being carried out. Selective inhibitors or agonists of the eicosanoid receptors may offer a second approach to modulating the contribution of eicosanoids to GI defense and injury.

REFERENCES

Appleyard CB, McCafferty DM, Tigley AW, Swain MG, Wallace JL. Tumor necrosis factor mediation of NSAID-induced gastric damage: role of leukocyte adherence. *Am J Physiol* 1996; 270: G42–G48.

Asako H, Kubes P, Wallace JL, Gaginella T, Wolf RE, Granger DN. Indomethacin induced leukocyte adhesion in mesenteric venules: role of lipoxygenase products. *Am J Physiol* 1992a; 262: G903–G908.

Asako H, Kubes P, Wallace JL, Wolf RE, Granger DN. Modulation of leukocyte adhesion in rat mesenteric venules by aspirin and salicylate. *Gastroenterology* 1992b; 103: 146–152.

Banerjee AK, Peters TJ. Experimental non-steroidal anti-inflammatory drug-induced enteropathy in the rat: similarities to inflammatory bowel disease and effect of thromboxane synthetase inhibitors. *Gut* 1990; 31: 1358–1364.

Befus AD, Fujimaki H, Lee TDG, Swieter M. Mast cell polymorphism: present concepts, future directions. *Dig Dis Sci* 1988; 33: 16S–24S.

Boughton-Smith NK, Hutcheson I, Whittle BJR. Relationship between PAF-acether and thromboxane A_2 biosynthesis in endotoxin-induced intestinal damage in the rat. *Prostaglandins* 1989; 38: 319–333.

Bukhave K, Laursen LS, Lauritsen K, Rask-Masden J, Naesdal J, Jacobsen O, et al. 5-lipoxygenase inhibition in double-blind trial with zileuton: how much is sufficient in active ulcerative colitis? *Gastroenterology* 1991; 100: A200.

Elliott SN, McKnight W, Cirino G, Wallace JL. Nitric oxide-releasing nonsteroidal anti-inflammatory drug accelerates gastric ulcer healing in rats. *Gastroenterology* 1995; 109: 524–530.

Flower RJ, Vane JR. Inhibition of prostaglandin synthetase in brain explains the anti-pyretic activity of paracetamol (4-acetamide-phenol). *Nature* 1972; 120: 412–411.

Ford-Hutchinson AW. Leukotriene B_4 in inflammation. *CRC Crit Rev Immunol* 1990; 10: 1–12.

Fretland D, Sanderson T, Smith P, Adams L, Carson R, Fuhr J, Tanner J, Clapp N. Oral efficacy of a leukotriene B_4 receptor antagonist in colitic cotton-top tamarins. *Gut* 1995; 37: 702–707.

Fretland DJ, Levin S, Tsai BS, Djuric SW, Widomski DL, Zemaitis JM, Shone RL, Bauer RF. Effect of leukotriene-B_4 receptor antagonist, SC–41930, on acetic acid-induced colonic inflammation. *Agents Actions* 1989; 27: 395–397.

Goldman G, Welbourn R, Valeri CR, Shepro D, Hechtman HB. Thromboxane A_2 induces leukotriene B_4 synthesis that in turn mediates neutrophil diapedesis via CD 18 activation. *Microvasc Res* 1991; 41: 367–375.

Gretzer B, Ehrlich K, Maricic N, Lambrecht N, Respondek M, Peskar BM. Selective cyclo-oxygenase-2 inhibitors and their influence on the protective effect of a mild irritant in the rat stomach. *Br J Pharmacol* 1998; 123: 927–935.

Grimbone MA, Brock AF, Schafer AI. Leukotriene B4 stimulates polymorphonuclear leukocyte adhesion to cultured vascular endothelial cells. *J Clin Invest* 1984; 74: 1552–1555.

Grisham MB, Granger DN. Neutrophil-mediated mucosal injury: role of reactive oxygen metabolites. *Dig Dis Sci* 1998; 33: 6S–15S.

Gryglewski RJ, Szczeklik A, Wandzilak M. Effect of six prostaglandins, prostacyclin and iloprost on generation of superoxide anions by human polymorphonuclear leukocytes stimulated by zymosan or formyl-methionyl-leucyl-phenylalanine. *Biochem Pharmacol* 1987; 36: 4209–4212.

Halushka PV, Mais DE, Mayeux PR, Morinelli TA. Thromboxane, prostaglandin and leukotriene receptors. *Annu Rev Pharmacol Toxicol* 1989; 29: 213–239.

Ham EA, Soderman DD, Zanetti ME, Dougherty HW, McCauley E, Kuehl FA. Inhibition by prostaglandins of leukotriene B_4 release from activated neutrophils. *Proc Natl Acad Sci USA* 1983; 80: 4349–4353.

Haurand M, Floh L. Leukotriene formation by human polymorphonuclear leukocytes from endogenous arachidonate. Physiological triggers and modulation by prostanoids. *Biochem Pharmacol* 1989; 38: 2129–2137.

Hawkey CJ. Synthesis of prostaglandin E_2, thromboxane B_2 and prostaglandin catabolism in gastritis and gastric ulcer. *Gut* 1986; 27: 1484–1492.

Hernandez LA, Grisham MB, Twohig B, Arfors KE, Harlan JM, Granger DN. Granulocytes: the culprit in ischemic damage to the intestine. *Am J Physiol* 1987; 253: H699–H703.

Higgs GA, Moncada S, Salmon JA, Seager K. Source of thromboxane and prostaglandins in experimental inflammation. *Br J Pharmacol* 1985; 89: 1162–1188.

Hogaboam CM, Bissonnette EY, Chin BC, Befus AD, Wallace JL. Prostaglandins inhibit inflammatory mediator release from rat mast cells. *Gastroenterology* 1993; 104: 122–129.

Hudson M, Chitolie A, Hutton RA, Smith MSH, Pounder RE, Wakefield AJ.

Thrombotic vascular risk factors in inflammatory bowel disease. *Gut* 1996; 38: 733–737.

Hudson N, Balsitis M, Everitt S, Hawkey CJ. Enhanced gastric mucosal leukotriene B_4 synthesis in patients taking non-steroidal anti-inflammatory drugs. *Gut* 1993; 34: 742–747.

Kanwar S, Johnston B, Kubes P. Leukotriene C_4/D_4 induces P-selectin and sialyl Lewis[x]-dependent alterations in leukocyte kinetics in vivo. *Circ Res* 1995; 77: 879–887.

Kanwar S, Wallace JL, Befus D, Kubes P. Nitric oxide synthesis inhibition increases epithelial permeability via mast cells. *Am J Physiol* 1994; 266: G222–G229.

Kaufmann HJ, Taubin HL. Nonsteroidal anti-inflammatory drugs activate quiescent inflammatory bowel disease. *Ann Intern Med* 1987; 107: 513–516.

Konturek SJ, Brzozowski T, Piastucki I, Radecki T, Dembinska-Kiec A. Role of prostaglandin and thromboxane biosynthesis in gastric necrosis produced by taurocholate and ethanol. *Dig Dis Sci* 1983; 28: 154–160.

Kubes P. Nitric oxide modulates epithelial permeability in the feline small intestine. *Am J Physiol* 1992; 262: G1138–G1142.

Kubes P, Kanwar S, Niu X-F, Gaboury JP. Nitric oxide synthesis inhibition induces leukocyte adhesion via superoxide and mast cells. *FASEB J* 1993; 7: 1293–1299.

Kubes P, Suzuki M, Granger DN. Nitric oxide: an endogenous modulator of leukocyte adhesion. *Proc Natl Acad Sci USA* 1991; 88: 4651–4655.

Kujubu DA, Fletcher BS, Varnum BC, Lim RW, Herschman HR. TIS10, a phorbol ester tumor promoter-inducible mRNA from swiss eTe cells, encodes a novel prostaglandin synthase/cyclooxygenase homologue. *J Biol Chem* 1991; 266 No. 20, 12,866–12,872.

Kunkel SL, Spengler M, May MA, Spengler R, Larrick J, Remick D. Prostaglandin E_2 regulates macrophage-derived tumor necrosis factor gene expression. *J Biol Chem* 1988; 263: 5380–5384.

Kunkel SL, Wiggins RC, Chensue SW, Larrick J. Regulation of macrophage tumor necrosis factor production by prostaglandin E_2. *Biochem Biophys Res Commun* 1986b; 137: 404–410.

Kunkel SL, Chensue SW. Arachidonic acid metabolites regulate interleukin-1 production. *Biochem Biophys Res Commun* 1985; 128: 892–897.

Kunkel SL, Chensue SW, Phan SH. Prostaglandins as endogenous mediators of interleukin 1 production. *J Immunol* 1986a; 136: 186–192.

Lindström P, Lerner R, Palmblad J, Patarroyo M. Rapid adhesive responses of endothelial cells and of neutrophils induced by leukotriene B4 are mediated by leucocytic adhesion protein CD18. *Scand J Immunol* 1990; 31: 737–744.

Lobos EA, Sharon P, Stenson WF. Chemotactic activity in inflammatory bowel disease. Role of leukotriene B$_4$. *Dig Dis Sci* 1987; 32: 1380–1388.

MacNaughton WK, Cirino G, Wallace JL. Endothelium-derived relaxing factor (nitric oxide) has protective actions in the stomach. *Life Sci* 1989; 45: 1869–1876.

Martich GD, Dannen RL, Ceska M, Saffredini AF. Detection of interleukin-8 and tumour necrosis factor in normal humans after intravenous endotoxin administration: the effect of anti-inflammatory agents. *J Exp Med* 1991; 173: 1021–1024.

Miller DK, Gillard JW, Vickers PJ, Sadowski S, Léveillé C, Mancini JA, et al. Identification and isolation of a membrane protein necessary for leukotriene production. *Nature* 1990; 343: 278–281.

Mizuno H, Sakamoto C, Matsuda K, Wada K, Uchida T, Noguchi H, Akamatsu T, Kasuga M. Induction of cyclooxygenase 2 in gastric mucosal lesions and its inhibition by the specific antagonist delays healing in mice. *Gastroenterology* 1997; 112: 387–397.

Nielsen OH, Ahnfelt-Ronne I, Thomsen MK, Kissmeyer A-M, Langholz E. Effect of the leukotriene LTD$_4$/LTE$_4$ antagonist, SR 2640, in ulcerative colitis: an open clinical study. *Prostaglandins Leukotrienes Essen Fatty Acids* 1991; 42: 181–184.

Perdue MH, Ramage JK, Burget D, Marshall J, Masson S. Intestinal mucosal injury is associated with mast cell activation and leukotriene generation during Nippostrongylus-induced inflammation in the rat. *Dig Dis Sci* 1989; 34: 724–731.

Peskar BM, Dreyling KW, Peskar BA, May B, Goebell H. Enhanced formation of sulfidopeptide-leukotrienes in ulcerative colitis and Crohn's disease: inhibition by sulfasalazine and 5-aminosalicylic acid. *Agents Actions* 1986; 18, 381–383.

Pounder R. Silent peptic ulceration: deadly silence or golden silence. *Gastroenterology* 1989; 96: 626–631.

Raud J. Vasodilatation and inhibition of mediator release represent two distinct mechanisms for prostaglandin modulation of acute mast cell-dependent inflammation. *Br J Pharmacol* 1990; 99: 449–454.

Reuter BK, Cirino G, Wallace JL. Markedly reduced intestinal toxicity of a diclofenac derivative. *Life Sci* 1994; 55, PL1–PL8.

Rioux KP, Wallace JL. Mast cell activation augments gastric mucosal injury through a leukotriene-dependent mechanism. *Am J Physiol* 1994; 266: G863–G869.

Robert A. Antisecretory, antiulcer, cytoprotective and diarrheogenic properties of prostaglandins. *Adv Prost Thrombox Res* 1976; 2: 507–520.

Roberts WG, Simon TJ, Berlin RG, Haggitt RC, Snyder ES, Stenson WF, et al. Leukotrienes in ulcerative colitis: results of a multicenter trial of a leukotriene biosynthesis inhibitor, MK-591. *Gastroenterology* 1997; 112: 725–732.

Santucci L, Fiorucci S, Giansanti M, Brunori PM, DiMatteo FN, Morelli A. Pentoxifylline prevents indomethacin induced acute mucosal damage in rats: role of tumour necrosis factor alpha. *Gut* 1994; 35: 909–915.

Schmassman A, Stettler C, Netzer P, Flogerzi B, Peskar BM, Halter F. L-745,337, a selective inhibitor of COX-2, delays healing of experimental gastric ulcers comparable to traditional NSAIDs. *Gastroenterology* 1996; 110: A252.

Schultz RM, Marder P, Spaethe SM, Herron DK, Sofia MJ. Effects of two leukotriene B_4 (LTB$_4$) receptor antagonists (LY255283 and SC-41930) on LTB$_4$-induced human neutrophil adhesion and superoxide production. *Prostaglandins Leukot Essent Fatty Acids* 1991; 43: 267–271.

Scott RB, Maric M. Limited role for leukotrienes and platelet-activating factor in food protein induced jejunal smooth muscle contraction in sensitized rats. *Can J Physiol Pharmacol* 1991; 69: 1841–1846.

Sharon P, Stenson WF. Metabolism of arachidonic acid in acetic acid colitis in rats: similarity to human inflammatory bowel disease. *Gastroenterology* 1985; 88: 55–63.

Sharon P, Stenson WF. Enhanced synthesis of leukotriene B_4 by colonic mucosa in inflammatory bowel disease. *Gastroenterology* 1984; 86: 453–460.

Shoda T, Hatanaka K, Saito M, Majima M, Ogino M, Harada Y, et al. Induction of cyclooxygenase type-2 (COX-2) in rat endometrium at the peak of serum estradiol during the estrus cycle. *Jpn J Pharmacol* 1995; 69: 289–291.

Skandalis N, Rotenberg A, Meuwissen S, De Groot GH, Ouwendijk RJT, Tan TG. Ridogrel for the treatment of mild to moderate ulcerative colitis. *Gastroenterology* 1996; 110: A1016.

Slater DM, Berger LC, Newton R, Moore GE, Bennett PR. Expression of cyclooxygenase types 1 and 2 in human fetal membranes at term. *Am J Obstet Gynecol* 1995; 172: 77–82.

Spatafora M, Chiappara G, d'Amico D, Volpes D, Melis M, Pace E, Merendino A. Effect of indomethacin on the kinetics of tumour necrosis factor alpha release and tumour necrosis factor alpha gene expression by human blood monocyte. *Pharmacol Res* 1991; 23: 247–257.

Stenson WF, Lauritsen K, Laursen LS, Rask-Madsen J, Jacobsen O, Naesdal J, et al. Clinical trial of Zileuton, a specific inhibitor of 5-lipoxygenase, in ulcerative colitis. *Gastroenterology* 1991; 100: A253.

Tepperman BL, Soper BD. Nitric oxide synthase induction and cytoprotection of rat gastric mucosa from injury by ethanol. *Can J Physiol Pharmacol* 1994; 72: 1308–1312.

Vaananen PM, Keenan CM, Grisham MB, Wallace JL. Pharmacological investigation of the role of leukotrienes in the pathogenesis of experimental NSAID-gastropathy. *Inflammation* 1992; 16: 227–240.

van Outryve M, Huble F, van Eeghem P, de Vos M. Comparison of ridogrel versus prednisolone, both administered rectally, for the treatment of active ulcerative colitis. *Gastroenterology* 1996; 110: A1035.

Vane JR. Inhibition of prostaglandin synthesis as a mechanism of action for aspirin-like drugs. *Nature New Biol* 1971; 231: 232–235.

Vilaseca J, Salas A, Guarner F, Rodriguez R, Malagelada J-R. Participation of thromboxane and other eicosanoid synthesis in the course of experimental inflammatory colitis. *Gastroenterology* 1990; 98: 269–277.

Viñals M, Martinez-Gonzalez J, Badimon JJ, Badimon L. HDL-induced prostacyclin release in smooth muscle cells is dependent on cyclooxygenase-2 (Cox-2). *Arterioscler Thromb Vasc Biol* 1997; 17: 3481–3488.

Wakefield AJ, Sankey EA, Dhillon AP, Sawyerr AF, More L, Sim R, et al. Granulomatous vasculitis in Crohn's disease. *Gastroenterology* 1995; 100: 1279–1287.

Wallace JL. Nonsteroidal anti-inflammatory drugs and gastroenteropathy: the second hundred years. *Gastroenterology* 1997; 112: 1000–1016.

Wallace JL, Bak A, McKnight W, Asfaha S, Sharkey KA, MacNaughton WK. Cyclooxygenase 1 contributes to inflammatory responses in rats and mice: implications for gastrointestinal toxicity. *Gastroenterology* 1998; 115: 101–109.

Wallace JL, Granger DN. Pathogenesis of NSAID gastropathy are neutrophils the culprits? *Trends Pharmacol Sci* 1992; 13: 129–131.

Wallace JL, Keenan CM. Orally active inhibitor of leukotriene synthesis accelerates healing in a rat model of colitis. *Am J Physiol* 1990a; 258: G527–G534.

Wallace JL, Keenan CM. Leukotriene B$_4$ potentiates colonic ulceration in the rat. *Dig Dis Sci* 1990b; 35: 622–629.

Wallace JL, Higa A, McKnight GW, Macintyre DE. Prevention and reversal of experimental colitis by a monoclonal antibody which inhibits leukocyte adherence. *Inflammation* 1992a; 16: 343–354.

Wallace JL, Keenan CM, Gale D, Shoupe TS. Exacerbation of experimental colitis by nonsteroidal antiinflammatory drugs is not related to elevated leukotriene B$_4$ synthesis. *Gastroenterology* 1992b; 101: 18–27.

Wallace JL, MacNaughton WK, Morris GP, Beck PL. Inhibition of leukotriene synthesis markedly accelerates healing in a rat model of inflammatory bowel disease. *Gastroenterology* 1989; 96: 29–36.

Wallace JL, McKnight GW, Keenan CM, Byles NIA, MacNaughton WK. (1990) Effects of leukotrienes on susceptibility of the rat stomach to damage and investigation of the mechanism of action. *Gastroenterology* 98: 1178–1186.

Walt RP, Kemp RT, Filipowicz B, Davies JG, Bhaskar NK, Hawkey CJ. Gastric mucosal protection with selective inhibition of thromboxane synthesis. *Gut* 1987; 28: 541–544.

Wertheim WA, Kunkel SL, Standiford TJ, Burdick MD, Becker FS, Wilke CA, Gilbert AR, Strieter RM. Regulation of neutrophil-derived IL-8: the role of prostaglandin E_2, dexamethasone, and IL-4. *J Immunol* 1993; 151: 2166–2175.

Whittle BJR. (1984) Cellular mediators in gastric damage: actions of thromboxane A_2 and its inhibitors, in *Mechanisms of Mucosal Protection in the Upper Gastrointestinal Tract,* Allen A, et al. eds. Raven, New York, 1994; pp. 295–301.

Whittle BJR, Kauffman GL, Moncada S. Vasoconstriction with thromboxane A_2 induces ulceration of the gastric mucosa. *Nature* 1981; 292: 472–474.

Whittle BJR, Oren-Wolman RN, Guth PH. Gastric vasoconstrictor actions of leukotriene C_4, $PGF_{2\alpha}$, and thromboxane mimetic U-46619 on rat submucosal microcirculation in vivo. *Am J Physiol* 1985; 248: G580–G586.

Wong K, Freund F. Inhibition of *n*-formylmethiony-leucyl-phenylalanine induced respiratory burst in human neutrophils by adrenergic agonists and prostaglandins of the E series. *Can J Physiol Pharmacol* 1981; 59: 915–920.

Woolverton CJ, White JJ, Sartor RB. Eicosanoid regulation of acute intestinal vascular permeability induced by intravenous peptidoglycan polysaccharide polymers. *Agents Actions* 1989; 26: 301–309.

Xie W, Chipman JG, Robertson DL, Erikson RL, Simmons DL. Expression of a mitogen-responsive gene encoding prostaglandin synthase is regulated by mRNA splicing. *Proc Natl Acad Sci USA* 1991; 88: 2692–2696.

Xie W, Robertson DL, Simmons DL. Mitogen-inducible prostaglandin G/H synthase: a new target for nonsteroidal antiinflammatory drugs. *Drug Dev Res* 1992; 25: 249–265.

Yoshida N, Takemura T, Granger DN, Anderson DC, Wolf RE, McIntire LV, Kvietys PR. Molecular determinants of aspirin-induced neutrophil adherence to endothelial cells. *Gastroenterology* 1993; 105: 715–724.

Zipser RD, Nast CC, Lee M, Kao HW, Duke R. In vivo production of leukotriene B_4 and leukotriene C_4 in rabbit colitis. Relationship to inflammation. *Gastroenterology* 1987; 92: 33–39.

2   Therapeutic Implications of the Nitric Oxide Pathway in Gastrointestinal Diseases

B. L. Tepperman and B. J. R. Whittle

CONTENTS

INTRODUCTION
PHYSIOLOGICAL ACTIONS OF NO ON THE GUT
THERAPEUTIC POTENTIAL OF NO DONORS
NO-NSAIDS
PATHOLOGICAL ACTIONS OF NO: ROLE OF iNOS
THERAPEUTIC POTENTIAL OF NOS INHIBITORS
CONCLUSIONS
REFERENCES

1. INTRODUCTION

Over the past decade, nitric oxide (NO) has been shown to play an unprecedented range of roles in biological systems. Diverse physiologic and pathophysiologic roles for NO have been identified, including those of a vasodilator, neurotransmitter, antimicrobial agent, immunomodulator, and intracellular signaling molecule (Moncada et al., 1991; Moncada and Higgs, 1995; Whittle, 1994). It can be formed in a wide

From: *Drug Development: Molecular Targets for GI Diseases*
Edited by: T. S. Gaginella and A. Guglietta © Humana Press Inc., Totowa, NJ

range of cell types, such as the endothelial cell, macrophage, neurons, hepatocytes, fibroblasts, epithelial cells, smooth muscle cells, and cardiac myocytes. In the gastrointestinal (GI) tract, NO can bring about changes in secretion, motility, blood flow, electrolyte and water absorption, mucosal protection, and inflammation, and many of these changes are transduced via activation of soluble guanylate cyclase (Moncada et al., 1991; Moncada and Higgs, 1995). This chapter reviews studies on the role of NO in the GI tract, especially as it relates to maintenance of physiological function and mucosal integrity; the therapeutic potential of agents that modulate the NO system will also be discussed.

1.1. Chemistry and Formation of NO in Biological Systems

NO is produced in biological systems following the five-electron oxidation of one of the chemically equivalent guanidine nitrogens of L-arginine by the family of nitric oxide synthase (NOS) enzymes, forming the free radical NO, and citrulline as byproduct (Palmer and Moncada, 1989; Palmer et al., 1987). The NOS isoforms share homology with cytochrome P_{450} reductase (Kerwin et al., 1995; Prince, 1993). NO is hydrophobic, and has a very short half-life, reacting rapidly with O_2, superoxide anion, thiols, and transition metals to form nitrogen dioxide, nitrite and nitrate ions, peroxynitrate, nitrosothiols, and metal–NO adducts (Stamler et al. 1992).

1.2. NOS Isoforms

Three distinct isoforms of the NOS enzyme have been isolated, and represent the products of three different genes (Kerwin et al., 1995; Moncada and Higgs, 1995). These isoforms are designated endothelial NOS (eNOS) (Lamas et al., 1992); neuronal NOS (nNOS) (Garthwaite et al., 1989), which describes their originally found location; and the inducible NOS (iNOS), originally described in inflammatory cells (Hevel et al., 1991). Both eNOS and nNOS are constitutively expressed, and are translated under physiological conditions; iNOS is transcriptionally regulated in response to an inflammatory challenge, both cytokines and endotoxin being potent stimuli. Neuronal-like NOS has also been detected in nonneural tissues, including gastric epithelial cells (Price et al., 1996). Similarly, iNOS has been detected in endothelial cells, hepatocytes, neutrophils, and smooth muscle cells. The nNOS and iNOS isoforms are predominantly soluble enzymes, but eNOS is more than 90% particulate (Forstermann et al., 1991).

The NOS isoforms utilize L-arginine as the substrate for NO production, as well as molecular oxygen and nicotinamide adenine dinucleotide phosphate (NADPH), in the catalyzed reactions. Moreover, the three isoenzymes contain a heme group and require tetrahydrobiopterin (BH_4), flavin adenine dinucleotide, and flavin mononucleotide as cofactors. Cytokines, such as interferon (IFN)-γ or tumor necrosis factor (TNF)-α, have been reported to markedly increase the concentrations of BH_4, which is a limiting cofactor for NOS activity. The nNOS and eNOS isoforms are Ca^{2+}- and calmodulin-dependent enzymes; iNOS is a Ca^{2+}- and calmodulin-independent enzyme. Inducible NOS can also bind calmodulin, and, indeed, in mouse macrophages, this binding is so strong that calmodulin can be considered a subunit of the enzyme. The iNOS isoform produces a greater and longer-lasting NO release than do eNOS and nNOS. The NOS isoforms are competitively inhibited by N^G-monomethyl-L-arginine (L-NMMA) and other L-arginine analogs; the expression of iNOS, but not the other isoforms, is inhibited by corticosteroids (Moncada and Higgs, 1995).

NOS isoenzymes have been purified and cloned from several sources. In humans, the presence of three different genes coding for nNOS, iNOS, and eNOS are located on chromosomes 12, 17, and 7, respectively (Marsden et al., 1993; Xu et al., 1993).

2. PHYSIOLOGICAL ACTIONS OF NO ON THE GUT

2.1. Blood Flow

NO has been shown to play an important role in vascular tone within the GI circulation. Different physiological stimuli may participate in NO release, such as shear stress, changes in Ca^{2+} concentration, or changes in oxygen tension (Klein-Nulend et al., 1998; Moncada et al., 1991; Nelin et al., 1996; Vanhoutte and Shimokawa, 1989). The shear stress produced on the endothelium luminal surface in response to increases in blood flow is suggested to be the most important physiological stimulus for endothelial NO release (Fleming and Busse, 1995).

Intravenous administration of the NOS inhibitor, L-NMMA, in a dose-dependent manner, reduces resting gastric mucosal blood flow in experimental studies (Pique et al., 1989, 1992a), suggesting the involvement of endogenous NO in modulating the resting gastric microcirculation. Similarly, L-NMMA or N^G-nitro-L-arginine methyl ester (L-NAME) have been shown to increase vascular resistance in the mesenteric circulation (Pique et al., 1992b), and can reduce blood flow in the small and large intestine (Alemayehu et al., 1994; Iwata et al., 1992).

In the stomach, the increase in gastric mucosal blood flow caused by secretagogues, such as pentagastrin, can be affected without any influence on acid secretion by administration of L-NAME, and an effect can be reversed by co-administration of L-arginine (Pique et al., 1992a; Kato et al., 1997). Similarly, hyperemia was reduced by the cyclo-oxygenase (COX) inhibitor, indomethacin, confirming earlier reports of the involvement of endogenous prostanoids (Tepperman and Whittle, 1992; Whittle and Tepperman, 1991). Similarly back-diffusion of H^+ leads to an increase in gastric blood flow, and this increase can be inhibited by L-NAME treatment, but not indomethacin (Pique et al., 1992a; Wachter et al., 1995), indicating the involvement of endogenous prostanoids. This compensatory increase in gastric mucosal blood flow is not apparent in cirrhotic animals (Ferraz and Wallace, 1996). Furthermore, the gastric blood flow, in response to a nitrovasodilator that acts through NO release, is impaired in these animals (Beck et al., 1993; Ferraz et al., 1995). Long term administration of a prostaglandin (PG) analog to cirrhotic rat restored the blood flow response to a nitrovasodilator. These findings suggest that NO and PGs can interact in the regulation of gastric blood flow in healthy and cirrhotic animals.

As in the stomach, the esophagus is also able to resist damage caused by refluxed acid, by increasing mucosal blood flow (Orlando, 1994). It has recently been demonstrated that this hyperemic response was preceded by luminal histamine release (Feldman et al., 1996). The hyperemia was thus attenuated by mast cell stabilization, histamine H_1 receptor blockade, and NOS inhibition. NOS inhibition also blocked histamine release, suggesting that mast-cell-derived histamine, acting via an NO-dependent mechanism, plays a role in this response.

In the intestine, NO also appears to play an interactive role in regulating blood flow. Sympathetic neurogenically mediated vasoconstriction of intestinal arterioles is increased during NOS inhibition (Nase and Boegehold, 1996), and this enhancement can be reversed by exposure to L-arginine. The most likely source of this NO, released during increased sympathetic nerve activity, was considered to be the microvascular endothelium (Nase and Boegehold, 1997).

NO also appears to be involved in intestinal hyperemia in response to luminal application of certain foodstuffs (Matheson et al., 1997). Glucose administration into rat ileal loops resulted in an increase in blood flow, which was blocked by L-NAME. It is not known if glucose causes direct production of NO, or whether epithelial cells transduce a vasodilator signal through vascular endothelial-derived NO during postprandial intestinal hyperemia.

2.2. NO and Cell Adhesion

Beyond its vasodilator activity, NO exerts a variety of effects at the blood and endothelial interface, including the inhibition of platelet aggregation, and attenuation of leukocyte and endothelial interaction (Davenpeck et al., 1994; Kubes et al., 1991). For a leukocyte to adhere, it must initially make a brief tethering interaction with endothelium, which then develops into a rolling interaction (Lawrence et al., 1994; Granger and Kubes, 1994). This rolling is mediated by a family of adhesion molecules termed selectins. P-selectin appears to play a role in the initial stages of inflammation; E-selectin and vascular cell adhesion molecule (V-CAM)-1-dependent leukocyte–endothelial cell interaction contribute to the rolling interaction during the chronic stages of inflammation (Bevilacqua et al., 1987; Granger and Kubes 1994). In surgically prepared experimental animals, administration of a NOS inhibitor is associated with enhanced leukocyte and endothelial interaction, with increased leukocyte adherence and emigration (Kubes et al., 1991; Ma et al., 1993).

Furthermore, inhibition of NO synthesis promotes P-selectin-dependent leukocyte rolling (Davenpeck et al., 1994), suggesting that NO may be a homeostatic regulator of leukocyte rolling, under normal conditions. Delivery of exogenous NO decreases leukocyte rolling in acute inflammation induced by a variety of conditions (Gaboury et al., 1993; Gauthier et al., 1994; Johnston et al., 1996).

2.3. NO and Gastric Acid Secretion

NOS inhibition does not directly modulate basal- or pentagastrin-stimulated acid secretion (Pique et al., 1992a). However, constitutively formed NO appears to be involved in the acute antisecretory action of agents such as lipopolysaccharide treatment and cytokines (Martinez-Cuesta et al., 1992; Esplugues et al., 1993), or by hypovolemia or moderate hypothermia, acting through mechanisms in the brain (Esplugues et al., 1996). It has also been observed that NOS inhibition could reduce acid secretion in response to a protein meal or pentagastrin infusion in dogs (Bilski et al., 1994).

Parenteral administration of NO donors has, however, also been shown to reduce vagally mediated acid secretion (Barrachina et al., 1994), as well as histamine-stimulated acid secretion (Takeuchi et al., 1994). It has also been reported that NO donors, such as FK 409, inhibited pentagastrin-stimulated acid secretion in doses that did not affect blood flow, and that the effect was probably mediated, to some extent, via suppression of histamine release from enterochromaffin-like cells (Kato et al., 1998). It has been demonstrated that high concentrations of NO donors can inhibit parietal cell activity in vitro, suggesting a direct action of NO on acid secretory activity (Brown et al., 1993a). Thus, the effects of endogenous and exogenous NO on acid secretion is complex, and appears to depend on the prevailing physiological or pathological conditions.

2.4. NO and Gastroduodenal Secretion
of Mucus and HCO_3^-

Gastric mucus forms a continuous viscoelastic layer over the mucosa (Allen et al., 1989). This layer is an important factor in mucosal protection against topical irritation by noxious agents in the lumen (Allen, 1981). Furthermore, HCO_3^- secreted from the duodenal epithelial cells into the mucous gel has been shown to establish a pH gradient in the gel, thereby providing a line of defense against gastric acid (Flemstrom and Kivilaakso, 1953; Williams and Turnberg, 1981). NO donors, such as isosorbide dinitrate and S-nitroso-*N*-acetyl-penicillamine (SNAP), have been shown to increase mucus gel thickness in rat stomach (Brown et al., 1992). NOS inhibitors have been shown to reduce the ability of mucosal cells to secrete and synthesize mucus (Takahashi et al., 1995). It has also been reported that L-arginine treatment could reverse the reduction in gastric cellular mucous secretion in response to hypoxia-reoxygenation in vitro (Kim and Kim, 1998). NO has been demonstrated to mediate mucus secretion in response to a number of stimulatory agents (Brown et al., 1993b; Ichikawa et al., 1998). Inhibition of NO synthesis reduced mucus secretion in vivo by approx 20%, although this is less than the stimulating influences of intraluminal acid and endogenous PGs (Sababi et al., 1995). Similarly, chronic L-NAME treatment in rats significantly affected gastric mucus output (Qui et al., 1996).

Inhibition of NOS activity has been shown to increase resting duodenal alkaline secretion to various degrees in experimental animals, suggesting that endogenous NO may modulate the basal secretion of HCO_3^- (Hällgren et al., 1995; Sababi et al., 1995; Takeuchi et al., 1993). This inhibition of alkaline output has been attributed to suppression of a stimulatory nicotinic receptor-dependent neural mechanism (Hällgren et al., 1995).

Using a technique that could simultaneously determine NO output and HCO_3^- secretion, it has been observed that luminal acid formation increased NO output, and thus was inhibited by L-NMMA treatment (Holm et al., 1998). Furthermore, L-NMMA also reduced the H^+-stimulated increase in alkaline secretion. Luminal administration of a NO donor has been shown to increase mucosal HCO_3^- secretion in the dog (Bilski and Konturek, 1994). The acid-induced increase in HCO_3^- secretion can be inhibited by an extract of *Helicobacter pylori,* and this effect could be overcome by L-arginine (Fändricks et al., 1997). Mucosal damage in response to a hyperosmotic challenge also increased gastroduodenal HCO_3^- secretion, and this effect was attenuated by L-NAME treatment (Takeuchi and Okabe, 1995). Thus, endogenous NO appears to mediate alkaline output in response to luminal acid, and as a consequence of an injurious challenge to the stomach; under more physiological conditions, endogenous NO may attenuate alkaline secretion.

2.5. NO and Intestinal Electrolyte and Water Secretion

In recent years, investigators have demonstrated that L-arginine, as well as NOS inhibitors, are able to influence intestinal secretion (Izzo et al., 1998), but results using these agents are contradictory and depend on the segment of intestine studied, the animal species involved, and other experimental conditions, including in vivo or in vitro conditions, intact or stripped tissues, and the type of challenge used. It is likely that, under physiological conditions, a NO-dependent proabsorptive tone exists. This conclusion is based on a number of findings that NOS inhibitors induce net fluid and electrolyte secretion in vivo in several animal species (Shirgi-Degen and Beubler, 1995; Mourad et al., 1996; Barry et al., 1994; Miller et al., 1993). However, in some pathophysiological states, including inflammatory bowel disease (IBD), in which NO may be produced at high concentrations (Whittle, 1994, 1995, 1997), such NO formation may be capable of evoking net secretion. A notable exception is the diarrhea produced by bacterial enterotoxin, in which NO may have a proabsorptive role. Thus, NO donors and L-arginine can reduce *Clostridium difficile* toxin A-induced secretion, as well as fluid secretion caused by cholera toxin (Qiu et al., 1996; Beubler and Shirgi-Degen, 1997).

Because NO appears to mediate both secretagogue and proabsorptive actions on the intestine, it will be necessary in future studies to identify more precisely the conditions under which NO exerts these diverse actions.

2.6. NO and GI Motility

NO has been shown to be an important mediator of relaxation in GI smooth muscle and sphincters (Sanders and Ward, 1992). Strong evidence has accumulated demonstrating that NO is one of the key transmitters of nonadrenergic, noncholinergic (NANC) nerve-induced relaxation of GI smooth muscle (Sanders and Ward, 1992; Stark and Szurszewski, 1992), and such nerves are now classified as nitrergic. The early evidence for such nitrergic innervation included the demonstration that NOS immunoreactivity can be detected in GI myenteric and submucosal neurons (Llewellyn-Smith et al., 1992), and that NO release in response to electrical field stimulation can be inhibited by tetrodotoxin (Boeckxstaens et al., 1990). NO as a mediator of NANC relaxation of basal tone, as well as following neuronal stimulation, has been demonstrated in rat and guinea pig stomach, duodenum, or ileum, the canine ileocecal junction or duodenum, the human colon, the rabbit jejunum, and the canine and human esophagus and lower esophageal sphincter (Martinez-Cuesta et al., 1996; Bayguinov et al., 1992; Izzo et al., 1996; Konturek et al., 1997, 1995b).

In the stomach and duodenum, NO has been postulated to play a physiological role in the regulation of gastric emptying in response to various luminal nutrients (Anvari et al., 1998; Orihata and Sarna, 1996; Sun et al., 1996). In the esophagus, NO plays an important role in the mediation of propulsive activity by regulating the period and gradient between the onset of a swallow and contractions of the esophageal circular muscle (Murray et al., 1991; Yamato et al., 1992). Similarly, NO has been suggested to play a role in the coordination of peristaltic activity in guinea pig intestine via a dual excitatory and inhibitory effect on intestinal motility. The excitatory effect involved cholinergic motor neurons; the inhibitory effect reflected relaxation of intestinal muscle (Holzer et al., 1997).

NO has also been linked with the slowly migrating, cyclic peristaltic wave associated with the interdigestive state in most mammals. This interdigestive migrating complex involves a number of components, including contraction originating in the stomach and propagating to the terminal colon. This latter component is regulated by the gut hormone, motilin (Mizumoto et al., 1997). NO has been proposed to influence these contractions, because NOS inhibition resulted in their appearance (Sarna et al., 1993), even in the fed animal (Maczka et al., 1993). Inhibition of NOS was also found to stimulate motilin release via cholinergic pathways independent of the vagus. The contractions induced by NO synthesis inhibition appeared to be mediated by activation of 5-hydroxytryptamine (5-HT) receptors (Bogers et al., 1991).

The mechanisms of NO-induced relaxation of GI smooth muscle is a subject of much investigation. A body of evidence suggests that NO may have some association with vasoactive intestinal peptide (VIP), a signaling peptide that has also been identified as a NANC mediator (Grider et al., 1992). However, other studies have also demonstrated that, although vagal activation evokes both VIP and NO release, there is no evidence for any interaction (Takahashi and Owyang, 1995; Willis et al., 1996), and the relaxation induced by VIP does not involve NO (Holzer-Petsche and Moser, 1996).

The contractile response of the duodenum to a NOS inhibitor can be suppressed by tetrodotoxin or hexamethonium, indicating a neural involvement (Martinez-Cuesta et al., 1996). Furthermore, NO relaxes circular muscle of the rat gastric corpus, both directly at a muscular site and indirectly via inhibition of acetylcholine release (Holzer-Petsche and Moser, 1996). A similar neural mechanism has been proposed for NO-mediated inhibition of duodenal motility (Hallgren et al., 1995). In contrast, it has been shown that NO does not inhibit acetylcholine release in guinea pig ileal circular muscle, but inhibits tachykinin release, which acts via neurokinin (NK)1 receptors (Yunker and Galligan, 1996).

Pathological conditions associated with ileus, in which complete or partial GI motor dysfunction can occur, may involve NO (Calignano et al., 1992). Studies of canine GI motility during periods of endotoxemia have shown that gastric emptying and colonic transit are slowed. Similarly the interdigestive migrating complex is delayed (Cullen et al., 1997). These changes have been attributed to NO production by endotoxin (Hellstrom et al., 1997; Wirthlin et al., 1996). The lipopolysaccharide-induced changes in intestinal transit were reversed by L-NAME treatment (Wirthlin et al., 1996), and the effects on the interdigestive complex were negated (Cullen et al., 1997).

3. THERAPEUTIC POTENTIAL OF NO DONORS

From the foregoing discussion, the therapeutic implications for drugs acting on the L-arginine–NO system within the gut are apparent. NOS inhibitors have been used extensively to uncover the physiological actions of NO, or to reverse disturbances resulting from excessive NO production. However, situations also occur in which a deficiency of NO has been identified, and this subheading deals with the potential therapeutic value of NO donors in these clinical situations.

3.1. Gallbladder and Sphincter of Oddi

Delivery of bile to the small intestinal lumen is controlled by hepatic bile secretion, gallbladder contraction, and the patency of sphincter of Oddi. The hormone, cholecystokinin, is believed to be the physiological stimulant for postprandial gallbladder contraction and sphincter relaxation. Recent studies have shown that the effect of cholecystokinin on the sphincter of Oddi is mediated through NANC nerves, and that NO is an important element in the pathway (Luman et al., 1997; Shima et al., 1998).

In human volunteers, administration of the NO donor, glyceryl trinitrate (GTN), has been shown to produce gallbladder dilatation in the fasting state, to reduce postprandial gallbladder dilatation in the fasting state, and in emptying (Greaves et al., 1998), and to inhibit sphincter of Oddi motility (Luman et al., 1997). It has been suggested that GTN would be useful during endoscopic retrograde cholingiopancreatography cannulation and gallstone extraction (Luman et al., 1997). Although it has been speculated that long-term nitrate therapy, and the resultant inhibition of gallbladder motility, may be a risk factor in the accelerated genesis of gall stones (Forgacs et al., 1984; Pomeranz and Shafter, 1985), the relaxant effect of GTN and other NO donors, such as isorbide dinitrate, have been shown to reduce the pain associated with acute biliary colic (Hassel, 1993).

3.2. Esophagus and Lower Esophageal Sphincter

Animal studies suggest that NO may play a role in the regulation of esophageal motility, being at least in part responsible for the onset of the swallow and coordinated occurrence of contractions in the circular smooth muscle (Murray et al., 1991; Yamato et al., 1992). In the esophagus, endogenous NO has been implicated in the development of a latency period and latency gradient, and in the regulation of the amplitude of esophageal body peristalsis (Konturek et al., 1995a, 1997; Yamato et al., 1992). Furthermore, NO has been shown to be a mediator of lower esophageal sphincter relaxation (Tottrup et al., 1991a, 1991b).

NO donors have been utilized in studies aimed at treating two disturbances in normal esophageal motility: diffuse esophageal spasm and achalasia. The former disturbance is a functional disorder (Vantrappen et al., 1979), in which the mechanisms responsible for the physiologic timing of contractions are dysfunctional. It has been shown that administration of GTN to patients with esophageal spasm significantly prolonged the latency period, restored normal peristaltic contractions, and reduced their duration, thus abolishing the adverse clinical symptoms. In contrast, treatment with L-arginine was ineffective, but this may not be unexpected, if there is a functional disruption of the NO pathway (Konturek et al., 1995a).

Achalasia is a motor disorder characterized by abnormal peristalsis, elevated pressure of the lower esophageal sphincter, and failure of sphincter relaxation in deglutition. A reduction in NOS-containing neurons has been associated with this disorder in humans (Mearin et al., 1993). In an opossum model of achalasia, a NO donor, sodium nitroprusside, has been shown to reduce resting lower esophageal pressure in the achalasia, as well as in a control group of animals (Singaram et al., 1996). Furthermore, in patients with achalasia, NO donors will induce relaxation of esophageal muscle (Gonzalez et al., 1997). These results suggest that NO donors may have an important therapeutic role in the treatment of esophageal motor disorders.

3.3. Gastric Emptying

NO donors have also been proposed in the treatment of functional disturbances of gastric motility and emptying. Studies in animals have demonstrated that NO suppresses fundic, antral, pyloric, and duodenal contractions (Bayguinov and Sanders, 1993; Anvari et al., 1998; Orihata and Sarna, 1994). In a study of the abnormalities of GI motility associated with diabetes in experimental animals, it was found that normal antral motility could be restored by the NO donor, nitroprusside (Martinez-Cuesta et al., 1995). In humans, NO donors have been shown to inhibit pyloric motility in response to intraduodenal triglyceride (Sun et al., 1996). Similarly, GTN administration slowed the rate of gastric emptying, and decreased antral motor activity (Konturek et al., 1995b). In addition, L-arginine administration reduced antral motility changes in humans in response to a liquid test meal (Fiorucci et al., 1995).

3.4. Intestinal Secretion and Absorption

Parenteral administration of NO-generating compounds stimulate water and electrolyte absorption in vivo in rabbit ileum and rat jejunum (Barry et al., 1994; Shirgi-Degen and Beubler, 1995). Luminal administration of L-arginine or the NO donor, SNAP, caused significant increases in water and electrolyte absorption. Furthermore, a NO donor attenuated the ileal secretion and permeability changes induced in rats by administration of *C. difficile* toxin A (Qui et al., 1996). Similarly, sodium nitroprusside treatment was shown to inhibit jejunal secretion in animals treated with *Escherichia coli* enterotoxin (Shirgi-Degen and Beubler, 1995).

These observations support the use of NO-generating compounds in the treatment of some pathologic hypersecretory states. Recent studies have examined the effect of NO donors as a class of absorption enhancers. Intrarectal administration of NO donors in rabbits induced increases in insulin absorption, as well as large-mol-wt (4000) dextran (Utogochi et al., 1998). Therefore, NO donors may have therapeutic potential to act as potent absorption enhancers in a clinical setting.

3.5. Mucosal Protection

Intragastric or parenteral administration of the GTN nitroprusside, and SNAP can protect against acute gastric mucosal injury induced by topical irritants, and by iv infusions of endothelin-1, endotoxin, or platelet-activating factor (Kitagawa et al., 1990; Wallace et al., 1989; MacNaughton et al., 1989; Boughton-Smith et al., 1990, 1992). Application of transdermal patches of nitroglycerin has been shown to reduce gastric injury provoked by nonsteroidal anti-inflammatory agents (Barrachina et al., 1995). NO donors have also been shown to be effective in reducing gastric lesions in response to water immersion stress (Hisanaga et al., 1996) and ischemia followed by reperfusion (Andrews et al., 1994). However, higher doses of NO donors, infused locally, have been shown to cause mucosal damage (Lopez-Belmonte et al., 1993).

In the intestine, administration of NO donors provides significant protection against the mucosal and microvascular dysfunction associated with ischemia–reperfusion (Payne and Kubes, 1993). Prophylactic administration of L-arginine improved intestinal barrier function after mesenteric ischemia in the rat (Schleiffer and Raul, 1996) and spermine–NO could attenuate the mucosal dysfunction associated with prolonged hypothermic ischemia and reperfusion (Villarreal et al., 1995). In addition, a NO donor has been shown to diminish thermal-injury-associated venule constriction within the GI tract (Yoshida et al., 1997).

4. NO–NSAIDs

Nonsteroidal anti-inflammatory drugs (NSAIDs) have been a mainstay in the treatment of pain, fever, and inflammation. However, the long-term use of these drugs is associated with significant adverse effects, most notably gastric ulceration, bleeding, and perforation, as well as an increased risk of bleeding from preexisting peptic ulcers (Soll et al., 1991). Both the beneficial (anti-inflammatory, analgesic) and detrimental (ulcerogenic) effects of NSAIDs are probably attributable to the ability of these drugs to suppress PGs. Suppression of PG synthesis leads to tissue damage via a reduction in mucosal blood flow and neutrophil infiltration, adherence, and activation (Wallace, 1993).

One experimental strategy being explored for the reduction of the detrimental effects of NSAIDs is the use of a derivative of the drug, flurbiprofen, which contains a moiety similar to the NO-releasing moieties found in many organic nitrates (Wallace et al., 1994b). This compound suppressed gastric PG synthesis, but caused significantly less mucosal hemorrhagic damage than flurbiprofen. Furthermore, flurbiprofen-NO did not reduce mucosal blood flow to the same extent as flurbiprofen (Wallace et al., 1995). This agent was also found to reduce platelet aggregation more potently than flurbiprofen (Cirino et al., 1995).

Similarly, a nitroxybutylester derivative of the NSAID, ketoprofen, also resulted in less acute gastric mucosal injury than did its parent compound, while demonstrating comparable anti-inflammatory activity (Wallace et al., 1994a). Likewise, nitroxybutylester derivatives of other NSAIDs did not elicit leukocyte adherence to the endothelium of the mucosal microvasculature. NO-releasing derivatives of aspirin have also been shown to reduce the susceptibility of the stomach to shock-induced damage, by inhibiting neutrophil adherence to the vascular endothelium (Wallace et al., 1997).

This class of NO-containing compounds was also found to be effective in reducing the extent of intestinal damage in response to endotoxic shock, although the changes in blood pressure and hematocrit were similar to that produced by the parent compound itself (Wallace et al., 1995). Nitroxybutylester derivatives of other NSAIDs (aspirin, naproxen, diclofenac, and ketorolec) have been shown to have similar GI-sparing properties (Cuzzolin et al., 1995; Cirino et al., 1996; Rishi et al., 1996). One of these agents, NO-naproxen, has recently been shown to prevent gastric damage resulting from chronic administration of a NOS inhibitor in rats (Muscara et al., 1998).

5. PATHOLOGICAL ACTIONS OF NO:
ROLE OF iNOS

5.1. Cytotoxic Actions of NO

High concentration of NO can interact with various target molecules, such as oxygen, thiol groups, and metals, within the prosthetic groups of various enzymes, resulting in their activation or inactivation. Utilizing murine macrophages, NO has been shown to react with nonsulfur centers of aconitase of the tricarboxylic acid cycles, as well as complexes I and II of the electron transport chain within target molecules. The inhibition of these essential components of cellular respiration resulted in depletion of cellular ATP stores, with consequent cytotoxicity (Stuehr and Nathan, 1989).

Additional mechanisms by which NO may mediate cytotoxicity include impairment of DNA synthesis (Kwon et al., 1991), direct toxicity through deamination reactions (Nguyen et al., 1992), and, possibly more importantly, via the potentiation of the toxicity of oxygen radicals. In this latter scheme, NO has combined with O_2^- to form the intermediate, peroxynitrite, which is then protonated to peroxynitrous acid under acidic conditions: Peroxynitrous acid yields the toxic products, hydroxyl radical and nitrogen dioxide (Beckman and Koppenol, 1996). Peroxynitrite can initiate cytotoxic oxidative reactions in vivo and in vitro. Initiation of lipid peroxidation, direct inhibition of mitochondrial respiratory chain enzymes, inactivation of glyceralderhyde-3-phosphate dehydrogenase, inhibition of membrane Na^+/K^+ adenosine triphosphatase (ATPase) and other oxidative protein modifications contribute to the cytotoxic effect of peroxynitrite (Beckman and Kippenol, 1996). In addition, peroxynitrite is a potent trigger of DNA strand breakage, with subsequent activation of the nuclear enzyme poly-adenosine diphosphate ribosyl synthetase, and eventual severe energy depletion of the cells (Szabo, 1996).

NO donors have been shown to exacerbate the cytotoxic effect of hydrogen peroxide in rabbit gastric mucosal cells (Hata et al., 1996), and to be necessary for induction of mucosal injury by various types of intestinal bacteria (Cuzzolin et al., 1997). High concentrations of NO have also been shown to injure rat intestinal epithelial cells, and this damage could be ameliorated by inhibitors of guanylate cyclase

(Tepperman et al., 1993, 1994, 1998). Excessive levels of NO from endogenous or exogenous sources result in a reduction in gastric cellular viability, and this response appears to be related causally to an increase in intracellular Ca^{2+} (Tripp and Tepperman, 1996). In isolated cells, the cytotoxic effect of NO was found to be caused by increased generation of oxidants, as a result of a decrease in glutathione production (Wakulich and Tepperman, 1997). Furthermore, it has been demonstrated that high levels of NO-inactivated glutatione peroxidase in isolated cells lead to increased accumulation of peroxides (Asahi et al., 1995).

Local intra-arterial infusion of NO donors, which release high concentrations of NO, can produce injury in rat gastric mucosa, and this damage appears to be related to peroxynitrite formation and lipid peroxidation (Lamarque and Whittle, 1995a, 1995b).

In intestinal epithelial monolayers, excessive NO production is associated with increased intercellular permeability (Salzman et al., 1995; Unno et al., 1997a, 1997b, 1995). The mechanism of this increased permeability appears to be associated with decreases in cellular cyclic adenosine monophosphate levels (Salzman et al., 1995), reduced levels of glutathione (Unno et al., 1997b), and the formation of peroxynitrous acid (Unno et al., 1997a).

In the GI tract, induction of iNOS has been observed in rat small intestinal and colonic epithelial cells and such expression is associated with a reduction in cell viability (Tepperman et al., 1993, 1994; Miller et al., 1993). Furthermore, administration of extracts of *H. pylori* have been shown to result in induction of NOS and injury in duodenal mucosal cells (Hahm et al., 1998; Lamarque et al., 1998); *Listeria* infection resulted in increased iNOS expression in monolayers of human colonic epithelial cells (Li et al., 1998). In cultured human epithelial cells, bacterial challenge resulted in iNOS activation, and that response could be ameliorated by pretreatment with a NOS inhibitor (Salzman et al., 1998).

5.2. iNOS and Inflammation

There is a vast amount of evidence causally linking the induction of calcium-independent NOS with gastric and intestinal mucosal inflammation in experimental animals and humans. A large number of studies have identified increased expression and activity of iNOS in experimental models of IBD, as well from human inflamed colonic, gastric, and esophageal tissue (Boughton-Smith et al., 1993a; Ferretti et al., 1995; Gupta et al., 1998; Kimura et al., 1997; Rachmilewitz et al., 1994). The increase in iNOS activity in experimentally induced colonic inflammation was found to be associated with an increase in neutrophil infiltration and subsequent tissue lipid peroxidation (Salzman et al., 1995; Kiss et al., 1997). The increase in neutrophil infiltration in the neonatal colon following endotoxin challenge was preceded by mast cell degranulation (Brown et al., 1998). In addition, iNOS has been reported to be upregulated in the gastric mucosa in response to 5-HT (Yasuhiro et al., 1997b) or compound 48/80 (Yasuhiro et al., 1997a) administration, and this was associated with an increase in mucosal injury.

The proinflammatory effect of increased levels of iNOS appear to be related to increased peroxynitrite activity. Thus, administration of superoxide or peroxyl scavengers reduces the extent of iNOS-mediated mucosal inflammation (Brown et al., 1998). Nitrotyrosine, an index of peroxynitrate and nitrosylated proteins, can be detected in inflamed tissue from experimental animals, and in humans with ulcerative colitis (Chamulitrat et al., 1996; Kimura et al., 1998; Singer et al., 1996).

Recently, it has been demonstrated that peroxynitrite formation, in a rat model of splanchnic artery occlusion shock, correlated with constitutive NOS rather than the inducible isoform (Cuzzocrea et al., 1998). Related to this is the observation that the overexpression of constitutive NOS plays a role in the increased susceptibility of the gastric mucosa to damage in portal hypertensive animals (Ohta et al., 1997). The mechanisms of this upregulation of constitutive NOS are not known, but may be related to the types of inflammatory challenge used in those studies. Thus, overproduction of NO, regardless of its source may provoke cellular injury, should the local environment be conducive to the cytotoxic mechanisms.

6. THERAPEUTIC POTENTIAL
OF NOS INHIBITORS

6.1. Isoform Selective vs Nonselective NOS Inhibitors

A number of strategies have emerged in order to control the physiological and pathophysiological levels of NO, and the inhibition of NOS has by far received the most attention. The consequences of preventing NOS synthesis are multifold, reflecting the diversity of NO as a signaling molecule. Because nonspecific blockade of NO synthesis, using competitive inhibitors such as L-NMMA or L-NAME, may, however, lead to unwanted effects caused by simultaneous inhibition of the constitutive and inducible isoforms of the enzyme, such agents are of limited therapeutic benefit.

An example of this difficulty is exemplified by the use of NOS inhibitors as therapy in sepsis. Although iNOS may contribute to cytotoxicity and circulatory failure, eNOS activity may be required to counteract the resultant vasoconstriction and platelet aggregation (Nava et al., 1991; Porsti and Paakkari, 1995). As a result, recent work has been directed at development of selective iNOS inhibitors. Drugs such as aminoguanidine and L-canavanine have been shown to be inhibitors of the inducible NOS in neutrophils and vascular tissue pancreatic insulinoma cells, as well as in intestine (Corbett et al., 1992; McCall et al., 1989; Umans and Samsel 1992; Liaudet et al., 1997a). However, their potency, selectivity, and profile of actions indicate that caution must exercised with the use of these agents. Thus, aminoguanidine has been shown to effectively inhibit eNOS, as well as iNOS in vivo, in a number of preparations (Laszlo and Whittle, 1997). Ursodeoxycholate can inhibit the induction of iNOS in vivo and in vitro, as well as reduce the extent of intestinal inflammation (Invernizzi et al., 1997). L-lysine, an inhibitor of L-arginine uptake, has been shown to exert beneficial hemodynamic effects, and to reduce organ dysfunction in endotoxic shock. Because L-lysine had no effects in the absence of endotoxin, the effects may reflect a selective action on iNOS (Liaudet et al., 1997b). However, since this essential amino acid will have other biochemical functions, its use as a therapeutic agent will be limited.

Glucocorticoids selectively inhibit induction of iNOS and cytotoxicity in many tissues, including gastrointestinal epithelium, after stimulation with endotoxin or cytokines, without affecting the constitutive form of the enzyme (Rees et al., 1990; Di Rosa et al., 1990). These glucocorticoids do not directly inhibit iNOS, but rather the effect is a result of reduced iNOS expression (Radomski et al., 1990). The contribution of the inhibition of iNOS to the profile of anti-inflammatory action of glucocorticoids has not been fully defined, because these corticosteroids also depress other inflammatory pathways, such as those involving phospholipase A_2 activation and cytokine release.

Other recently developed agents that can selectively modulate iNOS activity, at least in vitro, include 2,4-diamino-6-hydroxypyrinidine, which inhibits BH_4 synthesis (Bune et al., 1996); transforming growth factor β (TGF-β), which inhibits iNOS transcription and enhances iNOS degradation (Vodovotz et al., 1993); and α-melanocyte-stimulating hormone, which inhibits iNOS, and has potent anti-inflammatory properties on the liver (Chiao et al., 1996). However, these latter agents have not been evaluated for their effects on the GI tract, and in some cases TGF-β can cause untoward effects, possibly limiting its clinical use (Sanderson et al., 1995).

Recently, a new inhibitor of iNOS has been developed, which is effective under in vivo and in vitro conditions, and is 5000-fold selective for iNOS vs eNOS. This compound (N-(3-(aminomethyl) benzyl) acetamidine, or 1400W) was shown to be 50-fold more potent against iNOS than eNOS in a rat model of endotoxin-induced vascular injury (Garvey et al., 1997).

6.2. NOS Inhibition and Motility

Because excessive NO may play a role in functional disturbances of gastric and intestinal motility, such disorders potentially can be treated with inhibitors of NOS. The most common disorder in this respect is the rapid transit and disrupted GI motility of endotoxemia resulting from excessive NO (Wirthlin et al., 1996). *E. coli* lipopolysaccharide resulted in an increase in tissue iNOS activity, and in the rate of intestinal transit, which is reversed by L-NMMA or L-NAME, but not D-NAME. Dexamethasone was without effect, or reduced the rapid transit (Hellström et al., 1997), depending on experimental conditions. In contrast to the intestine, endotoxin treatment delayed gastric emptying, and this effect could be reversed by dexamethasone, perhaps suggesting the involvement of iNOS in this response (Takakura et al., 1997).

Although not a disorder of excess NO, the NO produced by eNOS facilitates gastric emptying, and this response can be inhibited by isoform nonselective NOS inhibitors (Anvari et al., 1998; Corak et al., 1997; Plourde et al., 1994). This may be clinically useful in the treatment of conditions associated with accelerated gastric emptying, such as those associated with gastroduodenal resective surgery.

6.3. NOS Inhibition and Diarrheal Disorders

Although it is likely that, under physiological conditions, a NO-dependent proabsorptive tone exists in the intestine, as reviewed in subheading 2.5, in some pathological states, NO can be produced at higher concentrations capable of evoking net secretion. Such NO appears to contribute to the diarrheal response in trinitrobenzene sulfonic acid (TNBS)-induced ileitis, and the spontaneous colitis seen in human leukocyte antigen (HLA)-B27 transgenic rats, and in a chronic colitis model in the rhesus monkey (Aiko et al., 1998; Miller et al., 1993; Ribbons et al., 1997).

Elevated activity of NOS is associated with the laxative action of several intestinal secretagogues, including castor oil, phenophtalein, bisacodyl, magnesium sulphate, bile salts, senna, and cascara. Studies using isoform selective and nonselective inhibitors have indicated that inhibition of NOS effectively ameliorates intestinal secretion, depending on the model evaluated. Thus, in studies using various colitis models, L-NAME effectively reduces TNBS-induced intestinal secretion (Miller et al., 1993); aminoguanidine, but not L-NAME, reduces the diarrheal response in HLA-B27 spontaneous colitis rats (Aiko et al., 1998). However, administration of a more selective iNOS inhibitor, L-N-6-(1-iminoethyl) lysine, orally to rhesus monkeys with chronic colitis, reduced tissue iNOS activation, yet did not provide any therapeutic benefit on the diarrhea (Ribbons et al., 1997). L-NAME or L-NMMA effectively reduce the diarrheal response to the laxatives listed above, but inhibitors of iNOS are only effective against bile salt and cascara-mediated secretion (Izzo et al., 1997; Mascolo et al., 1994).

6.4. iNOS Inhibition and Inflammation

In early studies, concurrent administration of NOS inhibitors, which are not isoform-selective with endotoxin challenge, substantially augmented the early phase of microvascular injury in the GI tract (Boughton Smith et al., 1993). By contrast, delay of administration of L-NMMA, until 3 h after endotoxin challenge, reduced the subsequent vascular leakage (Boughton-Smith et al., 1993b; Laszlo et al., 1995a, 1994, 1995b), at a time when inducible NOS activity becomes apparent. Thus, the beneficial effect of delayed administration of L-NMMA and

L-NAME is considered to be the result of their ability to inhibit iNOS activity. The therapeutic efficacy of delayed administration of isoform nonselective NOS inhibitors in intestinal injury models has been demonstrated in a number of laboratories (Hogaboam et al., 1995; Mishima et al., 1998). Aminoguanidine, a putative iNOS inhibitor, although reducing the late-phase vascular leakage induced by endotoxin (Kavuklu et al., 1998; Sorrells et al., 1996; Unno et al., 1997), also enhances the early phase of mucosal and microvascular dysfunction in a manner similar to that seen after administration of nonisoform-selective NOS inhibitors (Laszlo et al., 1995b; Laszlo and Whittle 1997). Other putative iNOS inhibitors have been shown to protect the intestine. Thus, L-canavanine protects the intestine against endotoxemia by maintaining oxidative metabolism and preserving tissue ATP stores (Liaudet et al., 1997). Such studies emphasize the importance of the development of highly selective inhibitors of iNOS in the therapeutic control of intestinal inflammation.

The putative iNOS-selective inhibitor, S-methylisothiourea, ameliorated endotoxin-induced reductions in intestinal hyperpermeability and mucosal mitochondrial function (Unno et al., 1997). More recently, 1400W was found to be a potent and highly selective inhibitor of iNOS in intestinal dysfunction (Laszlo and Whittle, 1997). In these studies, 1400W had no detrimental effects on the early phase following endotoxin challenge, but inhibited the late-phase injury. Administration of nonselective NOS inhibitors, such as L-NAME, or selective iNOS inhibitors, such as S-(2-aminoethyl)isothiouronium bromide, ameliorated experimentally induced colitis in the rat (Kiss et al., 1997; Rachmilewitz et al., 1995; Southey et al., 1997; Unno et al., 1997c).

In contrast to the prevailing attitude that iNOS is cytotoxic, a number of studies provide some opposing evidence. In iNOS knock-out mice, acetic-acid-induced mucosal injury was not attenuated, and healing appeared impaired (McCafferty et al., 1997). In other studies, the use of more selective iNOS antagonists did not appear to reduce experimentally induced colitis, although aminoguanidine also did not reduce NOS activity in that study (Ribbons et al., 1997). NO released from the NO donors, CAS 754 or SIN-1, did not cause breakdown of mucosal or microvascular barrier integrity under normal or inflammatory conditions (Kubes et al., 1995). These findings, however, contrast with studies with NO donors that have demonstrated a marked injurious action on the gastric mucosa following local infusion (Lopez-Belmonte et al.,

1993; Lamarque and Whittle, 1995a, 1995b). Exploration of dependency on the experimental setting for the production of tissue injury with NO donors may yield information on the mechanism of NO cytotoxicty.

The results of a number of studies have suggested that NO released via iNOS expression, following lipopolysaccharide administration, can protect the gastric mucosa from damage in response to luminal irritants or stress (Brzozowski et al., 1997; Konturek et al., 1998; Mercer et al., 1998; Tepperman and Soper, 1994; Yu et al., 1997), and can protect the intestinal mucosa from an inflammatory challenge via a reduction in leukocyte infiltration and adhesion (Binion et al., 1998). This iNOS-mediated protection has also been attributed to an increase in cytoprotective PGE_2 release (Franco and Doria, 1998), and, as an antioxidant, either directly for maintaining cellular glutathione or activating other antioxidants, such as manganese superoxide dismutase (Chamulitrat, 1998; Kim and Kim, 1998; Valentine et al., 1996).

In contrast to these studies, it has been demonstrated that the purified lipopolysaccharide derived from *H. pylori* is highly active in vivo in stimulating the expression of iNOS in duodenal epithelial cells, associated with cytotoxicity in these cells (Lamarque et al., 1998). This epithelial injury is inhibited by a selective inhibitor of iNOS, and by superoxide dismutase. Such findings again point to the involvement of NO, in combination with superoxide, to produce peroxynitrite, in epithelial injury associated with *H. pylori* infection. The control of such tissue damage with selective iNOS inhibitors may provide a complementary approach to peptic ulcer therapy.

The involvement of NO in the tissue injury associated with infectious diseases of the gut have also been explored. In a model of jejunal infection with *Trichinella spiralis*, oral treatment with L-NAME lowered bacterial count and myeloperoxidase levels, although effects on iNOS activity were complex (Hogaboam et al., 1996). In patients in the acute phase of shigellosis, inflammation in rectal biopsies was associated with expression of iNOS in the epithelium (Islam et al., 1997). A role for NO has also been proposed in necrotizing enterocolitis in infants (Ford et al., 1997).

There is also invovlement of iNOS in the chronic microvascular leakage and tissue inflammatory injury in the small intestine that follows the administration of nonsteroidal anti-inflammatory agents such as indomethacin (Whitle et al., 1995). This slowly developing enteropathy involves indigenous bacteria, and is attenuated by inhibition of iNOS, suggesting that, following ingress of bacteria, lipopolysaccharide is liberated in the intestinal mucosa, which brings about the induction of iNOS. As in these experimental studies, it is possible that such inflammatory conditions of the gut provoked by NSAIDs will respond to the therapeutic use of selective iNOS inhibitors.

7. CONCLUSIONS

It appears that the NO pathway offers a number of diverse therapeutic opportunities for diseases of the gut. The use of NO donors in a range of motility problems is currently under investigation, as is their use in protecting the gut mucosa from injury. Indeed, the therapeutic value of NO-containing NSAIDs is being actively pursued in experimental and clinical studies.

The use of inhibitors of NO production is also being evaluated, especially as anti-inflammatory agents in the gut, but it is likely that NO produced from iNOS, or its subsequent products, are not involved in all aspects of the inflammatory response in the gut. Because of their profile on leucocyte function, NO would not, for example, be expected to directly promote cellular infiltration. However, there is a wealth of literature supporting the cytotoxic actions of NO in many different inflammatory situations, both in and beyond the GI tract. The injurious effects of iNOS expression on microvascular injury that follows endotoxin challenge has been well characterized in many models. Such microvascular perturbation and plasma leakage are cardinal signs of inflammation, and point to the significant role of iNOS products in this pathological aspect.

It may be too early to dismiss NO or its subsequent products, produced by iNOS, as having any role in the complex inflammatory processes in the gut. The role of NO may well differ with the nature of the insult, the tissue and environment involved, and the local response and interaction with the other mediators involved. As with many other inflammatory mediators, it is entirely possible that a low level of expression of iNOS will reflect a positive host-defense response to challenge, but that exaggerated or uncontrolled expression of iNOS itself becomes detrimental. It is also feasible that the products of iNOS may have a greater role in the early phase of inflammation, such as following relapse in patients with IBD, but lower levels of iNOS activity could have a beneficial action in the process of resolution of the inflammatory response. The apparent paradox of conflicting beneficial and damaging roles of NO will require additional studies, but such events are well established in the field of inflammatory mediators, including the PG COX-1 and COX-2 pathways for protection and injury in the gut. The therapeutic potential of selective inhibitors of iNOS or its injurious products, such as peroxynitrite, should therefore to be considered further in a range of inflammatory conditions of the gut.

REFERENCES

Aiko S, Fuseler V, Grisham MB. Effects of nitric oxide synthase inhibition or sulfasalazine on the spontaneous colitis observed in HLA-B27 transgenic rats. *J Pharmacol Exp Ther* 1998; 284: 722–727.

Alemayehu A, Lock KR, Coatney RW, Chou CC. L-NAME, nitric oxide and jejunal motility, blood flow and oxygen uptake in dogs. *Br J Pharmacol* 1994; 111: 205–212.

Allen A. Structure and function of gastrointestinal mucus, in *Physiology of the Gastrointestinal Tract* (Johnson LR, ed.), Raven, New York, 1994, pp. 617–639.

Allen A, Hunter AC, Lenard AJ, Pearson JP, Sellers LA. Peptic activity and the mucus-bicarbonate barrier, in *Advances in Drug Therapy of Gastrointestinal Ulceration* (Garner A, Whittle BJR, eds.),Wiley, Chichester, 1989, pp. 139–151.

Andrews FJ, Malcontenti-Wilson C, O'Brien PE. Protection against gastric ischemia-reperfusion injury by nitric oxide generators. *Dig Dis Sci* 1994; 39: 366–373.

Anvari M, Paterson CA, Daniel EE. Role of nitric oxide mechanisms in control of pyloric motility and transpyloric flow of liquids in conscious dogs. *Dig Dis Sci* 1998; 43: 506–512.

Asahi M, Fujii J, Suzuki K, Seo HG, Kuzuya T, Hori M, Tada M, Fujii S, Taniguchi N. Inactivation of glutatione peroxidase by nitric oxide. Implication for cytotoxicity. *J Biol Chem* 1995; 270: 21,035–21,039.

Barrachina MD, Calatayud S, Canet A, Bello R, Diaz de Rojas F, Guth PH, Esplugues JV. Transdermal nitroglycerin prevents nonsteroidal anti-inflammatory drug gastropathy. *Eur J Pharmacol* 1995; 281: R3–R4.

Barrachina MD, Calatayud S, Esplugues J, Whittle BJR, Moncada S, Esplugues JV. Nitric oxide donors preferentially inhibit neuronally-mediated rat gastric acid secretion. *Eur J Pharmacol* 1994; 262: 181–183.

Barry MK, Aloisi JD, Pickering SP, Yeo CJ. Nitric oxide modulates water and electrolyte transport in the ileum. *Ann Surg* 1994; 219: 382–388.

Banyguinov O, Sanders KM. Role of nitric oxide as an inhibitory neurotransmitter in the canine pyloric sphincter. *Am J Physiol* 1993; 264: G975–G983.

Bayguinov O, Vogalis F, Morris B, Sanders KM. Patterns of electrical activity and neural responses in canine proximal duodenum. *Am J Physiol* 1992; 263: G887–G894.

Beck PL, McKnight GW, Kelly JK, Wallace JL, Lee SS. Hepatic and gastric cytoprotective effects of long-term prostaglandin E_1 administration in cirrhotic rats. *Gastroenterology* 1993; 105: 1483–1489.

Beckman JS, Koppenol WH. Nitric oxide, superoxide and peroxynitrite: the good, the bad and ugly. *Am J Physiol* 1996; 271: C1424–C1437.

Beubler E, Schirgi-Degen A. Nitric oxide counteracts 5-hydroxytryptamine and cholera toxin-induced fluid secretion and enhances the effect of oral rehydration solution. *Eur J Pharmacol* 1997; 326: 223–228.

Bevilacqua MP, Pober JS, Mendrick DL, Cotran RJ, Gimbrone MA. Identification of an inducible endothelial leukocyte adhesion molecule. *Proc Natl Acad Sci USA* 1987; 84: 9238–9242.

Bilski J, Konturek SJ. Role of nitric oxide in gastroduodenal alkaline secretion. *J Physiol Pharmacol* 1994; 45: 541–553.

Bilski J, Konturek SJ, Cieszkowski M, Czarnobilski K, Pawlik WW. Endogenous nitric oxide in the regulation of gastric acid secretion, gastrin release and blood flow. *Biomed Res* 1994; 15(Suppl, 2): 63–67.

Binion DG, Fu S, Ramanujam KS, Chai YC, Dweik RA, Drazha VA, et al. iNOS expression in human intestinal microvascular endothelial cells inhibits leukocyte adhesion. *Am J Physiol* 1998; 275: G592–G603.

Boeckxstaens GE, Pelckmans PA, Bogers JJ, Bult H, DeMan IG, Oosterbosch L, Herman AG, Van Maercke YM. Release of nitric oxide upon stimulation of nonadrenergic noncholinergic nerves in the rat gastric fundus. *J Pharmacol Exp Ther* 1990; 256: 441–447.

Bogers JJ, Pelckmans PA, Boeckxstaens GE, De Man JG, Herman AG, Van Maercke YM. Role of nitric oxide in serotonin-induced relaxations in the canine terminal ileum and ileocolonic junction. *Nauyn Schmiedebergs Arch Pharmcol* 1991; 344: 716–719.

Boughton-Smith NK, Evans SM, Hawkey CJ, Cole AT, Balsitis M, Whittle BJR, Moncada S. Differential changes in nitric oxide synthase activity in ulcerative colitis and Crohn's disease. *Lancet* 1993a; 342: 338–340.

Boughton-Smith NK, Evans SM, Laszlo F, Whittle BJR, Moncada S. Induction of nitric oxide synthase and intestinal vascular permeability by endotoxin in the rat. *Br J Pharmacol* 1993b; 110: 1189–1195.

Boughton-Smith NK, Deakin AM, Whittle BJR. Actions of nitric oxide on the acute gastrointestinal damage induced by PAF in the rat. *Agents Actions* 1992; 37(Special Conference Issue): C3–C9.

Boughton-Smith NK, Hutchenson I, Deakin AM, Whittle BJR, Moncada S. Protective effect of S-nitroso-N-acetyl-penicillamine in endotoxin-induced acute intestinal damage in the rat. *Eur J Pharmacol* 1990; 191: 485–488.

Brown JF, Chafee KA, Tepperman BL. Role of mast cells, neutrophils and nitric oxide in endotoxin-induced damage to the neonatal rat colon. *Br J Pharmacol* 1998; 123: 31–38.

Brown JF, Hanson PJ, Whittle BJR. Nitric oxide donors increase mucus gel thickness in rat stomach. *Eur J Pharmacol* 1992; 223: 103–104.

Brown JF, Hanson PJ, Whittle BJR. Nitric oxide donor, S-nitroso-N-acetyl-penicillamine, inhibits secretory activity in rat isolated parietal cells. *Biochem Biophys Res Commun* 1993a; 195: 1354–1359.

Brown JF, Keates AC, Hanson PJ, Whittle BJR. Nitric oxide generators and cGMP stimulate mucous secretion by rat gastric mucosal cells. *Am J Physiol* 1993b; 265: G418–G422.

Brzozowski T, Konturek PC, Sliwowski Z, Drozdowicz D, Pajdo R, Stachura J, Hahn EG. Lipopolysaccharide of *Helicobacter pylori* protects gastric mucosa via generation of nitric oxide. *J Physiol Pharmacol* 1997; 48: 699–717.

Bune AJ, Brand MP, Heales SJR, Shergill JF, Cammack R, Cook HT. Inhibition of tetrahydrobiopterin synthesis reduces in vivo nitric oxide production in experimental endotoxic shock. *Biochem Biophys Res Comm* 1996; 220: 13–19.

Calignano A, Whittle BJ, Di Rosa M, Moncada S. Involvement of endogenous nitric oxide in the regulation of rat intestinal motility in vivo. *Eur J Pharmacol* 1992; 229: 273–276.

Chamulitrat W. Nitric oxide inhibited peroxyl and alkoxyl radical formation with concomitant protection against oxidant injury in intestinal epithelial cells. *Arch Biochem Biophys* 1998; 355: 206–214.

Chamulitrat W, Skrepnik NV, Spitzer JJ. Nitrosyl complex formation during endotoxin-induced injury in the rat small intestine. *Shock* 1996; 5: 59–65.

Chiao H, Foster S, Thomas R, Lipton J, Star RA. Alpha-melanocyte-stimulating hormone reduces endotoxin-induced liver inflammation. *J Clin Invest* 1996; 97: 2038–2044.

Cirino G, Cicala C, Mancuso F, Baydoun AR, Wallace JL. Flurbinitroxy-butylester: a novel anti-inflammatory drug has enhanced antithrombotic activity. *Thromb Res* 1995; 79: 73–81.

Cirino G, Wheeler-Jones CP, Wallace JL, Del Soldato, P, Baydoun AR. Inhibition of inducible nitric oxide synthase expression by novel nonsteroidal anti-inflammatory derivatives with gastrointestinal-sparing properties. *Br J Pharmacol* 1996; 117: 1421–1426.

Corak A, Coskun T, Alican I, Kurtel H, Yegen BC. Effect of nitric oxide synthase blockade and indomethacin on gastric emptying and gastric contractility. *Pharmacology* 1997; 54: 298–304.

Corbett JA, Tilton RG, Chang K, Hasan K, Ido Y, Wang VL, et al. Aminoguanidine, a novel inhibition of nitric oxide formation prevents diabetic vascular dysfunction. *Diabetes* 1992; 41: 552–556.

Cullen JJ, Caropreso DK, Ikmann LL, Hinkhouse M, Conklin JH, Ephgrave KS. Pathophysiology of adynamic ileus. *Dig Dis Sci* 1997; 42: 731–737.

Cuzzolin L, Adami A, Crivellente F, Benoni G. Role of endogenous and exogenous nitric oxide on intestinal mucosa and microflora in the rat. *Inflammation* 1997; 21: 443–450.

Cuzzolin L, Conforti A, Adami A, Lussignoli S, Menestrina F, Del Soldato P, Benoni G. Anti-inflammatory potency and gastrointestinal toxicity of a new compound nitronaproxen. *Pharmacol Res* 1995; 31: 61–65.

Cuzzocrea S, Zingarelli B, Caputi AP. Role of constitutive nitric oxide synthase and peroxynitrate production in a rat model of splanchnic artery occlusion shock. *Life Sci* 1998; 63: 789–799.

Davenpeck KL, Gauthier TW, Lefer AM. Inhibition of endothelial-derived nitric oxide promotes P-selectin expression and actions in the rat microcirculation. *Gastroenterology* 1994; 107: 1050–1058.

Di Rosa M, Radomski M, Carnuccio R, Moncada S. Glucocorticoids inhibit the induction of nitric oxide synthase in macrophages. *Biochem Biophys Res Comm* 1990; 172: 1246–1252.

Esplugues JV, Barrachina MD, Beltran B, Calatayud S, Whittle BJR, Moncada J. Inhibition of gastric acid secretion by stress: a protective reflex mediated by cerebral nitric oxide. *Proc Natl Acad Sci USA* 1996; 93: 14,839–14,844.

Fändricks L, von Bothmer C, Johansson B, Holm M, Bölin I, Pettersson A. Water extracts of *Helicobacter pylori* inhibit duodenal mucosal alkaline secretion in anaesthetized rats. *Gastroenterology* 1997; 113: 1570–1575.

Feldman MJ, Morris GP, Dinda PK, Paterson WG. Mast cells mediate acid-induced augmentation of opossum esophageal blood flow via histamine and nitric oxide. *Gastroenterology* 1996; 110: 121–128.

Ferraz JGP, McKnight W, Sharkey KA, Wallace JL. Impaired vasodilatory responses in the gastric microcirculation of anaesthetized rats with secondary biliary cirrhosis. *Gastroenterology* 1995; 108: 1183–1191.

Ferraz JGP, Wallace JL. Prostaglandins modulate the responsiveness of the gastric microcirculation to sodium nitroprusside in cirrhotic rats. *Hepatology* 1996; 23: 123–129.

Ferretti M, Gionchetti P, Rizzello F, Venturi A, Stella P, Corti F, et al. Intracolonic release of nitric oxide during trinitrobenzene sulfonic acid colitis in the rat. *Dig Dis Sci* 1997; 42: 2606–2611.

Fiorucci S, Distrutti E, Quintieri A, Sarpi L, Sprichez Z, Gulla N, Morelli A.

L-arginine/nitric oxide pathway modulates gastric motility and gallbladder emptying induced by erythromycin and liquid meal in humans. *Dig Dis Sci* 1995; 40: 1365–1371.

Fleming I, Busse R. Control and consequence of endothelial nitric oxide formation. *Adv Pharmacol* 1995; 34: 187–206.

Flemstrom G, Kivilaakso E. Demonstration of a pH gradient at the luminal surface of rat duodenum and its dependence on mucosal alkaline secretion. *Gastroenterology* 1983; 84: 787–794.

Ford H, Watkins S, Reblock K, Rowe M. Role of inflammatory cytokines and nitric oxide in the pathogenesis of necrotizing enterocolitis. *J Pediatr Surg* 1997; 32: 275–82.

Forgacs IC, Maisley MN, Murphy GM, Dowling RH. Influence of gallstones and ursodeoxycholic acid on gallbladder emptying. *Gastroenterology* 1984; 87: 299–307.

Forstermann N, Schmidt HHH, Pollack JS, Sheng H, Mitchell JA, Warner TD, Nakane M, Murad F. Isoforms of nitric oxide synthase. Characterization and purification from different cell types. *Biochem Pharmacol* 1991; 42: 1849–1857.

Franco L, Doria D. Nitric oxide enhances prostaglandin production in ethanol-induced gastric mucosal injury in rats. *Eur J Pharmacol* 1998; 348: 247–256.

Gaboury J, Woodman RC, Granger DN, Reinhardt P, Kubes P. Nitric oxide prevents leukocyte adherence: role of superoxide. *Am J Physiol* 1993; 265: H862–H867.

Garthwaite J, Garthwaite G, Palmer RMJ, Moncada S. NMDA receptor activation induces nitric oxide synthesis in rat brain slices. *Eur J Pharmacol* 1989; 172: 413–416.

Garvey EP, Oplinger JA, Furfine ES, Kiff RJ, Laszlo F, Whittle BJR, Knowles RG. 1400 W is a slow tight binding and highly selective inhibitor of inducible nitric oxide in vitro and in vivo. *J Biol Chem* 1997; 272: 4959–4963.

Gauthier TW, Niu X-F, Kubes P. Nitric oxide attenuates leukocyte-endothelial interaction via P-selectin in splanchnic ischemia-reperfusion. *Am J Physiol* 1994; 267: G562–G568.

Gonzalez M, Mearin F, Vasconez C, Armengol JR, Malagelada JR. Oesophageal tone in patients with achalasia. *Gut* 1997; 41: 291–296.

Granger DN, Kubes P. Microcirculation and inflammation: modulation of leukocyte-endothelial cell adhesion. *J Leukoc Biol* 1994; 55: 662–675.

Greaves R, Miller J, O'Donnell L, McLean A, Farthing MJ. Effect of the nitric oxide donor, glyceryl trinitrate in human gall bladder motility. *Gut* 1998; 42: 410–413.

Grider JR, Murthy KS, Jin J-G, Makhlouf GM. Stimulation of nitric oxide from muscle cells by VIP: prejunctional enhancement of VIP release. *Am J Physiol* 1992; 262: G774–G778.

Gupta SK, Fitzgerald JF, Chong SK, Croffie JM, Garcia JG. Expression of inducible nitric oxide synthase (iNOS) mRNA in inflamed esophageal and colonic mucosa in a pediatric population. *Am J Gastroenterol* 1998; 93: 795–798.

Hahm KB, Lee KJ, Kim JH, Cho SW, Chung MH. *Heliobacter pylori* infection, oxidative DNA damage, gastric carcinogenesis and reversibility by rebamipide. *Dig Dis Sci* 1998; 43: 725–775.

Hällgren A, Flemström G, Sababi M, Nylander O. Effect of nitric oxide inhibition on duodenal function in the rat. Involvement of neural mechanisms. *Am J Physiol* 1995; 269: G246–G254.

Hassel B. Treatment of biliary colic with nitroglycerin. *Lancet* 1993; 342: 1305.

Hata Y, Ota S, Hiraishi H, Terano A, Ivey KJ. Nitric oxide enhances cytotoxicity of cultured rabbit gastric mucosal cells induced by hydrogen peroxide. *Biochim Biophys Acta* 1996; 1290: 257–260.

Hellstrom PM, al-Saffar A, Ljung T, Theodorsson E. Endotoxin actions on myoelectric activity, transit and neurpeptides in the gut. Role of nitric oxide. *Dig Dis Sci* 1997; 42: 1640–1651.

Hevel JM, White KA, Marletta MA. Purification of the inducible murine macrophage nitric oxide synthase. *J Biol Chem* 1991; 264: 22,789–22,791.

Hisanaga Y, Goto H, Tachi K, Hayakawa T, Sugiyama S. Implications of nitric oxide synthase activity in the genesis of water immersion stress-induced gastric lesions in rats: protective effect of FK506. *Aliment Pharmacol Ther* 1996; 10: 933–940.

Hogaboam CM, Colins SM, Blennerhassett MG. Effects of oral L-NAME during *Trichinella spiralis* infection in rats. *Am J Physiol* 1996; 271: G338–46.

Hogaboam CM, Jacobson K, Collins SM, Blennerhassett MG. Selective beneficial affects of nitric oxide inhibition in experimental colitis. *Am J Physiol* 1995; 268: G673–G684.

Holm M, Johansson B, Pettersson A, Fändriks L. Acid-induced duodenal mucosal nitric oxide output parallels bicarbonate secretion in the anaesthetized pig. *Acta Physiol Scand* 1998; 162: 461–468.

Holzer P, Lippe IT, Tabrizi AL, Lenard L, Barth L. Dual excitatory and inhibitory effect of nitric oxide on peristalsis in the guinea pig intestine. *J Pharmacol Exp Ther* 1997; 280: 154–161.

Holzer-Petsche U, Moser RL. Participation of nitric oxide in the relaxation of the rat gastric corpus. *Nauyn Schmiedebergs Arch Pharmacol* 1996; 354: 348–354.

Ichikawa T, Ishihara K, Kusakabe T, Kurihara M, Kawakami T, Saigenji K,

Hotta K. Distinct effects of tetragastrin, histamine and CCh on rat gastric mucin synthesis and contribution of NO. *Am J Physiol* 1998; 274: G138–G146.

Invernizzi P, Salzman AL, Szabo C, Ueta I, O'Connor M, Setchell KD. Ursodeoxycholate inhibits induction of NOS in human intestinal epithelial cells and in vivo. *Am J Physiol* 1997; 273: G131–G138.

Islam D, Veress B, Bardham PK, Lindberg AA, Christensson B. *In situ* characterization of inflammatory responses in the rectal mucosae of patients with shigellosis. *Infect Immun* 1997; 65: 739–49.

Iwata F, Joh T, Kawai T, Hoh M. Role of EDRF in splanchnic blood flow of normal and chronic portal hypertensive rats. *Am J Physiol* 1992; 263: G149–G154.

Izzo AA, Masolo N, Capasso F. Nitric oxide as a modulator of intestinal water and electrolyte transport. *Dig Dis Sci* 1998; 43: 1605–1620.

Izzo AA, Mascolo N, Maiolino P, Capasso F. Nitric oxide-donating compounds and cyclic GMP depress the spontaneous contractile activity of the isolated rabbit jejunum. *Pharmacology* 1996; 53: 109–113.

Izzo AA, Saubetin L, Rombola L, Capasso F. Role of constitutive and inducible nitric oxide synthase in senna- and cascara-induced diarrhea in the rat. *Eur J Pharmacol* 1997; 323: 93–97.

Johnston B, Kanwar S, Kubes P. Hydrogen peroxide induces leukocyte rolling: modulation by endogenous antioxidant mechanisms including nitric oxide. *Am J Physiol* 1996; 271: H614-H621.

Kato S, Hirata T, Takeuchi K. Nitric oxide, prostaglandin and sensory neurons in gastric mucosal blood flow response during acid secretion in rats. *Gen Pharmacol* 1997; 28: 513–519.

Kato S, Kitamura M, Korokiewicz RP, Takeuchi K. Role of nitric oxide in regulation of gastric acid secretion in rats: effects of NO donors and NO synthase inhibitor. *Br J Pharmacol* 1998; 123: 839–846.

Kavuklu B, Agalar C, Guc MO, Sayeh I. Evidence that aminoguanidine inhibits endotoxin-induced bacterial translocation. *Br J Surg* 1998; 85: 1103–1106.

Kerwin JF Jr, Lancaster JR Jr, Feldman PL. Nitric oxide: a new paradigm for second messengers. *J Med Chem* 1995; 38: 4343–4362.

Kim H, Kim KH. Role of nitric oxide in oxidative damage in isolated rabbit gastric cells exposed to hypoxia-reoxygeneration. *Dig Dis Sci* 1998; 43: 1042–1049.

Kimura H, Hobari R, Miura S, Shigematsu T, Hirokawa M, Akiba Y, et al. Increased expression of an inducible isoform of nitric oxide synthase and the formation of peroxynitrite in colonic mucosa of patients with active ulcerative colitis. *Gut* 1998; 42: 180–187.

Kimura H, Miura S, Shigematsu T, Ohkubo N, Tsuzuki Y, Kurose I, et al. Increased nitric oxide production and inducible nitric oxide synthase activity in colonic mucosa of patients with active ulcerative colitis and Crohn's disease. *Dig Dis Sci* 1997; 42: 1047–1054.

Kiss J, Lamarque D, Delchier JC, Whittle BJR. Time-dependent actions of nitric oxide synthase inhibition on colonic inflammation induced by trinitrobenzene sulfonic acid in rats. *Eur J Pharmacol* 1997; 336: 219–224.

Kitigawa H, Takeda F, Koheri H. Effect of endothelium-derived relaxing factor on the gastric lesion induced by HCl in rats. *J Pharmacol Exp Ther* 1990; 253: 1133–1137.

Klein-Nulend J, Helfrich MH, Sterck JG, MacPherson H, Joldersma M, Ralston SH, Semeins CM, Burger EH. Nitric oxide response to shear stress by human bone cells is endothelial nitric oxide synthase dependent. *Biochem Biophys Res Commun* 1998; 250: 108–114.

Konturek PC, Brzozowski T, Sliwowski Z, Pajdo R, Stachura J, Hahn EG, Konturek SJ. Involvement of nitric oxide and prostaglandins in gastroprotection induced by bacterial lipopolysaccharide. *Scand J Gastroenterol* 1998; 33: 691–700.

Konturek SJ, Gillessen A, Domschke W. Diffuse esophageal spasm: a malfunction that involves nitric oxide? *Scan J Gastroenterol* 1995a; 30: 1041–1045.

Konturek JW, Thor P, Domschke W. Effects of nitric oxide in antral motility and gastric emptying in humans. *Eur J Gastroenterol Hepatol* 1995b; 7: 97–102.

Konturek SJ, Thor P, Lukaszyk A, Gabryelewicz A, Konturek SJ, Domschke W. Endogenous nitric oxide in the control of esophageal motility in humans. *J Physiol Pharmacol* 1997; 48: 201–209.

Kubes P, Reinhardt PH, Payne O, Woodman RC. Excess nitric oxide does not cause cellular vascular or mucosal dysfunction in the cat small intestine. *Am J Physiol* 1995; 269: G34–G41.

Kubes P, Suzuki M, Granger, DN. Nitric oxide: an endogenous modulator of leukocyte adhesion. *Proc Natl Acad Sci USA* 1991; 88: 4651–4655.

Kwon NS, Stuehr DJ, Nathan CF. Inhibition of tumor cell ribonucleotide reductase by macrophage-derived nitric oxide. *J Exp Med* 1991; 174: 761–767.

Lamarque D, Kiss J, Tankovic J, Flejon JF, Delchier JC, Whittle, BJR. Induction of nitric oxide synthase in vivo and cell injury in rat duodenal epithelium by a water soluble extract of *Helicobacter pylori*. *Br J Pharmacol* 1998; 123: 1073–1078.

Lamarque D, Whittle BJR. Involvement of superoxide and xanthine oxidase in neutrophil-independent rat gastric damage induced by NO donors. *Br J Pharmacol* 1995a; 116: 1843–1846.

Lamarque D, Whittle BJR. Role of oxygen-derived metabolites in the rat gastric mucosal injury induced by nitric oxide donors. *Eur J Pharmacol* 1995b; 277: 187–194.

Lamas S, Marsden PA, Li GK, Tampst P, Michel T. Endothelial nitric oxide synthase: molecular cloning and characterization of a distinct constitutive enzyme isoform. *Proc Natl Acad Sci USA* 1992; 89: 6348–6352.

Laszlo F, Whittle BJR. Actions of isoform-selective and non-selective nitric oxide synthase inhibitors on endotoxin-induced vascular leakage in rat colon. *Eur J Pharmacol* 1997; 334: 99–102.

Laszlo F, Whittle BJ, Evans SM, Moncada S. Association of microvascular leakage with induction of nitric oxide synthase: effects of nitric oxide synthase inhibitors in various organs. *Eur J Pharmacol* 1995a; 283: 47–53.

Laszlo F, Whittle BJR, Moncada S. Time-dependent enhancement or inhibition of endotoxin-induced vascular injury in rat intestine by nitric oxide synthase inhibitors. *Br J Pharmacol* 1994; 111: 1309–1315.

Laszlo F, Whittle BJR, Moncada S. Attenuation by nitrosothiol NO donors of actue microvascular dysfunction in the rat. *Br J Pharmacol* 1995b; 115: 498–502.

Lawrence MB, Bainton DF, Springer TA. Neutrophil tethering to and rolling on E-selectin are separable by requirement for L-selectin. *Immunity* 1994; 1: 137–145.

Li CK, Seth R, Gray T, Bayston R, Mahida YR, Wakelin D. Production of proinflammatory cytokines and inflammatory mediators in human intestinal epithelial cells after invasion by *Trichinella spiralis*. *Infect Immun* 1998; 66: 2200–2206.

Liaudet L, Fishman D, Markert M, Perret C, Fiehl F. L-canavanine improves organ function and tissue adenosine triphosphate levels in rodent endotoxemia. *Am J Respir Crit Care Med* 1997a; 155: 1643–1648.

Liaudet L, Gnaeji A, Rosselet A, Markert BO, Perret C, Feihl F. Effect of L-lysine in nitric oxide overproduction in endotoxic shock. *Br J Pharmacol* 1997b; 122: 742–748.

Llewellyn-Smith IJ, Song ZM, Costa M, Bredt DS, Snyder SH. Ultrastructural localization of nitric oxide synthase immunoreactivity in guinea pig enteric neurons. *Brain Res* 1992; 577: 337–342.

Lopez-Belmonte J, Whittle BJR, Moncada S. Actions of nitric oxide donors in the prevention or induction of injury to the rat gastric mucosa. *Br J Pharmacol* 1993; 108: 73–78.

Luman W, Pryde A, Heading RC, Palmer KR. Topical glyceryl trinitrate relaxes the sphincter of Oddi. *Gut* 1997; 40: 541–543.

Ma X, Weyrich AJ, Lefer DJ, Lefer AM. Diminished basal nitric oxide release after myocardial ischemia and reperfusion promotes neutrophil adherence to coronary endothelium. *Circ Res* 1993; 72: 403–412.

MacNaughton K, Cirino G, Wallace JL. Endothelium-derived relaxing factor (nitric oxide) has protective actions in the stomach. *Life Sci* 1989; 45: 1869–1876.

Maczka M, Thor P, Lorens K, Konturek SJ. Nitric oxide inhibits the myoelectric activity of the small intestine in dogs. *J Physiol Pharmacol* 1993; 4: 31–42.

Maher MM, Gontarek JD, Jimenez RE, Cahill PA, Yeo CJ. Endogenous nitric oxide promotes ileal absorption. *J Surg Res* 1995; 58: 687–692.

Marsden PA, Heng HH, Scherer SW, Stewart RJ, Hall AV, Shi XM, Tsui LC, Schappert KT. Structure and chromosomal localization of the human constitutive endothelial nitric oxide gene. *J Biol Chem* 1993; 268: 17,478–17,488.

Martinez-Cuesta, MA, Barrachina MD, Pique JM, Whittle BJR, Esplugues J. Role of nitric oxide and platelet activating factor in the inhibition by endotoxin of pentagastrin-stimulated gastric acid secretion. *Eur J Pharmacol* 1992; 218: 351–354.

Martinez-Cuesta MA, Esplugues JV, Whittle BJR. Modulation by nitric oxide of spontaneous motility of the rat duodenum: role of tachykinins. *Br J Pharmacol* 1996; 118: 1335–1340.

Martinez-Cuesta MA, Massuda H, Whittle BJR, Moncada J. Impairment of nitrergic-mediated relaxation of rat isolated duodenum by experimental diabetes. *Br J Pharmacol* 1995; 114: 919–924.

Mascolo N, Gagnella TS, Izzo AA, Di Carlo G, Capasso F. Nitric oxide involvement in sodium choleate-induced fluid secretion and diarrhea in rats. *Eur J Pharmacol* 1994; 264: 21–26.

Matheson PJ, Wilson MA, Spain DA, Harris PD, Anderson GL, Garrison RN. Glucose-induced intestinal hyperemia is mediated by nitric oxide. *J Surg Res* 1997; 72: 146–154.

McCafferty DM, Mudgett JS, Swain MG, Kubes P. Inducible nitric oxide synthase plays a critical role in resolving intestinal inflammation. *Gastroenterology* 1997; 112: 1022–1027.

McCall TB, Boughton-Smith NK, Palmer RMJ, Whittle BJR, Moncada S. Synthesis of nitric oxide from L-arginine by neutrophils. *Biochem J* 1989; 261: 293–296.

Mearin F, Mourelle F, Guarner F, Salas A, Riveros-Moreno V, Moncada S, Malagelada JR. Patients with achalasia lack nitric oxide synthase in the gastroesophageal junction. *Eur J Clin Invest* 1993; 23: 724–728.

Mercer DW, Castaneda AA, Denning JW, Chang L, Russell DH. Effects of endotoxin in gastric injury from luminal irritants in rats: potential roles of nitric oxide. *Am J Physiol* 1998; 275: G449–G459.

Miller MJS, Sadowska-Krowicka S, Chatinuaruemol S, Kakis JL, Clark DA. Amelioration of chronic ileitis by nitric oxide synthase inhibition. *J Pharmacol Exp Ther* 1993; 264: 11–16.

Mishima S, Xu D, Lu Q, Deitch EA. Relationships among nitric oxide production, bacterial translocation and intestinal injury after endotoxin challenge in vivo. *J Trauma* 1998; 44: 175–182.

Mizumoto A, Muramatsu S, Yamada T, Itoh Z. Effect of nitric oxide synthase inhibition on plasma motilin release in fasted dogs. *Reg Peptides* 1997; 71: 9–14.

Moncada S, Higgs EA. Molecular mechanisms and therapeutic strategies related to nitric oxide. *FASEB J* 1995; 9: 1319–1330.

Moncada S, Palmer RMJ, Higgs EA. Nitric oxide: Physiology, pathophysiology and pharmacology. *Pharmacol Rev* 1991; 43: 109–142.

Mourad FH, O'Dennel LJD, Andre EA, Bearcroft CP, Owen RA. L-Arginine, nitric oxide and intestinal secretion: studies in rat jejunum in vivo. *Gut* 1996; 39: 539–544.

Murray C, Ledlow A, Bates JN, Conklin JL. Nitric oxide: mediator of nonadrenergic noncholinergic responses of opossum esophageal muscle. *Am J Physiol* 1991; 261: G401–G406.

Muscara MN, McKnight W, Del Soldato P, Wallace JL. Effect of a nitric oxide releasing naproxen derivative on hypertension and gastric damage induced by chronic nitric oxide inhibition in the rat. *Life Sci* 1998; 62: PL 235–240.

Nava E, Palmer RM, Moncada S. Inhibition of nitric oxide synthesis in peptic shock: how much is beneficial. *Lancet* 1991; 338: 1555–1557.

Nase GP, Boegehold MA. Nitric oxide modulates arteriolar responses to increased sympathetic nerve activity. *Am J Physiol* 1996; 271: H860–H869.

Nase GP, Boegehold MA. Endothelium-derived nitric oxide limits sympathetic neurogenic constriction in intestinal microcirculation. *Am J Physiol* 1997; 273: H426–H433.

Nelin LD, Thomas CJ, Dawson CA. Effect of hypoxia on nitric oxide production in neonatal pig lung. *Am J Physiol* 1996; 271: H8–H14.

Nguyen T, Brunson D, Crespi CL, Penman BW, Wishnok JS, Tannenbaum CR. DNA damage and mutations in human cells exposed to nitric oxide in vitro. *Proc Natl Acad Sci USA* 1992; 89: 3030–3034.

Ohta M, Tanoue K, Tarnawski AS, Pai R, Hani RM, Sander FC, Sugimache K, Sarfeh IJ. Overexpressed nitric oxide synthase in portal-hypertensive stomach of rat: a key to increased susceptibility to damage. *Gastroenterology* 1997; 112: 1920–1930.

Orlando RC. Esophageal epithelial defenses against acid injury. *Am J Gastroenterol* 1994; 89: S48–S52.

Orihata M, Sarna SK. Nitric oxide mediates mechano- and chemo-receptor-activated intestinal feedback control of gastric emptying. *Dig Dis Sci* 1996; 41: 1303–1309.

Palmer RMJ, Ferrige AG, Moncada S. Nitric oxide release accounts for the biological activity of endothelium derived relaxing factor. *Nature* 1987; 327: 524–526.

Palmer RMJ, Moncada S. Novel citrulline-forming enzyme implicated in the formation of nitric oxide by vascular endothelial cells. *Biochem Biophys Res Comm* 1989; 158: 348–352.

Payne D, Kubes D. Nitric oxide donors reduce the rise in reperfusion-induced intestinal mucosal permeability. *Am J Physiol* 1993; 265: G189–G196.

Pique JM, Esplugues JV, Whittle, BJR. Endogenous nitric oxide as a mediator of gastric mucosal vasodilatation during acid secretion. *Gastroenterology* 1992a; 102: 168–174.

Pique JM, Pizcueta MP, Bosch J, Fernandez M, Whittle BJR, Moncada S. Role of nitric oxide in the hyperdynamic splanchnic circulation of portal hypertensive rats, in Biology of Nitric Oxide, vol. 2 (Moncada S, et al., eds.), Portland, London, 1992b, pp. 60–64.

Pique JM, Whittle BJR, Espluges JV. Vasodilator role of endogenous nitric oxide in the rat gastric microcirculation. *Eur J Pharmacol* 1989; 174: 293–296.

Plourde V, Quintero E, Suto G, Coimbra C, Tache Y. Delayed gastric emptying induced by inhibitors of nitric oxide synthase in rats. *Eur J Pharmacol* 1994; 256: 125–129.

Pomeranz IS, Shaffer EA. Abnormal gall bladder emptying in a subgroup of patients with gallstones. *Gastroenterology* 1985; 88: 787–791.

Porsti I, Paakkari I. Nitric oxide-based possibilities for pharmacotherapy. *Ann Med* 1995; 27: 407–420.

Price KJ, Hanson PJ, Whittle BJ. Localization of constitutive isoforms of nitric oxide synthase in the gastric glandular mucosa of the rat. *Cell Tissue Res* 1996; 285: 157–163.

Prince RC. Rising interest in nitric oxide synthase. *Trends Biol Sci* 1993; 18: 35–36.

Qui B, Pothoulakis C, Castagliuolo I, Nikulasson Z, LaMont JT. Nitric oxide inhibits rat intestinal secretion by Clostridium difficile toxin but not *Vibrio cholerae* enterotoxin. *Gastroenterology* 1996; 111: 409–418.

Qiu BS, Pfeiffer CJ, Cho CH. Effects of chronic nitric oxide synthase inhibition in cold-restraint and ethanol-induced gastric mucosal damage in rats. *Digestion* 1996; 57: 60–66.

Rachmilewitz D, Karmeli F, Eliakim R, Stalnikowicz R, Ackerman Z, Amir G, Stamler JS. Enhanced gastric nitric oxide synthase activity in duodenal ulcer patients. *Gut* 1994; 35: 1394–1397.

Rachmilewitz D, Karmeli F, Okon E. Sulfhydryl blocker-induced rat colonic inflammation is ameliorated by inhibition of nitric oxide synthase. *Gastroenterology* 1995; 109: 98–106.

Radomski MW, Palmer RMJ, Moncada S. Glucocorticoids inhibit the expression of an inducible but not the constitutive nitric oxide synthase in vascular endothelial cells. *Proc Natl Acad Sci USA* 1990; 87: 10,043–10,047.

Rees DD, Collek S, Palmer RMJ, Moncada S. Dexamethasone prevents the induction by endotoxin of a nitric oxide synthase and the associated effects on vascular tone: an insight in endotoxin shock. *Biochem Biophys Res Commun* 1990; 173: 541–547.

Ribbons KA, Currie MG, Connor JR, Manning PT, Allen PC, Didier P, et al. Effect of inhibitors of inducible nitric oxide synthase on chronic colitis in the rhesis monkey. *J Pharmacol Exp Ther* 1997; 280: 1008–1015.

Rishi RK, Kishore K, Seth SD. Gastrointestinal protection by NO from NSAIDs induced injury. *Indian J Physiol Pharmacol* 1996; 40: 377–379.

Sababi M, Nilsson E, Holm L. Mucus and alkalai secretion in the rat duodenum: effects of indomethacin, N-omega-nitro-L-arginine and luminal acid. *Gastroenterology* 1995; 109: 1526–1534.

Salzman AL, Eaves-Pyles T, Linn JC, Denenberg AG, Szabo C. Bacterial induction of inducible nitric oxide synthase in cultured human intestinal epithelial cells. *Gastroenterology* 1998; 114: 93–102.

Salzman AL, Menconi MJ, Unno N, Ezzell RM, Casey DM, Gonzalez PK, Fink MP. Nitric oxide dilates tight junctions and depletes ATP in cultured CaCo–22BBe intestinal epithelial monolayers. *Am J Physiol* 1995; 268: G361–G373.

Sanders KM, Ward SA. Nitric oxide as a mediator of nonadrenergic noncholinergic neurotransmission. *Am J Physiol* 1992; 262: G379–G392.

Sanderson N, Factor V, Nagy P, Kopp J, Kondaiah P, Wakefield L, et al. Hepatic expression of mature transforming growth factor $\beta1$ in transgenic mice results in multiple tissue lesions. *Proc Natl Acad Sci USA* 1995; 2572–2576.

Sarna SK, Otterson MF, Ryan RP, Cowes VE. Nitric oxide regulates migrating motor complex cycling and its postprandial disruption. *Am J Physiol* 1993; 265: G749–G766.

Schleiffer R, Raul F. Prophylactic administration of L-arginine improves the intestinal barrier function after mesenteric ischemia. *Gut* 1996; 39: 194–198.

Shima Y, Mori M, Harano M, Tsugi H, Tanaka N, Yamazuto T. Nitric oxide mediates cerulein-induced relaxation of canine sphincter of Oddi. *Dig Dis Sci* 1998; 43: 547–553.

Shirgi-Degen A, Beubler E. Significance of nitric oxide in the stimulation of intestinal fluid absorption in the rat jejunum in vivo. *Br J Pharmacol* 1995; 114: 13–18.

Singaram C, Sweet MA, Gaumnitz EA, Bass P, Snipes RL. Evaluation of early events in the creation of an amyenteric opossum model of achalasia. *Neurogastroenterol Motil* 1996; 8: 351–361.

Singer II, Kawka DW, Scott S, Weidner JR, Mumford RA, Riehl TE, Stenson WF. Expression of inducible nitric oxide synthase and nitrotyrosine in colonic epithelium in inflammatory bowel disease. *Gastroenterology* 1996; 111: 871–885.

Soll AH, Weinstein WM, Kurata J, McCarthy D. Non-steroidal antiinflamma-tory drugs and peptic ulcer disease. *Ann Intern Med* 1991; 114: 307–319.

Sorrells DL, Friend C, Koltukusuz U, Courcoulas A, Boyle P, Garrett M, et al. Inhibition of nitric oxide with aminoguanidine reduces bacterial translocation after endotoxin challenge in vivo. *Arch Surg* 1996; 131: 1155–1163.

Southey A, Tanaka S, Murakami T, Miyoshi H, Ishizuka T, Sugiura M, Kawashima K, Sugita T. Pathophysiological role of nitric oxide in rat experimental colitis. *Int J Immunopharmacol* 1997; 19: 669–676.

Stamler JS, Singel DJ, Loscalzo J. Biochemistry of nitric oxide and its redox-activated forms. *Science* 1992; 253: 1898–1992.

Stark ME, Szurszewski JA. Role of nitric oxide in gastrointestinal and hepatic function and disease. *Gastroenterology* 1992; 103: 1928–1949.

Stuehr DJ, Nathan CF. Nitric oxide: a macrophage product responsible for cytostasis and respiratory inhibition in human target cells. *J Exp Med* 1989; 169: 1543–1555.

Sun WM, Doran J, Lingenfelser T, Hebbard GS, Morley JE, Dent J, Horowtiz M. Effects of glyceryl trinitrate on the pyloric motor responses to intraduo-denal triglyceride infusion in humans. *Eur J Clin Invest* 1996; 26: 657–664.

Szabo C. The pathophysiological roles of peroxynitrite in shock, inflammation and ischemia reperfusion injury. *Shock* 1996; 6: 79–88.

Takahashi S, Nakamura E, Okabe S. Stimulatory effect of leminoprazole on secretion and synthesis of mucus by rabbit gastric mucosal cells. *J Pharmacol Exp Ther* 1995; 275: 1396–1401.

Takahashi T, Owyang C. Vagal control of nitric oxide and vasoactive intestinal polypeptide release in the regulation of gastric relaxation in the rat. *J Physiol* (London) 1995; 484: 481–492.

Takakura K, Hasegawa K, Goto Y, Muramatsu I. Nitric oxide produced by inducible nitric oxide synthase delays gastric emptying in lipopolysaccha-ride-treated rats. *Anesthesiology* 1997; 87: 652–657.

Takeuchi K, Ohuchi T, Miyabe H, Niki S, Okabe S. Effects of nitric oxide synthase inhibitors on duodenal alkaline secretion in anesthetized rats. *Eur J Pharmacol* 1993; 231: 135–138.

Takeuchi K, Ohuchi T, Okabe S. Endogenous nitric oxide in gastric alkaline re-sponse in the rat stomach after damage. *Gastroenterology* 1994; 106: 367–374.

Takeuchi K, Okabe S. Mechanism of gastric alkaline response in the stomach after damage. Roles of nitric oxide and prostaglandins. *Dig Dis Sci* 1995; 40: 865–871.

Tepperman BL, Abrahamson TD, Soper BD. Role of cyclic guanylate mono-phosphate in nitric oxide-induced injury to rat small intestinal epithelial cells. *J Pharmacol Exp Ther* 1998; 284: 929–933.

Tepperman BL, Brown JF, Korolkewicz R, Whittle BJR. Nitric oxide synthase activity, viability and cyclic GMP levels in rat colonic epithelial cells: effect of endotoxin challenge. *J Pharmacol Exp Ther* 1994; 271: 1477–1482.

Tepperman BL, Brown JF, Whittle BJR. Nitric oxide synthase induction and intestinal epithelial cell viability in rats. *Am J Physiol* 1993; 265: G214–G218.

Tepperman BL, Soper BD. Nitric oxide synthase induction and cytoprotection of rat gasric mucosa from injury by ethanol. *Can J Physiol Pharmacol* 1994; 72: 1308–1311.

Tepperman BL, Whittle BJR. Endogenous nitric oxide and sensory neuropeptides interact in the modulation of the rat gastric microcirculation. *Br J Pharmacol* 1992; 105: 121–175.

Tottrup A, Svane D, Forman A. Nitric oxide mediating NANC inhibition in oppossum lower esophageal sphincter. *Am J Physiol* 1991a; 260: G385–G389.

Tottrup A, Knudsen MA, Gregersen H. Role of the L-arginine-nitric oxide pathway in relaxation of the lower esophageal sphincter. *Br J Pharmacol* 1991b; 104: 113–116.

Tripp MA, Tepperman BL. Role of calcium in nitric oxide-mediated injury to rat gastric mucosal cells. *Gastroenterology* 1996; 111: 65–72.

Umans JG, Samsel RW. L-canavanine selectively augments contraction in aortas from endotoxemic rats. *Eur J Pharmacol* 1992; 210: 343–346.

Unno N, Menconi MJ, Fink MP. Nitric oxide-induced hyperpermeability of human intestinal epithelial monolayers is augmented by inhibition of the amiloride-sensitive Na^+-H^+-antiport: potential role of peroxynitrous acid. *Surgery* 1997a; 122: 485–491.

Unno N, Menconi MJ, Smith M, Aguirre DE, Fink MP. Hyperpermeability of intestinal epithelial monolayers is induced by NO: effect of low extracellular pH. *Am J Physiol* 1997b; 272: G923–G934.

Unno N, Menconi MJ, Smith M, Fink MP. Nitric oxide mediates interferon-gamma-induced hyperpermeability in cultured human intestinal epithelial monolayers. *Crit Care Med* 1995; 23: 1170–1176.

Unno N, Wang H, Menconi MJ, Tytgat SH, Larkin V, Smith M, et al. Inhibition of inducible nitric oxide synthase ameliorates endotoxin-induced gut mucosal barrier dysfunction in rats. *Gastroenterology* 1997c; 113: 1246–1257.

Valentine JF, Tannahill CL, Stevenot SA, Sallustio JE, Nick HS, Eaker EY. Colitis and interleukin 1 beta upregulate inducible nitric oxide synthase and superoxide dismutase in rat myenteric neurons. *Gastroenterology* 1996; 111: 56–64.

Vanhoutte PM, Shimokawa H. Endothelium-derived relaxing factor and coronary vasospasm. *Circulation* 1989; 80: 1–9.

Vantrappen G, Janssens HO, Hellmans J, Coremans G. Achalasia, diffuse esophageal spasm and related motility disorders. *Gastroenterology* 1979; 76: 450–457.

Villarreal D, Grisham MB, Granger DN. Nitric oxide donors improve gut function after prolonged hypothermic ischemia. *Transplantation* 1995; 59: 685–689.

Vodovotz V, Bogdan C, Paik J, Xie Q, Nathan C. Mechanisms of suppression of macrophage nitric oxide release by transforming growth factor β. *J Exp Med* 1993; 178: 605–613.

Wachter C, Heinemann A, Jocic M, Holzer P. Visceral vasodilation and somatic vasoconstriction evoked by acid challenge of the rat gastric mucosa: diversity of mechanisms. *J Physiol* (London) 1995; 486: 505–516.

Wakulich CA, Tepperman BL. Role of glutathione in nitric oxide-mediated injury to rat gastric mucosal cells. *Eur J Pharmacol* 1997; 319: 333–341.

Wallace JL. Gastric ulceration: critical events at the neutrophil-endo thelium interface. *Can J Physiol Pharmacol* 1993; 71: 98–102.

Wallace JL, Cirino G, De Nucci G, McKnight W, MacNaughton WK. Endo-thelin has potent ulcerogenic and vasoconstrictor actions in the stomach. *Am J Physiol* 1989; 256: G661–G666.

Wallace JL, Cirino G, McKnight GW, Elliott SN. Reduction of gastrointestinal injury in acute endotoxic shock by flurbiprofen nitroxybutylester. *Eur J Pharmacol* 1995; 280: 63–68.

Wallace JL, McKnight W, Wilson TL, DelSoldato P, Cirino G. Reduction of shock-induced gastric damage by a nitric oxide-releasing aspirin derivative: role of neutrophils. *Am J Physiol* 1997; 273: G1246–G1251.

Wallace JL, Reuter, BK, Cicala C, McKnight W, Grisham MB, Cirino G. Novel anti-inflammatory drug derivatives with markedly reduced ulcero-genic properties in the rat. *Gastroenterology* 1994a; 107: 173–179.

Wallace JL, Reuter BK, Cirino. Nitric oxide-releasing non-steroidal anti-inflammatory drugs: a novel approach for reducing gastrointestinal toxicity. *J Gastroenterol Hepatol* 1994b; 9(Suppl 1): 540–544.

Whittle BJR. Nitric oxide in gastrointestinal physiology and pathophysiology, in *Physiology of the Gastrointestinal Tract,* 3rd ed. (Johnson LR, ed.), Raven, New York, 1994, pp. 267–294.

Whittle BJR. Nitric oxide in physiology and pathology. *Histochem J* 1995; 27: 727–737.

Whittle BJR. Nitric oxide—a mediator of inflammation or mucosal defence. *Eur J Gastroenterol Hepatol* 1997; 9: 1026–1032.

Whittle BJR, Laszlo F, Evans SM, Moncada S. Induction of nitric oxide synthase and microvascular injury in the rat jejunum provoked by indometh-acin. *Br J Pharmacol* 1995; 116: 2286–90.

Whittle BJR, Tepperman BL. Role of endogenous vasoactive mediators, nitric oxide, prostanoids and sensory neuropeptides in the regulation of gastric blood flow and mucosal integrity, in *Mechanisms of Injury, Protection and Repair of the Upper Gastrointestinal Tract* (Garner A, O'Brien PE, eds.), John Wiley, Chichester, 1991, pp. 127–137.

Williams SE, Turnberg LA. Demonstration of a pH gradient across mucus adherent to rabbit gastric mucosa: evidence for a mucus-bicarbonate barrier. *Gut* 1981; 22: 94–96.

Willis S, Allescher HD, Weigert N, Schusdziarra V, Schumpelick V. Influence of the L-arginine-nitric oxide pathway on vasoactive intestinal polypeptide release and motility in the rat stomach in vitro. *Eur J Pharmacol* 1996; 315: 59–64.

Wirthlin DJ, Cullen JJ, Spates ST, Conklin JL, Murray J, Caropreso DK, Ephgrave KS. Gastrointestinal transit during endotoxemia: the role of nitric oxide. *J Surg Res* 1996; 60: 307–311.

Xu W, Charles I, Moncada S, Gorman P, Liu L, Emson P. Chromosomal assignment of the inducible NOS gene and endothelial NOS gene to human chromosome 17p11–17q11 and chromosome 7, respectively. *Endothelium* 1993; 1: S24.

Yamato S, Spechler SJ, Goyal RK. Role of nitric oxide in esophageal peristalsis in the opossum. *Gastroenterology* 1992; 103: 197–204.

Yasuhiro T, Korolkewicz RP, Kato S, Takeuchi KC.Role of nitric oxide in pathogenesis of serotonin-induced gastric lesions in rats. *Pharmacol Res* 1997a; 36: 333–338.

Yasuhiro T, Konaka A, Ukawa H, Kato S, Takeuchi K. Role of nitric oxide in pathogenesis of gastric mucosal damage induced by compound 48/80 in rats. *J Physiol* (Paris) 1997b; 91: 131–138.

Yoshida M, Kurose I, Wakbayashi G, Hokari R, Ishikawa H, Otani Y, et al. Suppressed production of nitric oxide as a cause of irregular constriction of gastric venules induced by thermal injury in rats. *J Clin Gastroenterol* 1997; 25(Suppl 1): S56–S60.

Yu H, Sato EF, Minamiyama Y, Arakawa T, Kobayashi K, Inoue M. Effect of nitric oxide on stress-induced gastric mucosal injury in the rat. *Digestion* 1997; 58: 311–318.

Yunker AM, Galligan JJ. Endogenous NO inhibits NANC but not cholinergic neurotransmission to circular muscle of guinea pig leum. *Am J Physiol* 1996; 271: G904–G912.

3 Cytokines

Opportunities for Therapeutic Intervention

Alan D. Levine and Claudio Fiocchi

CONTENTS

1. INTRODUCTION

The gastrointestinal (GI) tract is a major target organ for a number of infectious, inflammatory, neoplastic and functional diseases in humans. Cytokines (CKs) are involved in essentially all of these GI disorders, but they play a particularly dominant role in illnesses whose clinical symptoms are the result of immune-mediated, persistent inflammatory processes. Typical examples include chronic gastritis, celiac disease (gluten-sensitive enteropathy), Crohn's disease (CD), and ulcerative colitis (UC). The pathogenesis of the last two entities, collectively named inflammatory bowel disease (IBD) because of common clinical

From: *Drug Development: Molecular Targets for GI Diseases*
Edited by: T. S. Gaginella and A. Guglietta © Humana Press Inc., Totowa, NJ

and pathological manifestations, has been intensively investigated (Fiocchi, 1998), specifically regarding the role CKs play in mediating the chronic inflammation that damages the small or large bowel of affected individuals (Fiocchi, 1996). In addition, the explosion in the field of animal models of IBD that has occurred in the past decade has considerably expanded the involvement of CKs in intestinal inflammation. Therefore, IBD represents the ideal clinical and experimental model to describe CK abnormalities in the inflamed GI system, and to discuss the related opportunities for therapeutic intervention. In doing so, this chapter focuses primarily on classical CKs, defined as glycoproteins secreted by activated immune cells, with occasional references to other classes of mediators, such as chemokines, growth factors, and eicosanoids.

2. GENERAL PROPERTIES

Communication among immune and nonimmune cells is a critical component in initiating, modulating, and terminating an immune or inflammatory response. Secreted and cell bound proteins, termed cytokines, regulate many of these biological responses. In the past decade, there has been an explosion in the number of CKs identified, and in the array of immunological functions attributed to CKs that are synthesized by, or target, inflammatory cells. In spite of the enormity and complexity of the CK network, a limited number of specific properties may be attributed to these proteins.

1. Pleiotropy: A single CK may be synthesized by multiple cell types, induce a biological response in multiple target cells, and mediate multiple stimulatory and/or inhibitory signals within a single or multiple cell lineages.
2. Redundancy: Multiple CKs are capable of eliciting the same biological response in vitro, yet not all of these activities appear to be manifest when the same CK is studied in vivo. In addition, genetic or immunological deletion of a given CK is not always associated with an expected or observable phenotype, which may be because of the implementation of alternate regulatory pathways with overlapping function.

3. Synthesis: CK production, commonly regulated at the transcriptional and mRNA stability level, is inducible and self-limiting, requiring continuous antigenic or inflammatory activation.
4. Crossregulation: CKs function not only by directly activating immune and inflammatory cells to a higher state of preparedness, but they also modulate host defense by interacting in a network-like complex with one another. These interactions with another CK may be additive, saturable, synergistic, or antagonistic. For example, a single CK may enhance or inhibit the synthesis, release, or function of a second CK, either directly or indirectly.
5. Local vs endocrine activity: The vast majority of immune CKs, which regulate lymphocytes, macrophages, eosinophils, mast cells, and neutrophils, act locally. These CKs exhibit autocrine or paracrine activity within a narrow region of injury, infection, or inflammation. One exception are chemokines, which function as chemoattractants for leukocytes, and must, by design, establish a medium-distance gradient to direct the appropriate migration of inflammatory cells to the damaged tissue. Some proinflammatory and anti-inflammatory CKs (*see* Subheading 3.4.) function in a manner similar to classical endocrine molecules, in which they enter the circulation and modulate the activity of distal organs. Despite the endocrine analogy, the half-life of most CKs in serum is less than 5 min.

3. CATEGORIES

CKs are grouped according to common characteristics, to facilitate understanding the roles of individual molecules as therapeutic agents and targets in GI inflammation. Because of the pleiotropy of these proteins, the classification process itself is somewhat artificial, in which a significant amount of overlap between categories is apparent. This subheading will provide information describing functional properties of CKs that most readily impact physiological or pathological mucosal immune responses.

3.1. Immunoregulatory: IL-2, IL-7, IL-12, IL-18

These CKs play a primary role in activating, modulating, and expanding the immunoregulatory T-cell population, yet also exert unique

Table 1
Immunoregulatory Cytokines

Cytokine	Main cellular source	Main target cells	Dominant functions[a]
IL-2	T-cells	T-cells, all IL-2R-bearing cells	T-cell activation, proliferation, clonal expansion, and differentiation
IL-7	Stromal cells	Leukocyte differentiation	T-cell proliferation and cytotoxicity
IL-12	Phagocytes, B-cells, dendritic cells	T-cells	Th-1 differentiation, mediation responses, induction of IFN-γ
IL-18	Macrophages, dendritic cells	T-cells	IL-12-like

[a]Relevant to mucosal immunity and intestinal inflammation.

activities on other immune and nonimmune target cells (Table 1). Interleukin (IL)-2 is produced by T-cells and stimulates their activation, proliferation, clonal expansion, and differentiation in an autocrine and paracrine manner (Theze et al., 1996). IL-7, a stromal cell-derived protein, influences the differentiation of a variety of leukocytes, but, in the context of intestinal inflammation, functions as an inducer of T-cell cytotoxicity and the proliferation of thymic and mature T-cells (Costello and Duffaud, 1992). IL-12 is the only known heterodimeric CK and is produced by antigen-presenting cells, such as dendritic cells, macrophages, and B-cells. IL-12 functions not only to enhance the cytotoxicity and interferon (IFN)-γ synthesis by natural killer cells and T-cells, but also as a key regulator of the differentiation of naïve T-cells into IFN-γ-producing cells (Trinchieri and Scott, 1994). IL-12 plays an important role in regulating immune responses to infectious agents and in initiating intestinal inflammation. IL-18 is a newly identified CK that shares with IL-12 the ability to induce IFN-γ synthesis by T-cells and natural killer cells. IL-18 is secreted by the same population of cells that synthesize IL-12, in addition to epidermal, adrenal, and epithelial cells (Kohno and Kurimoto, 1998). Because of the importance played by IL-12 in intestinal inflammation, the interest in IL-18 is currently high.

Table 2
Counterregulatory Cytokines

Cytokine	Main cellular source	Main target cells	Dominant functions[a]
IL-4	T-cells, mast cells, basophils	Multiple cell types	Th-2 differentiation, mediation of allergy, immuno-suppression, and anti-inflammatory activity
IL-10	Monocyte, macrophages, T- and B-cells, nonimmune cells	Multiple cells	Anti-inflammatory activity and immunosuppression
IL-13	T-cells	Multiple cells (except T-cells)	IL-4-like
TGF-β	Multiple cells	Epithelial, stromal and immune cells	Epithelial restitution, neutrophil chemotaxis, IgA switching, T-cell immunosuppression

[a]Relevant to mucosal immunity and intestinal inflammation.

3.2. Counterregulatory: IL-4, IL-10, IL-13, TGF-β

Within the mature, effector T-cell population, the production of CKs is relatively restricted. T-cells tend to express only one or two CKs per cell, and, during an immune response, the pattern of CKs produced by the T-cell population as a whole is polarized. One profile of CKs, typified by IFN-γ, is modulated by the immunoregulatory CKs discussed above. The other profile of CKs is known as counterregulatory (Table 2). Each cascade of CKs inhibits the synthesis and activity of the other, and leads to distinct and recognizable effector mechanisms in an immune response. IL-4 is the prototypic counterregulatory CK, which not only initiates this T-cell-dependent cytokine cascade, but also stimulates B-cell antibody-class switch, and eosinophil and mast cell activation critical to allergic reactions, and has potent immunosuppressive and anti-inflammatory activities (Chomarat and Bancherau, 1997). These latter activities of IL-4 make it a worthy target for further investigation in regulating mucosal immune and inflammatory responses. IL-13 is structurally and functionally related to IL-4, sharing components of its receptor and all biological activities, except IL-13 does not modulate T-cell differentiation (deVries and Zurawski, 1995). IL-10 influences, and is produced by, a wide variety of immune and nonimmune cells, but its potent anti-inflammatory and immunosuppressive activity on macrophages and dendritic cells, similar in fact to IL-4 and IL-13, have stimulated clinical trials in IBD (deVries, 1995). Transforming growth factor (TGF)-β, a member of a large family of growth factors, is a potent immunoregulatory protein, which initiates immunoglobulin (IgA)-class switching in B-cells (Sonoda et al., 1989), is chemotactic for neutrophils, and inhibits CK production by T-cells (Chantry et al., 1989). Because of the dual immunostimulatory and immunosuppressive activities of TGF-β, its potential role in mucosal immunity, and as a therapeutic target in IBD, is complex, yet promising.

3.3. Immunoeffector: IFN-γ, GM-CSF, IL-3, IL-5, IL-9, IL-11, IL-15

CKs, which function during the effector phase of the immune response, have an immediate impact on immune and nonimmune cells that directly function to eliminate the pathogen or perpetuate inflammation (Table 3). IFN-γ, a product of IL-12- or IL-18-stimulated T-cells and natural killer cells, has a broad spectrum of immunoeffector activities, which include the induction of major histocompatibility complex (MHC) class II on monocytes, macrophages, dendritic cells, and epithelial cells, activation of macrophage differentiation and phagocytosis, and, as mentioned earlier, inhibition of the IL-4-initiated CK cascade (Young and Hardy, 1995). Granulocyte macrophage-colony-stimulating factor (GM-CSF) and IL-3 are members of a family of colony-stimulating factors that primarily regulate the growth and differentiation of hematopoietic cells, yet also influence the activation of mature leukocytes in the periphery (Doe and Grimm, 1996). IL-5, secreted by T-cells and mast cells, promotes the growth, differentiation, and activation of eosinophils, basophils, and mast cells (Koike and Takatsu, 1994). IL-9 is a poorly characterized cytokine synthesized by activated T-cells and probably affects the proliferation and differentiation of mast cells, B-cells, and hematopoietic precursor cells (Demoulin and Renauld, 1998). IL-11, produced by stromal cells, exhibits a broad

Table 3
Immunoeffector Cytokines

Cytokine	Main cellular source	Main target cells	Dominant functions[a]
IFN-γ	T-cells, natural killer cells	Most cells	Induction of MHC class II antigens, monocyte activation, Th-1 differentiation, and IL-4 suppression
GM-CSF	Phagocytes, B-cells	Hematopoietic cells	Leukocyte differentiation
IL-3	Multiple cells	Hematopoietic cells	Leukocyte differentiation
IL-5	T-cells, mast cells	Eosinophils	Mediation of allergic and parasitic diseases
IL-9	Th2 cells	T-cells, mast cells	Undefined
IL-11	Hematopoietic stromal cells	Multiple cells	Stimulation of intestinal crypt cells
IL-15	Most cells	IL-2R-bearing cells	T-cell expansion, epithelial cell differentiation

[a]Relevant to mucosal immunity and intestinal inflammation.

spectrum of activities, including effects on platelets, leukocytes, bone marrow progenitor cells, intestinal epithelial cells, and hepatocytes (Du and Williams, 1994). IL-15 is produced by many cell types, including epithelial cells and fibroblasts, and appears to duplicate many of the activities of IL-2, because they share two chains of a trimeric receptor complex. IL-15 also stimulates the activation and chemotaxis of T-cells, maturation and isotype switching of B-cells, chemotaxis of neutrophils, proliferation of mast cells, and the cytotoxicity of natural killer cells (McInnes and Liew, 1998).

3.4. Proinflammatory: IL-1α, IL-1β, TNF-α, TNF-β, IL-6

The above groups of cytokines initiate and modulate acquired immune responses; proinflammatory CKs activate the innate immune

Table 4
Pro-inflammatory Cytokines

Cytokine	Main cellular source	Main target cells	Dominant functions[a]
IL-1α, -1β	Monocytes, macrophages	Most cells	Mediation of infectious and inflammatory responses
IL-6	Multiple cells	Most cells	Enhancement of immunoglobulin production, and immunoregulation
TNF-α	Macrophages	Multiple cells	Mediation of inflammatory and cytotoxic responses

[a]Relevant to mucosal immunity and intestinal inflammation.

system, and play a significant role in chronic intestinal inflammation (Table 4). Both members of the IL-1 family are produced by monocytes, macrophages, fibroblasts, and epithelial cells, stimulate a wide spectrum of inflammatory cells, and participate in all aspects of the response to infectious agents (Dinarello and Wolf, 1993). A natural antagonist of IL-1 (IL-1 receptor antagonist [IL-Ra]) competes for IL-1 binding to its receptors, and blocks all IL-1 biological activities. IL-1Ra has been effective in preventing colitis in some, but not all, animal models. Tumor necrosis factor (TNF)-α and TNF-β share many properties with each other and IL-1, including its cellular source and target cell population. In addition, TNF-α is secreted by T-cells, and induces tissue injury and apoptosis (Rink and Kirchner, 1996). IL-6 is produced by a broad spectrum of cell types, and modulates the activity of an equally broad spectrum of target cells. IL-6's primary function as an immunomodulatory protein is to enhance the synthesis of immunoglobulin by mature B-cells and to stimulate their final differentiation into plasma cells. Although classically categorized as a proinflammatory member of the IL-1–TNF–IL-6 triad, each sharing many activities with the others, more recently a number of anti-inflammatory functions, similar in fact to IL-10, have also been attributed to IL-6. For instance, IL-6 does not stimulate eicosanoids, nitric oxide, metalloproteinases, or adhesion molecule expression; inhibits the synthesis of IL-1 and TNF-α; and protects tissue from inflammatory injury (Barton, 1997).

3.5. Chemokines: IL-8, IL-16, RANTES,
MIP-1α, MIP-1β, and MCP-1

A large and growing family of chemotactic peptides are known as chemokines, which are subdivided by the presence of either a CXC or CC (C, cysteine; X, any amino acid) sequence in their primary structure. Chemokines are produced by a variety of cell types, and function to attract leukocytes to sites of infection or inflammation. Because many chemokines share a common set of receptors on the target-cell surface, there appears to be an enormous amount of redundancy in this system (Luster, 1998). It is likely that many chemokines contribute to the amplification of the chronic inflammation observed in human IBD and experimental animal models of enterocolitis.

4. CYTOKINES IN IBD

4.1. CK Abnormalities in Patients with IBD

4.1.1. IMMUNOREGULATORY, COUNTERREGULATORY, AND IMMUNOEFFECTOR CKS

Within the systemic and mucosal immune systems, the task of maintaining a state of local immune homeostasis, or health, is the primary responsibility of $CD4^+$ T-cells, classified as T-helper 1 (Th1) or Th2, depending on their CK secretory patterns (Th1: IL-2, IFN-γ, and so on; Th2: IL-4, IL-5, IL-10, and so on) (Mosmann and Sad, 1996). According to this artificial but convenient classification into Th1 or Th2 CKs, inflammatory diseases may result from an imbalance between Th1, (delayed-type hypersensitivity) and Th2 (allergic type) reactivity. Using this paradigm, numerous abnormalities of Th1 and Th2 CKs have been reported in IBD (Fiocchi, 1996).

The study of IL-2, primarily a Th1 CK, has shown a differential activity in CD and UC. Mucosal levels of IL-2 protein and mRNA are consistently higher in CD than in UC, as are levels of the IL-2Rα chain (Matsuura et al., 1996). In both adult and pediatric CD patients, mucosal immune cells exhibit a hyperreactivity to IL-2, compared to cells from UC patients (Kugathasan et al., 1998; Kusugami et al., 1989), and exacerbation of CD can be induced by the administration of IL-2

(Sparano et al., 1993). The Th1 connotation of CD is strongly supported by the enhanced spontaneous production of IFN-γ by CD mucosal mononuclear cells (Pallone et al., 1996). In addition, both protein and mRNA for IL-12, a CK essential for IFN-γ induction, are expressed at higher levels in CD- than UC-affected tissues (Monteleone et al., 1997). Finally, low production of IL-4, a prototypical Th2 CK, by lamina propria mononuclear cells and T-cell clones of CD patients (West et al., 1996), also reinforces the concept that this is a condition with a prominent Th1-like profile. The classification of UC as a Th2-like condition, however, is much less clear. In support of this possibility are lower levels of IFN-γ produced by mucosal mononuclear cells, and higher IL-5 levels in UC than CD mucosa (Fuss et al., 1996; Mullin et al., 1996). Limited and incomplete information exists on mucosal levels of IL-10 in IBD, although circulating levels of this Th2 CK are elevated in both CD and UC patients (Kucharzik et al., 1995), probably reflecting a nonspecific response to gut inflammation. Mucosal production of IL-15, a CK with many of the biological activities of IL-2, is enhanced in both forms of IBD (Sakai et al., 1998). From the above, it is evident that only limited information is available on the production and function of several CKs in human IBD. A full understanding of all immune abnormalities occurring in IBD is still beyond reach, but this has not impeded the development of novel therapeutic interventions based on CK manipulations aimed at reestablishing intestinal immune homeostasis and downregulating intestinal inflammation.

4.1.2. PROINFLAMMATORY CKS

Levels of proinflammatory CKs are predictably elevated in tissues involved by IBD. High concentrations of IL-1α and -β are found in both CD and UC intestine (Mahida et al., 1989; Youngman et al., 1993), but their local effects are mostly determined by the relative concentration of its natural antagonist, IL-1Ra. A mucosal imbalance between IL-1Ra and IL-1 has been reported in IBD, showing a relative deficiency of IL-1Ra, which could contribute to chronicity of inflammation (Casini-Raggi et al., 1995). IL-6 is also consistently elevated in IBD mucosa, which primarily derives from macrophages and epithelial cells (Kusugami et al., 1995; Stevens et al., 1992). In contrast to IL-1 and IL-6, protein and mRNA levels of TNF-α have been inconsistently reported as both normal and elevated in IBD. High TNF-α concentrations are found in the stools of children with CD and UC (Braegger et al., 1992), and production of TNF-α is higher in cultures of CD, rather than UC, mucosal mononuclear cells (Reinecker et al., 1993). *In situ* hybridization reveals elevated TNF-α mRNA in macrophages infiltrating IBD tissues (Cappello et al., 1992), but some studies found no differences in TNF-α mRNA expression in normal and IBD biopsies (Isaacs et al., 1992; Stevens et al., 1992). Obviously, proinflammatory CKs are prime targets for therapeutic intervention in IBD, as they are in many other inflammatory conditions affecting other systems.

4.1.3. CHEMOKINES

Chemokines are major players in IBD pathogenesis (MacDermott et al., 1998), but, because only few of this extremely large class of molecules have been investigated in CD or UC, their exact role in intestinal inflammation is incompletely understood. Levels of IL-8, a neutrophil-attractant chemokine, are greatly increased in the mucosa of CD and UC patients (Izzo et al., 1992, 1993), and they generally correlate with the degree of gut inflammation. Macrophages are a major source of IL-8 in the inflamed gut, but the contribution of epithelial cells to IL-8 production is still unclear. However, epithelial cells from both CD and UC patients produce considerable amounts of ENA-78 (Keates et al., 1997; Z'Graggen et al., 1997), also a potent neutrophil chemoattractant, which may explain the infiltration of polymorphonuclear leukocytes in the epithelium and the formation of crypt abscesses. Other chemokines, including monocyte chemotactic protein (MCP)-1, RANTES, macrophage inflammatory protein (MIP)-1α, MIP-1β, and IP-10, are also elevated in IBD mucosa (Grimm and Doe, 1996; Reinecker et al., 1995). In principle, all these chemokines are potential targets for anti-inflammatory intervention in IBD.

4.1.4. GROWTH FACTORS AND EICOSANOIDS

Growth factors and eicosanoids represent different classes of CKs, but they will be briefly mentioned, because they also contribute to the pathogenesis of IBD. Growth factors, particularly TGF-β, are crucially involved in mucosal injury and healing. This factor, in addition to displaying the previously mentioned anti-inflammatory and down-regulatory functions, is a preeminent mediator of intestinal epithelial restitution and defense (Dignass and Podolsky, 1993). Trefoil peptide, another molecule with mucosal protective properties, is secreted in large amounts by epithelial cells in IBD (Wright et al., 1993), and production of keratinocyte growth factor, a stromal cell-derived mitogen specific for epithelial cells, is also enhanced in IBD (Finch et al., 1996). TGF-β production is high in active CD and UC lesions, but, in inactive stages, only TGF-α is elevated (Babyatsky et al., 1996; Eberhart and Dubois, 1995). Eicosanoids are products of the arachidonic acid pathway, and they are intimately involved in mucosal cytoprotection and regeneration. Their role in intestinal inflammation is discussed in Chapter 1 of this book. Although modulation of eicosanoid synthesis and secretion is currently the focus of intense investigation aimed at preventing mucosal injury and controlling inflammation, growth factors are considered as substances with wound healing potential, rather than as true anti-inflammatory agents.

4.2. CK Abnormalities in Animal Models of IBD

4.2.1. EXPERIMENTAL MODELS OF IBD

In the past 6 yr, there has been a dramatic increase in the number of animal models of experimental enterocolitis. In order to remain focused on the therapeutic messages gleaned from these models, the models currently under investigation will be only briefly described. A more complete description of these models may be found in a variety of excellent reviews (Elson et al., 1995; Podolsky, 1997; Sartor, 1997). Experimental animals that exhibit colitis may be divided into chemically induced and immunological models in genetically and cellularly manipulated rodent strains. Colitis may be induced by direct damage to the epithelium with acetic acid, trinitrobenzene sulfonic acid (TNBSA)/ ethanol, indomethacin, carrageenan, dextran sulfate sodium, and peptidoglycan-polysaccharide, or by housing the primate cotton-top tamarin in captivity. Some of these models are species- or mouse-strain-dependent, which indicates that the genetics of the host is critical to establishing gut inflammation. Therefore, with the emergence of transgenic technology in the mouse and rat, animals deficient in specific gene products, or those that overexpress or aberrantly express a single protein product, develop colitic disease. Gene-deficiency models include IL-2 (IL-2$^{-/-}$), IL-10 (IL-10$^{-/-}$), T-cell receptor-α, T-cell receptor-β, and G$_{\alpha i2}$

receptor complex. Colitis resulting from altering the genetic background of an animal include the human leukocyte antigen (HLA)-B27/β_2-microglobulin transgenic rat, the human CD3-transgenic thymic-deficient mouse, N-cadherin dominant-negative chimeric mouse, C3H/HeJBir mouse, adoptively transferred CD45RB^{hi} T-cells into severe combined immunodeficiency strain of mouse, and the IL-7 transgenic mouse. In normal animals colitis is induced by the introduction of a chemical or immunostimulatory agent; therefore, in these genetically manipulated mice, the presence of intestinal flora is critically important for the onset of inflammation.

4.2.2. CHANGES IN EXPRESSION IN INFLAMED COLON

The current body of literature that has defined changes in local and systemic CK synthesis (mRNA) and production (protein) is extensive. Many immunoregulatory and proinflammatory CKs increase in the inflamed tissue, yet the pattern of increase is not consistent among models. This observation has two important consequences for therapeutic strategies in human IBD. First, if different subsets of CKs can be elevated in experimental colitis, it is likely that these CKs participate in secondary proinflammatory events that are not critical to disease initiation or perpetuation. The redundancy of CK networks would predict this observation, and suggests that strategies focused on late-acting mediator are likely to fail. Second, if each model yields a distinct profile of CK elevation, which profile mimics human UC and CD, two distinct diseases on their own account? In addition to increases or decreases in immunoregulatory, immunoeffector, or proinflammatory CKs and chemokines, counterregulatory and anti-inflammatory cytokine levels vary in each model, as well. Thus, an important distinction must be ascertained in order to develop a therapeutic strategy. Is the increase in the expression of a CK, either a pro- or anti-inflammatory mediator, a direct cause of the observed inflammation or a failed counterregulatory effort by the mucosal immune system?

4.2.3. IMPACT OF TARGET GENE DISRUPTION ON INFLAMMATION

Because the answer to this last question varies with each animal model, and has not been fully addressed in vivo, how can one focus on those CKs with the highest likelihood of therapeutic intervention?

Although the list of genetically altered animals that develop enterocolitis is long, not all under- and overexpression of CKs in the gut leads to disease. For instance, colitis in IL-1, IL-3, IL-4, IL-5, IL-6, IL-12, IL-13, IL-15, IFN-γ, TNF, and CSF-deficient and transgenic mice has not been reported. Therefore, the chapter now focuses on those CKs whose altered expression in vivo, mediated by genetic or immunological techniques, effects intestinal inflammation.

5. THERAPEUTIC IMPLICATIONS

5.1. CK Modulation for Therapeutic Intervention

Two general approaches may be envisioned to normalize CK activities in the inflamed intestine: One is to reestablish the equilibrium among immunoregulatory CKs (the balance between Th1 and Th2 CKs), and the second is to directly counteract the excessive production of CKs that promote or sustain inflammation. Both approaches are appealing, but major differences exist on the practical point of implementing one or the other. In animal models of IBD, the direct administration of immunoregulatory or counterregulatory CKs is feasible, as is the administration of blockers of proinflammatory CKs and chemokines. Both have been shown to be effective, and have generated new insights into the mechanisms of experimental intestinal inflammation. Unfortunately, the same is not always the case in humans, in whom issues of availability, safety, and selection of the most appropriate and effective CKs or anti-CKs greatly limit the current ability to intervene therapeutically. The following subheadings will illustrate how CKs are manipulated in animal models of IBD, and which clinical studies are currently under way, or are under consideration, for treatment of CD and UC patients.

5.2. CK Therapy in Experimental Models of IBD

5.2.1. IL-10

The efficacy of treatment with murine recombinant IL-10 for 5 wk, in rats transgenic for HLA-B27 and human β_2-microglobulin with established disease, was studied. After IL-10 administration, mesenteric lymph nodes remained hyperplastic, and colonic cellularity, myeloperoxidase, and inducible nitric oxide synthetase activities in the colonic mucosa increased with advancing disease. Despite a lack of effect on disease expression, IL-10 strikingly reduced the level of IFN-γ mRNA in gut mucosa, suggesting that IFN-γ may exert a critical role at an earlier stage of the disease, rather than in the maintenance of the lesions (Bertrand et al., 1998). In contrast, when colitis was induced with dextran sulfate sodium in mice, treatment with IL-10 resulted in a marked improvement in intestinal inflammation, and blocking endogenous IL-10 was found to cause a modest exacerbation of inflammation (Tomoyose et al., 1998). An anti-inflammatory role for IL-10 was demonstrated indirectly, using a newly described human regulatory T-cell (Tr1) (Groux et al., 1997). An antigen-specific human Tr1 cell clone, producing high levels of IL-10, low levels of IL-2, and no IL-4, was shown to prevent the colitis induced in severe combined immunodeficiency (SCID) mice by the adoptive transfer of CD4$^+$CD45RB^{hi} splenic T-cells only in those mice stimulated with the cognate antigen for this human T-cell clone (Asseman and Powrie, 1998; Groux et al., 1997). Finally, mice genetically deficient in functional IL-10 production develop spontaneous enterocolitis, which exhibits mononuclear cell infiltration of focal lesions with occasional transmural infiltration, crypt abscesses, and ulceration (Spencer and Levine, 1998). When these mice are treated with recombinant IL-10 and neutralizing antibodies to IL-12 (an immunoregulatory CK counterregulated by IL-10), the colitis in young animals is improved (Davidson et al., 1998; Rennick et al., 1997; Spencer and Levine, 1998). Together, these results suggest that IL-10 plays a major role in the control of gut inflammation, and justify the current clinical trials.

5.2.2. IL-11

The potential effect of recombinant human IL-11, at SC doses of 300 or 1000 µg/kg daily for 7 d, or 1000 µg/kg for 3 d, on TNBSA-induced colitis, was investigated in rats. IL-11 when given after TNBSA significantly decreased lesion formation and severity, reduced colonic fecal blood loss, and reduced colonic mucosal myeloperoxidase levels, without affecting the mucosal levels of prostaglandin E_2, leukotriene TB_4, and thromboxane B_2. It appears that IL-11 was protective against TNBSA-induced colitis, and that these responses were not mediated through modulation of eicosanoid metabolism products (Qiu et al., 1996).

5.2.3. TGF-β

In a variety of induced models of colitis, it was demonstrated that, by neutralizing TGF-β activity, inflammation worsened, suggesting that endogenous TGF-β exhibited an immunosuppressive activity in the gut. The colitis developed in SCID mice, reconstituted with CD45RB[hi] CD4[+] splenic T-cells, can be prevented by co-transfer of CD45RB[lo] CD4[+] T-cells. Inhibition of disease activity by the CD45RB[lo] T-cell population was reversed in vivo by an anti-TGF-β antibody, suggesting that TGF-β is a critical component of natural mucosal immunity, which prevents the development of pathogenic responses in the gut (Powrie et al., 1996). In another model, oral administration of TNB-haptenized colonic proteins (HCP), before rectal administration of TNBSA, effectively suppresses the ability of the latter to induce colitis (Neurath et al., 1996a). This suppression appears to be caused by the generation of mucosal T-cells producing TGF-β after oral HCP administration. Peyer's patch and lamina propria T-cells, from HCP-fed animals stimulated with anti-CD3/anti-CD28, had a 5–10-fold increase in their production of TGF-β from control animals. The suppressive effect of orally administered HCP was abrogated by the concomitant systemic administration of anti-TGF-β, suggesting a role for TGF-β on tolerance induction in TNBSA-induced colitis, and that TGF-β production can abrogate experimental granulomatous colitis, even after such colitis is established. Finally, when severe experimental colitis was induced by a single injection of 2,4,6-trinitrophenol (TNP)-substituted protein plus adjuvant in IL-2[−/−] mice, mucosal T-cells failed to produce TGF-β, compared to healthy wild-type mice (Ludviksson et al., 1997a). The critical importance of local TGF-β production was further substantiated when colitic mice, which were administered anti-TGF-β, exhibited pockets of colonic mononuclear cell infiltrates, suggesting that the disposition of IL-2[−/−] mice to develop chronic colonic inflammation results from an immune response that is not appropriately counter-regulated by the production of TGF-β (Ludviksson et al., 1997a).

5.2.4. IL-4

Two injections of recombinant human type 5 adenovirus (Ad5) vector expressing IL-4, into rats with colitis induced by TNBSA/ethanol, caused the overexpression of IL-4, and significantly inhibited tissue damage, serum and colon IFN-γ levels, and myeloperoxidase activity in the distal colon (Hogaboam et al., 1997). The therapeutic effect of IL-4 was associated with an inhibition of inducible nitric oxide expression and a reduction in nitric oxide synthesis. No therapeutic effect was observed in rats injected once with this vector, or with control vector injected twice. Thus, IL-4, introduced by Ad5, is therapeutic during acute inflammation in the rat colon.

5.3. CK Therapy in Human IBD

IL-1Ra is one of the naturally produced molecules that counteracts the proinflammatory actions of IL-1 (Dinarello and Thompson, 1991). In view of the excessive production of IL-1 and the relative deficiency of IL-1Ra in the mucosa of IBD patients (Casini-Raggi et al., 1995), administering IL-1Ra seems a reasonable approach to downregulation of intestinal inflammation. Trials with IL-1Ra have been attempted, but not completed, and it remains unknown whether the theoretical advantages of IL-1Ra-therapy would have resulted in practical benefits for IBD patients. Prominent among IL-10 multiple biological functions are immunosuppressive and anti-inflammatory activities. Positive results in some IBD animal models suggest potential efficacy in human IBD, and preliminary studies in patients with steroid-refractory CD, receiving iv IL-10, also show some beneficial effects (VanDeventer et al., 1997). The mechanisms of the apparent anti-inflammatory activity of IL-11 in some animal models of intestinal inflammation is still incompletely understood (Qiu et al., 1996). Nevertheless, preliminary studies in CD patients show that this CK can induce a significant drop of clinical activity (Bank et al., 1997).

5.4. CKs as Therapeutic Targets in Animal Models of IBD

The explosion in the past 6 yr in the number of transgenic, immunodeficient murine models of experimental colitis demonstrates the delicate immunological balance that normally exists in the antigen-rich environment of the GI lumen. As the characterization of these models evolves, two important concepts become apparent: A variety of immunodeficiencies can initiate acute, and at times chronic, enterocolitis in murine and other rodent models; a variety of alternate immunological CK networks can be activated in these models. Therefore, predicting which CK pathway to attack therapeutically becomes difficult, and the mechanistic connection between each of these models and human IBD becomes more tenuous. Despite these words of caution, summarized below are potentially novel CK targets whose overexpression in the gut has led to or been associated with the onset or maintenance of colitis.

5.4.1. IL-1

In experimental formalin–immune complex colitis, rabbit IL-1α is dramatically increased in tissue levels, and IL-1Ra also increases 3–4-fold. Treatment of colitic rabbits with corticosteroids significantly suppressed IL-1Ra, but not IL-1α mRNA steady-state levels, suggesting that IL-1 and IL-1Ra synthesis is differentially regulated in healthy and inflamed intestinal tissue (Cominelli et al., 1994). Recombinant IL-1Ra blocks the proinflammatory activity of endogenous IL-1 in rabbit immune colitis (Cominelli et al., 1992). These promising results with IL-1Ra have, however, not been as successful in other animal models of colitis.

5.4.2. IFN-γ

In murine models of colitis, increased expression of IFN-γ in inflamed tissue is almost universally observed, hence, this CK is a likely target for experimental immunotherapy. Using two strategies, either administering neutralizing antibodies to murine IFN-γ or developing the disease in genetically IFN-γ-deficient strains, the majority of the results have been equivocal, at best, and negative, in other cases. Anti-IFN-γ therapy for 12 wk in the CD45RB[hi]/SCID adoptive transfer model prevented colitis (Powrie et al., 1994), and CD45RB[hi] cells, derived from genetically IFN-γ-deficient strains of mice, transferred to SCID mice, were free of disease, with no evidence of the wasting syndrome (Ito and Fathman, 1997). In contrast, when Simpson et al. (1998) transferred cells from IFN-γ-deficient mice, in either the CD45RB[hi] model or the CD3ϵ thymic deficiency model, large numbers of IFN-γ deficient reconstituted mice developed wasting and colitis, which in many cases was of comparable severity to that seen in animals reconstituted with wild-type cells. In the IL-10[-/-] colitis model, neutralizing antibodies to IFN-γ

prevented disease in young mice, yet had no effect in older mice, or in immunodeficient mice reconstituted with cells from a diseased IL-10$^{-/-}$ mouse (Berg et al., 1996; Davidson et al., 1998). In aggregate, these results indicate that although IFN-γ is expressed at high levels in inflamed intestines, other pathological mechanisms must contribute to the initiation and maintenance of disease.

5.4.3. IL-12

Increased expression of IFN-γ in an inflamed colon may be regulated by the overexpression of IL-12. The effects of neutralizing IL-12 on the development and perpetuation of colitis in these models have been both promising and disappointing, respectively. Administering anti-IL-12 prophylactically, and early in the disease process, has completely prevented the clinical and immunological appearance of inflammation in the TNBSA-induced colitis model (Neurath et al., 1996a, 1996b, 1995), in the CD45RB^{hi}/SCID adoptive transfer model (Simpson et al., 1998), in IL-2$^{-/-}$ mice exhibiting spontaneous or TNP-induced colitis (Ehrhardt et al., 1997; Ludviksson et al., 1997), in the CD3ε thymic reconstitution model (Simpson et al., 1998), and in the IL-10$^{-/-}$ model (Davidson et al., 1998; Rennick et al., 1997; Spencer and Levine, 1998). Furthermore, when colitis in the TNBSA-induced model is prevented by oral administration of haptenated proteins (*see* subheading 5.2.3.), treatment of these mice with recombinant IL-12 inhibits the induction of tolerance (Kelsall et al., 1996; Neurath et al., 1996a). However, anti-IL-12 therapy delivered to chronically inflamed IL-10$^{-/-}$ mice does not ameliorate disease or alter the inflammatory response, probably because IL-12 is no longer expressed locally (Davidson et al., 1998; Spencer and Levine, 1998).

5.4.4. IL-18

IL-18 shares functional similarity to IL-12, and may therefore contribute to the synthesis of intestinal IFN-γ and initiate colonic inflammation, either alone or in collaboration with IL-12. Intensive efforts are under way in a number of laboratories to investigate whether blocking IL-18, alone and together with IL-12, may increase the efficacy of the anti-IL-12 therapy in chronically inflamed animal models.

5.4.5. IL-7

Intestinal epithelial cells produce IL-7, which serves as a potent regulatory factor for proliferation of intestinal mucosal lymphocytes. Transgenic expression of IL-7 cDNA by the SRα promoter in the mucosa leads to development of chronic colitis at 4–12 wk of age, with histopathological similarity to ulcerative colitis. The lymphoid infiltrates in the lamina propria and the epithelium were dominated by CD4+ T-cells, suggesting that chronic inflammation in the colonic mucosa may be mediated by dysregulation of colonic epithelial cell-derived IL-7 (Watanabe et al., 1998).

5.5. TNF-α

As discussed above, the number of pro-inflammatory cytokines that are directly involved in IBD pathogenesis is large, but only some of them are considered as practical targets for blockade, and even fewer have reached the stage of clinical trials. Despite the still undefined role of TNF-α in IBD pathogenesis, the rationale for neutralizing TNF-α is reasonably solid, and two different monoclonal antibodies (cA2 and CDP571) have been developed and given to patients with moderate-to-severe, treatment resistant CD (Stack et al., 1997; Targan et al., 1997). The beneficial effects of these antibodies are much more prolonged than their in vivo half-life, raising the question of whether direct neutralization of TNF-α is truly responsible for the observed effects.

6. FUTURE THERAPEUTIC OPPORTUNITIES

From the above considerations on therapeutic implications, it is evident that modulation of cytokine activity is far easier to carry out, and more likely to succeed in experimental models of gut inflammation than in actual IBD patients. On the other hand, the potential for various CK and anti-CK strategies to be effective in humans is real, and eventually some of them will result in human clinical trials. Some of these strategies will be mentioned as an indication of the wide range of theoretical and practical opportunities to become reality in the near future.

Among many CKs with anti-inflammatory function, IL-4 is one of the most potent suppressors of immune reactivity. However, its toxicity in humans may be a crucial limiting factor, and its potential as a therapeutic agent for IBD is uncertain. TGF-β is another agent with anti-inflammatory potential that is uniquely appealing, because of its role in mediating oral tolerance and switching off antigen-specific immune responses (Weiner, 1997). Induction of oral tolerance is an alternate approach to the management of autoimmune diseases, but whether TGF-β has a place in the therapeutic armamentarium against CD or UC requires additional investigation.

The potential to blockade CK with proinflammatory activity in IBD patients is even greater than that of administering anti-inflammatory CKs. Beside monoclonal antibodies against TNF-α, alternative strategies can be used to block its biological activity, including administration of soluble TNF-α receptors, TNF-α receptor fusion protein, TNF-α-converting enzyme, and type IV phosphodiesterase inhibitors. Additional strategies may include the use of monoclonal antibodies against soluble IL-1 or the IL-1 surface receptor. In addition to TNF-α and IL-1, at least two other CKs can be targeted for neutralization in IBD patients: IL-12 and IFN-γ. Respectively, they induce and mediate Th1 responses thought to be especially relevant to the immunopathogenesis of CD, and clinical trials with neutralizing antibodies are in a planning phase. Chemokines and their receptors should also targeted for blockade, but this will represent a particularly daunting enterprise, because of the extremely large number of chemoattractant molecules described so far. Finally, perhaps the use of signaling cascade inhibitors could be more broadly effective targeting downstream activation events triggered by the binding of CKs to their respective receptors.

REFERENCES

Asseman C, Powrie F. Interleukin 10 is a growth factor for a population of regulatory T cells. *Gut* 1998; 42: 157–8.

Babyatsky MW, Rossiter G, Podolsky DK. Expression of transforming growth factor α and β in colonic mucosa in inflammatory bowel disease. *Gastroenterology* 1996; 110: 975–984.

Bank S, Sninsky C, Robinson M, Katz S, Singleton J, Miner P, et al. Safety and activity evaluation of rhIL-11 in subjects with active Crohn's disease. *Gastroenterology* 1997; 112: A927.

Barton BE. IL-6: insights into novel biological activities. *Clin Immunol Immunopathol* 1997; 5: 16–20.

Berg DJ, Davidson N, Kuhn R, Muller W, Menon S, Holland G, et al. Enterocolitis and colon cancer in interleukin-10-deficient mice are associated with aberrant cytokine production and CD4(+) TH1-like responses. *J Clin Invest* 1996; 98: 1010–1020.

Bertrand V, Quere S, Guimbaud R, Sogni P, Chauvelot-Moachon L, Tulliez M, et al. Effects of murine recombinant interleukin-10 on the inflammatory disease of rats transgenic for HLA-B27 and human beta 2 microglobulin. *Eur Cytokine Netw* 1998; 9: 161–170.

Braegger CP, Nicholls S, Murch SH, Stephens S, Macdonald TT. Tumour necrosis factor alpha in stool as a marker of intestinal inflammation. *Lancet* 1992; 339: 89–91.

Cappello M, Keshav S, Prince C, Jewell DP, Gordon S. Detection of mRNA for macrophage products in inflammatory bowel disease by *in situ* hybridization. *Gut* 1992; 33: 1214–1219.

Casini-Raggi V, Kam L, Chong YJT, Fiocchi C, Pizarro TT, Cominelli F. Mucosal imbalance of interleukin-1 and interleukin-1 receptor antagonist in inflammatory bowel disease: a novel mechanisms of chronic inflammation. *J Immunol* 1995; 154: 2434–2440.

Chantry D, Turner M, Abney E, Feldman M. Modulation of cytokine production by transforming growth factor-β1. *J Immunol* 1989; 142: 4295–4300.

Chomarat P, Bancherau J. Update on interleukin-4 and its receptor. *Eur Cytokine Netw* 1997; 8: 333–344.

Cominelli F, Bortolami M, Pizarro TT, Monsacchi L, Ferretti M, Brewer MT, Eisenberg SP, Ng RK. Rabbit interleukin-1 receptor antagonist. Cloning, expression, functional characterization, and regulation during intestinal inflammation. *J Biol Chem* 1994; 269: 6962–6971.

Cominelli F, Nast CC, Duchini A, Lee M. Recombinant interleukin-1 receptor antagonist blocks the proinflammatory activity of endogenous interleukin-1 in rabbit immune colitis. *Gastroenterology* 1992; 103: 65–71.

Costello R, Duffaud F. Pleiotropic effects of interleukin 7 and their pathologic and therapeutic implications. *Eur J Med* 1992; 2: 119–120.

Davidson NJ, Hudak SA, Lesley RE, Menon S, Leach MW, Rennick DM. IL-12, but not IFN-gamma, plays a major role in sustaining the chronic phase of colitis in IL-10-deficient mice. *J Immunol* 1998; 161: 3143–3149.

Demoulin JB, Renauld JC. Interleukin 9 and its receptor: an overview of structure and function. *Inter Rev Immunol* 1998; 16: 345–364.

De Vries JE. Immunosuppressive and anti-inflammatory properties of interleukin 10. *Ann Med* 1995; 27: 537–541.

De Vries JE, Zurawski G. Immunoregulatory properties of IL-13: Its potential role in atopic disease. *Int Arch Allergy Immunol* 1995; 106: 175–179.

Dignass AU, Podolsky DK. Cytokine modulation of intestinal epithelial cell restitution: central role of transforming growth factor β. *Gastroenterology* 1993; 105: 1323–1332.

Dinarello CA, Thompson RC. Blocking IL-1: interleukin 1 receptor antagonist in vivo and in vitro. *Immunol Today* 1991; 12: 404–410.

Dinarello CA, Wolf SM. Role of interleukin-1 in disease. *N Engl J Med* 1993; 328: 106–113.

Doe WF, Grimm MC. Colony-stimulating factors in inflammatory bowel disease, in *Cytokines in Inflammatory Bowel Disease*, Fiocchi C (ed.) R.G. Landes, Austin 1996, 119–136.

Du XX, Williams DA. Interleukin-11: a multifunctional growth factor derived from the hematopoietic microenvironment. *Blood* 1994; 83: 2023–2030.

Eberhart CE, Dubois RN. Eicosanoids and the gastrointestinal tract. *Gastroenterology* 1995; 109: 285–301.

Ehrhardt RO, Ludviksson BR, Gray B, Neurath M, Strober W. Induction and prevention of colonic inflammation in IL-2-deficient mice. *J Immunol* 1997; 158: 566–73.

Elson CO, Sartor RB, Tennyson GS, Riddell RH. Experimental models of inflammatory bowel disease. *Gastroenterology* 1995; 109: 1344–67.

Finch PW, Pricolo V, Wu A, Finkelstein SD. Increased expression of keratinocyte growth factor messenger RNA associated with inflammatory bowel disease. *Gastroenterology* 1996; 110: 441–451.

Fiocchi C. *Cytokines in Inflammatory Bowel Disease*. R.G. Landes, Austin 1996.

Fiocchi C. Inflammatory bowel disease: etiology and pathogenesis. *Gastroenterology* 1998; 115: 182–205.

Fuss IJ, Neurath M, Boirivant M, Klein JS, Delamotte C, Strong SA, Fiocchi C, Strober W. Disparate CD4+ lamina propria (LP) lymphokine secretion profiles in inflammatory bowel disease. Crohn's disease LP manifest increased secretion of IFN-γ, whereas ulcerative colitis LP cells manifest increased secretion of IL-5. *J Immunol* 1996; 157: 1261–1270.

Grimm MC, Doe WF. Chemokines in inflammatory bowel disease mucosa: expression of RANTES, macrophage inflammatory protein (MIP)-1α, MIP-1β, and γ-interferon-inducible protein 10 by macrophages, lymphocytes, endothelial cells, and granulomas. *Inflamm Bowel Dis* 1996; 2: 88–96.

Groux H, O'Garra A, Bigler M, Rouleau M, Antonenko S, De Vries JE, Roncarolo MG. CD4+ T-cell subset inhibits antigen-specific T-cell responses and prevents colitis. *Nature* 1997; 389: 737–742.

Hogaboam CM, Vallance BA, Kumar A, Addison CL, Graham FL, Gauldie J, Collins SM. Therapeutic effects of interleukin-4 gene transfer in experimental inflammatory bowel disease. *J Clin Invest* 1997; 100: 2766–2776.

Isaacs KL, Sartor RB, Haskill S. Cytokine messenger RNA profiles in inflammatory bowel disease mucosa detected by polymerase chain reaction amplification. *Gastroenterology* 1992; 103: 1587–1595.

Ito H, Fathman CG. CD45RBhigh CD4+ T cells from IFN-gamma knockout mice do not induce wasting disease. *J Autoimmun* 1997; 10: 455–459.

Izzo RS, Witkon K, Chen AI, Hadjiyane C, Weinstein MI, Pellecchia C. Interleukin-8 and neutrophil markers in colonic mucosa from patients with ulcerative colitis. *Am J Gastroenterol* 1992; 87: 1447–1452.

Izzo RS, Witkon K, Chen AI, Hadjiyane C, Weinstein MI, Pellecchia C. Neutrophil-activating peptide (interleukin-8) in colonic mucosa from patients with Crohn's disease. *Scand J Gastroenterol* 1993; 28: 296–300.

Keates S, Keates AC, Mizoguchi E, Bhan A, Kelly CP. Enterocytes are the primary source of the chemokine ENA-78 in normal colon and ulcerative colitis. *Am J Physiol* 1997; 273: G75–G82.

Kelsall BL, Stuber E, Neurath M, Strober W. Interleukin-12 production by dendritic cells. The role of CD40–CD40L interactions in Th1 T-cell responses. *Ann NY Acad Sci* 1996; 795: 116–126.

Kohno K, Kurimoto M. Interleukin 18, a cytokine which resembles IL-1 structurally and IL-12 functionally but exerts its effects independently of both. *Clin Immunol Immunopathol* 1998; 86: 11–15.

Koike M, Takatsu K. IL-5 and its receptor: which role do they play in the immune response. *Int Arch Allergy Immunol* 1994; 104: 1–9.

Kucharzik T, Stoll R, Lugering N, Domschke W. Circulating antiinflammatory cytokine IL-10 in patients with inflammatory bowel disease (IBD). *Clin Exp Immunol* 1995; 100: 452–456.

Kugathasan S, Willis J, Dahms BB, O'Riordan MA, Hupertz V, Binion DG, Boyle JT, Fiocchi C. Intrinsic hyperreactivity of mucosal T-cells to interleukin-2 in pediatric Crohn's disease. *J Pediatr* 1998; 133: 675–681.

Kusugami K, Fukatsu A, Tanimoto M, Shinoda M, Haruta J-I, Kuroiwa A, et al. Elevation of interleukin-6 in inflammatory bowel disease is macrophage- and epithelial cell-dependent. *Dig Dis Sci* 1995; 40: 949–959.

Kusugami K, Youngman KR, West GA, Fiocchi C. Intestinal immune reactivity to interleukin 2 differs among Crohn's disease, ulcerative colitis and control. *Gastroenterology* 1989; 97: 1–9.

Ludviksson BR, Ehrhardt RO, Strober W. TGF-beta production regulates the development of the 2,4,6-trinitrophenol-conjugated keyhole limpet hemocyanin-induced colonic inflammation in IL-2-deficient mice. *J Immunol* 1997a; 159: 3622–3628.

Ludviksson BR, Gray B, Strober W, Ehrhardt RO. Dysregulated intrathymic development in the IL-2-deficient mouse leads to colitis-inducing thymocytes. *J Immunol* 1997b; 158: 104–111.

Luster AD. Chemokines: Chemotactic cytokines that mediate inflammation. *N Engl J Med* 1998; 338: 436–445.

Macdermott RP, Sanderson IR, Reinecker H-C. Central role of chemokines (chemotactic cytokines) in the immunopathogenesis of ulcerative colitis and Crohn's disease. *Inflamm Bowel Dis* 1998; 4: 54–67.

Mahida YR, Wu K, Jewell DP. Enhanced production of interleukin 1-β by mononuclear cells isolated from mucosa with active ulcerative colitis and Crohn's disease. *Gut* 1989; 30: 835–838.

Matsuura T, Kusugami K, Morise K, Fiocchi C. Interleukin-2 and interleukin-2 receptor in inflammatory bowel disease, in *Cytokines in Inflammatory Bowel Disease* Fiocchi C (ed.) R.G. Landes, Austin, 1996, pp. 41–55.

Mcinnes IB, Liew FY. Interleukin 15: a proinflammatory role in rheumatoid arthritis synovitis. *Immunol Today* 1998; 19: 75–79.

Monteleone G, Biancone L, Marasco R, Morrone G, Marasco O, Luzza F, Pallone F. Interleukin 12 is expressed and actively released by Crohn's disease intestinal lamina propria mononuclear cells. *Gastroenterology* 1997; 112: 1169–1178.

Mosmann TR, Sad S. Expanding universe of T-cell subsets: Th1, Th2 and more. *Immunol Today* 1996; 17: 138–146.

Mullin GE, Maycon ZR, Braun-Elwert L, Cerchia R, James SP, Katz S, et al. Inflammatory bowel disease mucosal biopsies have specialized lymphokine mRNA profiles. *Inflamm Bowel Dis* 1996; 2: 16–26.

Neurath MF, Fuss I, Kelsall B, Meyer Zum Buschenfelde KH, Strober W. Effect of IL-12 and antibodies to IL-12 on established granulomatous colitis in mice. *Ann NY Acad Sci* 1996b; 795: 368–370.

Neurath MF, Fuss I, Kelsall BL, Presky DH, Waegell W, Strober W. Experimental granulomatous colitis in mice is abrogated by induction of TGF-beta-mediated oral tolerance. *J Exp Med* 1996a; 183: 2605–2616.

Neurath MF, Fuss I, Kelsall BL, Stuber E, Strober W. Antibodies to interleukin 12 abrogate established experimental colitis in mice. *J Exp Med* 1995; 182: 1281–1290.

Pallone F, Fais S, Boirivant M. Interferon system in inflammatory bowel disease, in *Cytokines in Inflammatory Bowel Disease* Fiocchi C (ed.) R.G. Landes, Austin, 1996, pp. 57–67.

Podolsky DK. Lessons from genetic models of inflammatory bowel disease. *Acta Gastroenterol Belg* 1997; 60: 163–165.

Powrie F, Carlino J, Leach MW, Mauze S, Coffman RL. Critical role for transforming growth factor-beta but not interleukin 4 in the suppression of T helper type 1-mediated colitis by CD45RB(low) CD4+ T cells. *J Exp Med* 1996; 183: 2669–2674.

Powrie F, Leach MW, Mauze S, Menon S, Caddle LB, Coffman RL. Inhibition of Th1 responses prevents inflammatory bowel disease in SCID mice reconstituted with CD45RBhi CD4+ T cells. *Immunity* 1994; 1: 553–562.

Qiu BS, Pfeiffer CJ, Keith JC, Jr. Protection by recombinant human interleukin-

11 against experimental TNB-induced colitis in rats. *Dig Dis Sci* 1996; 41: 1625–1630.

Reinecker H-C, Loh EY, Ringler DJ, Metha A, Rombeau JL, Macdermott RP. Monocyte-chemoattractant protein 1 gene expression in intestinal epithelial cells and inflammatory bowel disease mucosa. *Gastroenterology* 1995; 108: 40–50.

Reinecker H-C, Steffen M, Witthoeft T, Pflueger I, Schreiber S, Macdermott RP, Raedler A. Enhanced secretion of tumour necrosis factor-alpha, IL-6, and IL-1β by isolated lamina propria mononuclear cells from patients with ulcerative colitis and Crohn's disease. *Clin Exp Immunol* 1993; 94: 174–181.

Rennick DM, Fort MM, Davidson NJ. Studies with IL-10$^{-/-}$ mice: an overview. *J Leukoc Biol* 1997; 61: 389–396.

Rink L, Kirchner H. Recent progress in the tumor necrosis-α field. *Int Arch Allergy Immunol* 1996; 111: 199–209.

Sakai T, Kusugami K, Nishimura H, Ando T, Yamaguchi T, Ohsuga M, et al. Interleukin 15 activity in the rectal mucosa of inflammatory bowel disease. *Gastroenterology* 1998; 114: 1237–1243.

Sartor RB. How relevant to human inflammatory bowel disease are current animal models of intestinal inflammation? *Aliment Pharmacol Ther* 1997; 11 (Suppl 3): 89–96; discussion 96–97.

Simpson SJ, Shah S, Comiskey M, De Jong YP, Wang B, Mizoguchi E, Bhan AK, Terhorst C. T cell-mediated pathology in two models of experimental colitis depends predominantly on the interleukin 12/Signal transducer and activator of transcription (Stat)-4 pathway, but is not conditional on interferon gamma expression by T cells. *J Exp Med* 1998; 187: 1225–1234.

Sonoda E, Matsumoto R, Hitoshi Y, Ishii T, Sugimoto M, Araki S, et al. Transforming growth factor β induces IgA production and acts additively with interleukin 5 for IgA production. *J Exp Med* 1989; 170: 1415–1420.

Sparano JA, Brandt LJ, Dutcher JP, Dubois JS, Atkins MB. Symptomatic exacerbation of Crohn disease after treatment with high-dose interleukin-2. *Ann Intern Med* 1993; 118: 617, 618.

Spencer D, Levine A. Local production of IL-12 by lamina propria mononuclear cells is triggered with the onset of colitis and subsides during chronic disease. *Gastroenterology* 1998; 114: A-1089.

Stack WA, Mann SD, Roy AJ, Heath P, Sopwith M, Freeman J, et al. Randomised controlled trial of CDP571 antibody to tumour necrosis factor-α in Crohn's disease. *Lancet* 1997; 349: 521–524.

Stevens C, Walz G, Singaram C, Lipman ML, Zanker B, Muggia A, et al. Tumor necrosis factor-α, interleukin-1β, and interleukin-6 expression in inflammatory bowel disease. *Dig Dis Sci* 1992; 37: 818–826.

Targan SR, Hanauer SB, Vandeventer SJH, Mayer L, Present DH, Braakman

T, et al. Short-term study of chimeric monoclonal antibody cA2 to tumor necrosis factor a for Crohn's disease. *N Engl J Med* 1997; 337: 1029–1035.

Theze J, Alzari PM, Bertoglio J. Interleukin 2 and its receptors: recent advances and new immunological functions. *Immunol Today* 1996; 17: 481–486.

Tomoyose M, Mitsuyama K, Ishida H, Toyonaga A, Tanikawa K. Role of interleukin-10 in a murine model of dextran sulfate sodium-induced colitis. *Scand J Immunol* 1998; 33: 435–440.

Trinchieri G, Scott P. Role of interleukin 12 in the immune response, disease, and therapy. *Immunol Today* 1994; 15: 460–463.

Vandeventer SJH, Elson CO, Fedorak RN. Multiple doses of intravenous interleukin 10 in steroid-refractory Crohn's disease. *Gastroenterology* 1997; 113: 383–389.

Watanabe M, Ueno Y, Yajima T, Okamoto S, Hayashi T, Yamazaki M, et al. Interleukin 7 transgenic mice develop chronic colitis with decreased interleukin 7 protein accumulation in the colonic mucosa. *J Exp Med* 1998; 187: 389–402.

Weiner HL. Oral tolerance: immune mechanisms and tratment of autoimmune diseases. *Immunol Today* 1997; 18: 335–343.

West GA, Matsuura T, Levine AD, Klein JS, Fiocchi C. Interleukin-4 in inflammatory bowel disease and mucosal immune reactivity. *Gastroenterology* 1996; 110: 1683–1695.

Wright NA, Poulsom R, Stamp G, Vannoorden S, Sarraf C, Elia G, et al. Trefoil peptide gene expression in gastrointestinal epithelial cells in inflammatory bowel disease. *Gastroenterology* 1993; 194: 12–20.

Young HA, Hardy KJ. Role of interferon-γ in immune cell regulation. *Immunol Today* 1995; 58: 373–381.

Youngman KR, Simon PL, West GA, Cominelli F, Rachmilewitz D, Klein JS, Fiocchi C. Localization of intestinal interleukin 1 activity, protein and gene expression to lamina propria cells. *Gastroenterology* 1993; 104: 749–758.

Z'Graggen K, Walz A, Mazzucchelli L, Strieter RM, Mueller C. C-X-C chemokine ENA-78 is preferentially expressed in intestinal epithelium in inflammatory bowel disease. *Gastroenterology* 1997; 113: 808–816.

4 Peptide Growth Factors in Gastrointestinal Disorder Therapeutics

Antonio Guglietta and Marija Veljača

CONTENTS

1. INTRODUCTION

The term "peptide growth factors" (PGFs) refers to a group of compounds with peptidic structure that share the ability to regulate cell proliferation and differentiation. In contrast to the classical hormones that are produced and secreted by specific cells, PGFs are usually synthesized by cells of a variety of different tissues, and often exert their pharmacological effects on target cells located not far from the site of release (paracrine response), and sometimes even on the same

From: *Drug Development: Molecular Targets for GI Diseases*
Edited by: T. S. Gaginella and A. Guglietta © Humana Press Inc., Totowa, NJ

PGFs-producing cells (autocrine response) (Pimentel, 1994). The list of such compounds is very long and includes well characterized substances, along with others whose characteristics have not been completely elucidated (Pimentel, 1994). The regulation of cell proliferation and differentiation may, however, be just one of several pharmacological effects of PGFs: epidermal growth factor (EGF) and transforming growth factor-α (TGF-α), for example, in addition to stimulating proliferation of epithelial cells of the gastrointestinal (GI) tract, are also potent inhibitors of gastric acid secretion (Elder et al., 1975; Koffman et al., 1982; Guglietta and Lesch, 1993; Guglietta et al., 1994). Because several PGFs are synthesized in, and exert their pharmacological effects on, the GI tract, under both normal or pathologic conditions, this ability of regulating cell proliferation and differentiation could actually be exploited therapeutically in several pathologic conditions of the GI tract. The pharmacological effects of selected PGFs not related to cellular growth may also contribute to their beneficial GI activity.

This chapter deals with those PGFs that regulate proliferation/differentiation of the constituent cells of the GI tract (i.e., mucosal cells, endothelial cells, and so on), and mostly with those for which strong preclinical and, in some cases, clinical evidence of beneficial activity in GI disorders exists. Other PGFs, which exert their cell-proliferation/ differentiation effect primarily on liver and pancreas, or on cells not belonging to the GI system (i.e., on lymphocytes such as interleukins), will not be considered in this review, nor will peptides, such as trefoil peptides, which stimulate repair of GI lesions through mechanisms not affecting cell proliferation (Sands and Podolsky, 1996; Otto and Wright 1994), although they are potentially useful in the treatment of GI and hepatic disorders.

2. ROLE OF PGFs IN HEALTH AND PATHOLOGIC PROCESSES OF GI TRACT

For the maintenance of normal trophism and function, the GI tract depends on the production of its own PGFs. Experimentally, this can be demonstrated by observing the effect of the removal of the major source of a specific PGF. In rats, removal of the salivary glands, in which most rat EGF is synthesized (Heinz et al., 1978, Gresik et al.,

1979; Carpenter and Wahl, 1990), causes a reduction in gastric content of immunoreactive EGF and a delay in the healing of gastric and duodenal ulcerations (Konturek et al.,1988). A human equivalent of this condition can be seen in Sjögren's syndrome, the autoimmune disease of salivary glands, sometimes associated with atrophy of gastric mucosa and other GI problems (Takasugi et al., 1979; Kjellen et al., 1986; Sheikh and Shaw-Stiffel, 1995).

On the other hand, much data exists also suggesting a role for some of these PGFs in the normal repair process of several pathologic conditions of the GI tract. Unlike normal GI tissue, in biopsies taken from inflammatory bowel disease (IBD) patients, a novel cell lineage that reacts with anti-EGF antibody appears associated with ulcerative lesions, suggesting a reparative activity of EGF-like material (Wright et al., 1990a, 1990b). Furthermore, altered synthesis/expression of several PGFs and their receptors has been demonstrated in various experimental and clinical conditions characterized by GI damage (Hansson et al., 1990; Tarnawski et al., 1992a; Jankowski et al., 1993; Alexander et al., 1995; Chowdhury et al., 1996; Romano et al., 1996; Hoffmann et al., 1997; Konturek et al., 1997). Interference has also been demonstrated between *Helicobacter pylori,* whose colonization of GI mucosa is associated with gastritis, peptic ulcer disease, and cancer, and PGFs, which could result in a disturbance of the delicate balance that controls the renewal, maintenance, and repair of the gastroduodenal mucosa (Ascencio et al., 1995).

There is even an indication that the therapeutic effect of some common drugs used to treat GI disorders might be mediated through synthesis of some PGFs. Actually, several antiulcer agents, such as sucralfate, ebrotidine, sulglycotide, rebamipide, and sucrose octasulfate, have been shown to stimulate the expression or bind to several PGFs receptors (Slomiany et al., 1992; Tarnawski et al., 1992b, 1998; Zhu et al., 1993, Piotrowski et al., 1995).

3. PGFs WITH POTENTIAL THERAPEUTIC USE IN GI DISEASES

3.1. Epidermal Growth Factor Family of Peptides

EGF is a 6-kDa peptide that was first discovered as a contaminant of nerve growth factor, and was then purified and characterized from

Table 1
Peptide Growth Factor Families with Potential Clinical Use in
Gastrointestinal Disorders

EGF Family (Groenen et al., 1994)	FGF Family (Galzie et al., 1997)	PDGF Family (Meyer-Ingold and Eichner, 1995)	TGF-β Family[a] (Lawrence 1996)
EGF	FGF-1 (Acidic fibroblast growth factor)	PDGF-AA	TGF-β_1
TGF-α	FGF-2 (Basic fibroblast growth factor)	PDGF-AB	TGF-β_2
Amphiregulin	FGF-3 (Oncogene int2)	PDGF-BB	TGF-β_3
HB-EGF	FGF-5 (Oncogene fibroblast growth factor 5)		
SDGF	FGF-6 (Oncogene hst2)		
Betacellulin	FGF-7 (Keratinocyte growth factor)		
VGF	FGF-8 (Androgen-induced growth factor)		
SFGF	FGF-9 (Glial-activating factor)		
MGF			
NDF			
HRG-α			
HRG-β_1			

[a]Mammalian peptides.

mouse salivary glands (Cohen, 1960; Levi-Montalcini and Cohen 1960; Cohen, 1962; Savage et al.,1972). A few years later, the human equivalent of mouse EGF, urogastrone, was isolated from urine (Gregory, 1975) and Brunner's glands of the duodenum (Elder et al., 1978; Heinz et al., 1978). Several other members of the EGF family (Table 1) were subsequently discovered (Carpenter and Wahl, 1990). All members of the EGF family share the EGF motif (six cysteine residues forming three disulfide bonds), bind to a specific cellular receptor, and mimic the pharmacological actions of mouse EGF (Carpenter and Wahl, 1990; Groenen et al., 1994).

The EGF receptor is a transmembrane glycoprotein consisting of a single polypeptide chain and N-linked carbohydrates. The receptor has an external domain, a transmembrane domain, and a cytoplasmic domain with tyrosine kinase activity (TKA) (Pringent and Lemoine, 1992). Binding of the ligand causes receptor dimerization, which increases the catalytic activity of its tyrosine kinase and leads to phosphorylation of the receptor, and of a number of substrates, such as phospholipase C gamma, mitogen-activated protein kinase, and ras guanosine triphosphatase-activating protein (Pringent and Lemoine, 1992). With the exception of a few cell types, the activated receptor–ligand complex is then endocytosed and degraded by lysosomes, or recycled to the cell membrane (Pringent and Lemoine, 1992).

EGF was named for its ability to accelerate the eruption of incisors and the opening of eyelids in newborn mice, which appeared to be caused by an increase in the growth rate of epidermal tissue (Cohen, 1962). It is now clear, however, that the proliferative activity of EGF is not limited to epithelial tissue, and that, in addition, members of this family possess other pharmacological properties (Elder et al., 1975; Koffman et al., 1982; Guglietta and Lesch, 1993; Guglietta et al., 1994).

3.2. Fibroblast Growth Factors

The term "fibroblast growth factors" (FGF) refers to a family of peptides consisting of at least nine members, designated FGF-1–FGF-9, some of which, however, are also known by alternative names (i.e., acidic FGF [aFGF] and basic FGF [bFGF], for FGF-1 and FGF-2, respectively, or keratinocyte growth factor, for FGF-7) (Table 1). Their amino acid lengths vary from 155 to 246, with 30–50% sequence homology and conservation of two cysteine residues. Multiple molecular forms exist for some members of the family, such as FGF-2 or FGF-8 (Galzie et al., 1997). FGFs have been isolated from brain, hypothalamus, retina, cartilage and solid tumors (Ross et al., 1974; Gospodarowitz et al., 1978; Shing et al., 1984).

At least four distinct receptors for FGFs have been described (FGFR-1, FGFR-2, FGFR-3, and FGFR-4) as a subgroup of the TK receptor family (Partanen et al., 1992; Galzie et al., 1997). Although not all possible FGF-FGFR interactions have been studied, it appears that one FGF receptor can bind several members of the FGF family, and one type of FGF can similarly bind to several different FGF receptors (Galzie et al., 1997). Following a general scheme thought to be common to the entire family of TK receptors, binding of the ligand to the FGF receptor(s) induces dimerization of the receptor(s), followed by activation of the TK function and phosphorylation of the receptor, which leads to activation of the binding sites for proteins that are targets of the receptor TK, and to internalization of the receptor via receptor-mediated endocytosis (Ullrich and Schlessinger 1990; Fantl et al., 1993; Galzie et al., 1997). FGF-2 is also known to bind to a variety of molecules, such as heparin and heparin sulphate proteoglycans, which are thought to protect the peptide from inactivation by proteolytic enzymes present in tissues (Galzie et al., 1997). Some members of the FGF family (FGF-1, FGF-2, and FGF-9) lack a secretory signal sequence, and are probably not secreted by the conventional endoplasmic reticulum–Golgi pathway (Burgess and Maciag, 1989). It has therefore been suggested that these molecules are intracellular under normal conditions, and are released from dying or dead cells during cell injury (Galzie et al., 1997).

Generally, FGF molecules have been shown to modulate cell proliferation, differentiation, and cell function, and to play an important role in normal development of wound healing, as well as in tumorogenesis and metastasis (Galzie et al., 1997).

3.3. Platelet-Derived Growth Factor

Platelet-derived growth factor (PDGF), originally isolated from platelets, and later found to be synthesized also by endothelial cells, vascular smooth muscle cells, activated monocytes, and macrophages (Meyer-Ingold, 1995), is a peptide consisting of two different, but closely related, polypeptide chains (A and B) joined by disulfide bonds (Antoniades, 1981; Antoniades and Hunkapiller, 1983). Different arrangements of the two chains give rise to three different isomers of the molecule, known as PDGF-AA (two A chains), PDGF-AB (one A chain and one B chain), and PDGF-BB (two B chains), all of which are natural cell products (Meyer-Ingold and Eichner, 1995).

Two receptors that bind PDGF molecules have been identified: PDGF-α, which binds all three isoforms, and PDGF-β, which displays higher affinity for the PDGF-BB isoform (Hart et al., 1988; Heldin et al., 1988). The PDGF receptors are members of the TK family of receptors; as is the case of other similar receptors, binding of the ligand causes dimerization of the receptors, autophosphorylation, and kinase activation, which results in the transduction of the signal (Claesson-Welsh, 1994).

PDGF is a potent mitogen for a variety of cell types, including fibroblasts, osteoblasts, and arterial smooth muscle and glial cells. It possesses chemotactic activity for fibroblast and arterial smooth cells, and is thought to play a major physiological role in wound healing and embryogenesis (Pimentel, 1994).

3.4. Transforming Growth Factor β

Initially discovered as a product of retrovirally transformed fibroblasts (De Larco and Todaro, 1978), transforming growth factor β (TGF-β) was subsequently also shown to be secreted by cells transformed by other viruses or chemicals, as well as normal cells of embryonic and adult tissues (Proper et al., 1982; Lawrence, 1996). The TGF-β family is composed of over 30 different molecules found in a variety of animal species. Mammalian TGF-β, however, comes in three isoforms (TGF-$β_1$, TGF-$β_2$ and TGF-$β_3$) of about 25 kDa each; these are secreted as much larger molecules, from which the active form is then cleaved (Lawrence, 1996).

TGF-βs bind to two major transmembrane receptors (type I and type II) associated with intracellular kinase activity (Derynck, 1994; Chen et al., 1995). Two type II receptors have been identified, and several members of the type I receptor exist (Lawrence, 1996). TGF-$β_1$ and TGF-$β_3$ show a higher affinity than TGF-$β_2$ for the first type II receptor (Derynck, 1994). Although the signaling pathways for TGF-βs have not been completely elucidated, it is likely that multiple pathways exist to transduce the signal of different TGF-β molecules (Derynck, 1994; Lawrence, 1996). A number of soluble proteins, such as α-fetoprotein and the proteoglycan, decorin, are also known to bind TGF-β (Miyazono et al., 1993).

The TGF-βs exert a variety of biological effects. These molecules play an essential role in regulation of cellular proliferation (inhibiting proliferation of most cells, stimulating the growth of some mesenchymal cells), in immunologic response (immunosuppressive role), and in the formation of extracellular matrix (Lawrence 1996). In the early phase of tissue repair, TGF-β is a potent chemotactic factor for cells that stimulate the inflammatory and granulation phase of wound healing, in the remodeling phase of wound healing, it directly stimulates new matrix synthesis by fibroblasts (Lawrence, 1996).

3.5. Vascular Endothelial Growth Factor

A family of polypetides with endothelial cell mitogenic activity (vascular endothelial cell growth factors [VEGFs]), structurally related to PDGF, has recently been identified (Keck et al., 1989). VEGFs exist in four isoforms (VEGF-121, VEGF-165, VEGF-189, and VEGF-206), which contain identical aminoterminal residues (Pimentel 1994). VEGF-189 and VEGF-206 are chiefly cell-associated; VEGF-121 and VEGF-165 are secreted by cells in the surrounding environment (Pimentel, 1994).

The VEGF gene is expressed in a variety of normal adult organs and tissues, as well as in tumors (Pimentel 1994). In rats, the highest density of VEGF binding sites is found in brain, spinal cord, lung, adrenal cortex, glandular stomach, spleen, and pancreas (Pimentel, 1994). The receptor mediating the effects of VEGF appears to be a protein with associated TKA (Pimentel, 1994), and postreceptor events may include phosphorylation of the receptor and other cellular proteins, entry of Ca^{2+} into the cells, activation of phospholipase C, and hydrolysis of phosphoinositides (Pimentel, 1994). The primary biological effect of VEGF is the stimulation of proliferation of endothelial cells and angiogenesis. This mitogenic activity appears to be restricted to the secreted forms of VEGF (Pimentel, 1994).

4. GI DISORDERS THAT COULD BENEFIT FROM TREATMENT WITH PGFs

In theory, all GI disorders characterized by a disturbance of cell proliferation, or those conditions in which a stimulation of proliferation of different cell types (mucosal cells, fibroblasts, endothelial cells, and so on) is desired, could benefit from treatment with PGFs. These include a variety of conditions: esophagitis, gastric ulcer, and inflammatory bowel disease. For some of them, experimental data exist to support the therapeutic use of PGFs; for others, this is only speculative, and based on theoretical considerations. From a practical point of view, however, treatment of these disorders with PGFs is not always necessary or advisable, for a variety of reasons: fast spontaneous healing; the possibility of removing the cause of ulceration, thus promoting spontaneous healing; or unfavorable risk:benefit ratio. Nevertheless, PGF treatment may be appealing in many of these cases.

4.1. Gastrointestinal Ulcers

Mucosal erosions or frank ulceration occur throughout the GI tract in a variety of disorders, such as microbial infections, drug treatment, trauma, chemical poisoning, and peptic ulcer disease. Whatever the cause of the ulcer, in order to heal the damage, cell migration (restitution) and proliferation (regeneration) must occur. In the case of superficial mucosal damage (i.e., erosions), healing is achieved through restitution and proliferation of the mucosal cells; in the case of a deep ulceration, the damage is first repaired by granulation tissue, consisting of fibroblasts, collagen, capillaries, and chronic inflammatory cells, which eventually becomes a fibrous framework, providing the basis for re-epithelialization by restitution and regeneration (Szabo et al., 1995a). In order to promote spontaneous healing, in some cases, it is sufficient to remove the factor(s) associated with ulcer formation. Eradication of *H. pylori,* a microorganism thought to be involved in the development of gastroduodenal ulcers, is, for instance, sufficient to promote healing of the ulcer associated with *H. pylori* infection (Salcedo and Al-Kawas, 1998). However, in situations in which it is not possible to remove the cause(s) of the ulcer, or when a faster and better healing is required, it may be desirable to pharmacologically intervene with compounds that act directly on the healing process. Certain PGFs have indeed been shown to stimulate proliferation of cell types involved in the repair of GI ulcer, achieving a faster and enhanced healing characterized by a more vascularized granulation tissue (Tarnawski et al., 1991, Szabo et al., 1995a, 1995b; Szabo and Sandor 1996). Treatment of a GI ulceration with PGFs may be particularly appealing in those patients who might have impaired healing because of inadequate endogenous level of PGFs. Data showing reduced levels of EGF in the saliva of patients with active or healing peptic ulcer, compared to levels in healthy individuals, indicate that this may indeed be the case, at least, in some patients (Ohmura et al., 1987; Maccini and Veit, 1990).

Data exist showing that PGFs accelerate and enhance the healing of experimental ulcers. Preclinical data have shown that EGF and TGF-α stimulate the activity of ornithine decarboxylase, a step required for polyamine synthesis, the production of which is closely related to the burst of intracellular activity preceding cell division (Feldman et al., 1978), and the prevention and repair of GI ulceration (Konturek et al., 1988; Romano et al., 1992, 1994). These effects are clearly seen after systemic administration of EGF, but, although less often, they have also been reported after oral delivery of the compound (Skov-Olsen et al.,1986). A clinical study has confirmed the healing effect of EGF in gastric ulcer patients. Treatment with iv EGF (6 µg twice weekly for 8 wk) resulted in a significantly better healing rate, compared to a control group that received the active placebo, cetraxate hydrochloride (200 mg orally 4×/d) (Itoh and Matsuo, 1994). In another clinical trial, duodenal ulcer patients treated with oral hEGF (450 or 600 mg/d for 6 wk) showed a healing rate comparable to the one obtained with 200 mg cimetidine 4×/d (Haedo et al., 1996).

bFGF (FGF-2) has also been shown to accelerate the healing of experimental ulcers. Oral treatment with bFGF or its acid-resistant form (bFGF-CS-23) (100 ng/100 g twice a day for 3 wk) accelerated the healing of cystamine-induced duodenal ulcer in rat (Szabo et al., 1991, 1994). On a molar basis, the antiulcer effect of bFGF-CS-23 (100 ng/100 g) was about 7 million times more potent than that of 10 mg/100 g cimetidine. A similar stimulation of healing was seen in acetic acid-induced gastric ulcers in rats (Satoh et al., 1991). bFGF-CS-23 had no effect on the development of cystamine-induced duodenal ulcer or ethanol-induced gastric damage. This suggests that the reduction of gastric and duodenal damage seen after chronic administration of bFGF-Cs-23 is indeed the result of an accelerated healing, probably caused by stimulation of proliferation of the cell types involved in repair of a GI ulcer, (particularly to an effect on angiogenesis) (Szabo and Sandor 1996), rather than by a preventive effect on the formation of the ulcer. The safety and efficacy of the acid-resistant form of bFGF was also tested clinically. Four-week oral treatment of patients with bFGF-CS-23 (10 µg/d or 50–100 µg twice daily) resulted in a rapid healing of gastric and duodenal ulcers resistant to standard antiulcer therapy, without any adverse effect (Wolfe et al., 1994). Similarly, oral bFGF-CS23 (0.1 mg twice daily) treatment of patients suffering from nonsteroidal anti-inflammatory drug-associated gastropathy, refractory to conventional treatment, had, after 4 wk, led to either complete healing of four ulcers or reduction of the ulcer area in five ulcers (Hull et al., 1995).

Several other PGFs have also been shown to accelerate the healing of experimental GI ulcers and/or prevent their development. Although additional data and clinical evidence of their efficacy should be collected, PGFs may also represent an alternative to future treatment of GI ulcers. PDGF-BB, for instance, has also been shown to stimulate proliferation of several cell types involved in the repair of GI ulcer. Oral administration of PDGF-BB resulted in prevention and/or accelerated healing of experimentally induced duodenal ulcers (100 and 500 ng/ 100 g twice a day for 3 wk) (Vattay et al., 1991) or indomethacin-induced gastric damage in rats (0.1 nmol/kg) (Guglietta et al., 1992), without affecting gastric acid secretion (Vattay et al., 1991).

Members of the TGF-β family have also been shown to accelerate the healing of experimentally induced GI ulcers. Local infiltration of TGF-β_1 into a surgical incision of the rabbit stomach resulted in a faster ulcer healing (Mustoe et al., 1990), although a similar effect was seen after local injection of neutralizing antibody to TGF-β_1 (Ernst et al., 1996). Similar results were also obtained with local infiltration (1–50 μg/kg) or systemic administration (500 μg/kg) of the isomer TGF-β_3 in a cryoprobe-induced model of gastric ulcer in rats (Coerper et al., 1997). Finally, oral treatment with VEGF (1 μg/100 g/d for 21 d) has also been reported to accelerate healing of experimentally induced duodenal ulcer, which, histologically, was associated with prominent angiogenesis and granulation tissue production (Szabo et al., 1998).

4.2. Inflammatory Bowel Disease

IBD is a chronic inflammatory disease of unknown etiology, which, in the majority of cases, affects the colon and terminal ileum. Although mixed forms have been described, IBD actually refers to two distinct pathologic entities, ulcerative colitis and Crohn's disease, distinguishable chiefly on the basis of localization and histopathology. Despite the fact that several etiopathogenic hypotheses have been proposed (Fiocchi, 1998), the etiology and pathogenesis of this disease remain obscure, and treatment remains mostly empirical. Because one of the morphologic features of IBD is the development of mucosal ulcerations, a rationale for the use of agents that stimulate ulcer repair, such as PGFs, exists, and, indeed, several PGFs have been shown to accelerate healing and/or to ameliorate experimentally induced IBD lesions.

EGF has been shown to ameliorate experimental colitis in rats. Given by repeated sc injections (25 and 100 µg/kg/12 h) or by iv infusion (50 and 200 µg/kg/24 h) for 7 d, EGF significantly reduced trinitrobenzene sulfonic acid (TNBS)-induced colonic ulceration and inflammation (Luck and Bass, 1994). This beneficial effect was seen after systemic administration of the peptide, and there was no effect whatsoever after intrarectal administration (Luck and Bass, 1994). This effect, which is shared by other members of the EGF family of peptides (Guglietta et al., 1993, 1997), and which is also seen in several other models of colitis (Guglietta et al., 1996), seems to be even more pronounced when EGF treatment is started before the induction of colitis (Guglietta et al., 1993; Procaccino et al., 1994). The protective effect of EGF on experimental colitis is mediated through its TK-linked receptor, because pretreatment with specific TK inhibitors completely abolishes it (Lesch and Guglietta, 1995). Rapidity of action is perhaps the most remarkable feature of EGF efficacy in this particular model of colitis. In the authors' hands, rats treated intraperitoneally with 10 nmol/kg (62 µg/kg) of human EGF 1 h prior to a single intracolonic administration of 50 mg/ kg of TNBS dissolved in 50% EtOH, showed a significant reduction in the area of colonic damage as early as 1 h after TNBS challenge (Fig.1; unpublished data). This suggests that mechanisms other than stimulation of cell proliferation might be responsible for the beneficial effect of EGF on TNBS colitis.

A beneficial effect on the course of experimental colitis is also seen after repeated administration of other PGFs. Intracolonic administration of PDGF-BB (100 and 500 ng/100 g twice daily), initiated 2 d after induction of colitis with the sulphydril alkylator, iodoacetamide, and continued for 10 d, resulted in a significant and dose-dependent reduction of the rat colon weight and colonic area damaged (Sandor et al., 1995; Szabo and Sandor, 1996). A similar effect in the same model of colitis was also reported with bFGF (FGF-2) (Szabo and Sandor, 1996).

A significant reduction in macroscopic and histologic damage scores, as well as in colon weight, was observed in TNBS-treated rats 14 d after im injection of 200 µg TGF-β_1 cDNA, subcloned to the pRSV

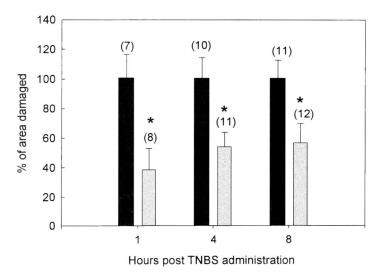

Fig. 1. Effect of EGF on TNBS-induced colitis in rats. Animals were pretreated with 10 nmol/kg (62 μg/kg) EGF, given intraperitoneally. One h later they received intracolonic injection of 50 mg/kg TNBS dissolved in 50% EtOH. Animals were sacrificed 1, 4, or 8 h after TNBS administration, and the extent of colonic damage was measured using computerized image analysis. ■, TNBS, untreated; ▨, TNBS/EGF treated. *, $P < 0.05$ based on Student's t test, and compared to the respective untreated group. Numbers in parenthesis refer to the number of animal/group (unpublished data).

expression vector (Giladi et al., 1995). Compounds that stimulate generation of TGF-β in the colonic mucosa have also been shown to ameliorate experimental colitis. Oral administration of haptenized colonic proteins, before rectal administration of hapten TNBS, stimulates in rats the generation of mucosal T-cells producing TGF-β, and suppresses the ability of TNBS to induce colitis. Moreover, this suppressive effect of haptenized colonic proteins was abrogated by TGF-β antibody (Neurath et al., 1996).

Recently, it has also been reported that intracolonic treatment with VEGF (10–500 ng/100 g) decreased the area and severity of iodacetamide-induced colitis in rats, and reduced the severity of associated clinical signs, such as diarrhea and lethargy (Sandor et al., 1998).

Table 2
Clinical Experience with PGFs in Gastrointestinal Disorders

Condition	PGF	Main effects	Ref.
GU and DU	EGF	Ulcer healing	Itoh and Matsuo, 1994
	EGF	Ulcer healing, decreased acid secretion	Heado et al., 1996
			Koffman et al., 1982
	bFGF-CS23	Ulcer healing	Wolfe et al., 1995
			Hull et al., 1995
NEC	EGF	Increase in cell mitotic activity	Sullivan et al., 1991
CMA	EGF	Increase in crypt-cell proliferation	Walker-Smith et al., 1985
			Drumm et al., 1988
Z-E syndrome	EGF	Decreased gastric acid secretion	Elder et al., 1975

GU, Gastric ulcer; DU, Duodenal ulcer; NEC, Necrotizing enterocolitis; CMA, Congenital microvillus atrophy; Z-E syndrome, Zollinger-Ellison syndrome.

4.3. Therapeutic Use of PGF in Miscellaneous Conditions of GI Tract

Clinical data also support the use of PGFs in GI diseases, such as necrotizing enterocolitis and congenital microvillus atrophy (Table 2). Six-day iv infusion of EGF (100 ng/kg/h), to a 9-mo-old girl suffering from extensive necrotizing enteritis, resulted in a significant increase in crypt-cell mitotic activity, associated with recovery of villus architecture (Sullivan et al., 1991). Furthermore, when intravenously infused to three children affected by congenital microvillus atrophy, at a dose of 100 ng/kg/h for two 6-d periods, with a 5-day rest period between the two courses, EGF caused an increased crypt cell production rate, accompanied by an increase in crypt cell population size and the proliferation fraction (Walker-Smith et al., 1985; Drumm et al., 1988).

In addition to the disorders mentioned above, and, on the basis of some theoretical considerations or preliminary experimental data, a variety of other GI pathologies could also benefit from treatment with PGFs. These include disorders such as esophagitis, other atrophic conditions of the GI tract, small bowel resection, and even cancer (Guglietta, 1993; Guglietta and Sullivan, 1995). As in the case of the disorders discussed above, time and additional experimental and clinical studies will tell whether these diseases represent good targets for pharmacotherapy with PGFs.

5. PROBLEMS ASSOCIATED WITH DEVELOPMENT OF PGFs AS DRUGS

The development of PGFs as therapeutic agents is associated with several problems, some of which are related to the peptide structure of these molecules, the others to their pharmacological activity.

5.1. Problems Associated with Peptide Nature of PGFs

Development of any peptide as a therapeutic agent presents special problems, and challenges.

5.1.1. PRODUCTION

The cost of production of PGFs may be very high, to the point of discouraging their development for the treatment of diseases with a relatively small number of patients. Depending on the size of the peptide and other considerations, a PGF may be produced either by conventional chemical synthesis or, more commonly, by recombinant DNA technology. Although the conventional synthesis is probably suitable only for very small peptides, it has the advantage that the contaminants of the final product are usually known and can be removed to the point of acceptable chemical purity. For large peptides, however, conventional chemical synthesis may not be feasible or cost effective. In this case, the use of recombinant DNA technology has major advantages, although extra care should be taken to assure that the finished product is free of other biological contaminants. In the future, technical advances may further improve this technique, and bring down the cost PGF production.

5.1.2. DELIVERY/DEGRADATION

Peptides are usually quickly degraded by the enzymes present in the GI tract, making the oral route of administration not feasible for PGFs. Luckily, among PGFs, there are a few interesting exceptions to this rule. PDGF, for instance, is an acid-resistant molecule (Szabo and Sandor, 1996), which could therefore be suitable for oral administration. In order to solve the degradation problem, it is otherwise possible to synthesize PGF analogs that would, unlike their original counterparts, be able to resist degradation in the GI tract, while retaining their original pharmacological activity. The synthesis of an acid-stable and bioactive mutant of bFGF, in which two Cys were replaced by two Ser in positions 70 and 88, is a successful example of this strategy (Seno et al., 1988). Another approach is the administration of an acid-labile PGF in specially designed acid/protease-resistant formulations (Ganderton, 1991), which would deliver the active ingredient to distant sites (i.e., colon). Intracolonic delivery of PGFs by the rectal route, may also be suitable for treatment of diseases of the colon, such as IBD. This, however, faces similar problems of degradation of the active pharmacologic agent, for example, the degradation by the intestinal flora.

Although oral delivery may in general be the most practical way of administering a drug, and may almost be a requirement for long-term treatment, this is not necessarily the best possible route of administration for certain GI indications. Disorders like necrotizing enterocolitis or a flare-up of IBD may be more efficiently treated with an iv infusion of such a drug. In these conditions, GI degradation of PGFs may not present a problem. Finally, a more futuristic approach, suitable also for long-term therapy, could be delivery of PGFs through gene therapy (Giladi et al., 1995).

5.1.3. ABSOPTION

Generally speaking, proteins and peptides are poorly absorbed by the intact GI tract. Because many GI disorders amenable to treatment with PGFs are characterized by inflamed and ulcerated mucosa, conditions that are known to facilitate the GI absorption of compounds, including peptides, this may not present a major problem. Furthermore, because of the favorable anatomic localization, an oral or intrarectally delivered peptide may, in certain GI disorders, already be at the site where it is supposed to exert its pharmacological effect (i.e., stomach or colon). Therefore, absorption into the blood stream may not even be required for the achievement of therapeutic efficacy. If, on the other hand, in order to elicit a beneficial pharmacologic effect, the PGF needs to be absorbed into the blood stream and transported to the site of action, special strategies may be employed to enhance its GI absorption (Gangwar et al., 1997).

Obviously, all the problems related to the peptidic nature of PGFs could be avoided if nonpeptide analogs of these compounds could be identified. Although difficult to achieve, modern chemistry approaches have made this a reasonably promising option (Rohrer et al., 1998).

5.2. Problems Related to Pharmacological Activity of Peptide Growth Factors

One of the major concerns that have been encountered during development of PGFs as therapeutic agents is related to their proliferative activity (Playford, 1997). Because PGFs act as mitogens for a variety of tumor cells, there is a reasonable concern that administration of PGFs could stimulate the growth of an existing tumor, or even induce the formation of a new one (Guglietta, 1993; Guglietta and Sullivan, 1995). Selecting the right patient populations, and the right pathologic conditions, could, however, minimize this theoretical risk. Making sure that patients do not have any growing tumors seems to be an obvious recommendation. Furthermore, oral or rectal administration of a PGF that is not absorbed into the blood stream represents a safer choice, compared to a PGF that reaches the blood stream (either by injection/infusion directly into a blood vessel, or by absorption following oral or rectal administration), and is therefore transported to various tissues of the body, exposing them to unwanted effects. Perhaps the most important point is to limit the use of these compounds only to the pathologies that require short-term treatment, hence avoiding long exposure of cells to the proliferative activity (Guglietta, 1993; Guglietta and Sullivan, 1995).

6. CONCLUSIONS

PGFs have a variety of pharmacological effects that could be exploited in the treatment of several GI diseases. Their potential beneficial effects in these pathologic conditions are supported by preclinical and, in some cases, also clinical data. Development of PGFs as therapeutic agents presents certain practical problems, and raises potential biological risks, but these compounds may represent a valid alternative for future treatment of several GI disorders.

REFERENCES

Alexander RJ, Panja A, Kaplan-Liss E, Mayer L, Raicht RF. Expression of growth factor receptor-encoded mRNA by colonic epithelial cells is altered in inflammatory bowel disease. *Dig Dis Sci* 1995; 40: 485–494.

Antoniades HN. Human platelet-derived growth factor (PDGF): purification of PDGF-I and PDGF-II and separation of their reduced subunits. *Proc Natl Acad Sci USA* 1981; 78: 7314–7317.

Antoniades HN, Hunkapiller MW. Human platelet-derived growth factor (PDGF): amino-terminal amino acid sequence. *Science* 1983; 220: 963–965.

Ascencio F, Hansson HA, Larm O, Wadstrom T. 1995; *Helicobacter pylori* interacts with heparin and heparin dependent growth factors. *FEMS Immunol Med Microbiol* 1995; 12: 265–272.

Burgess WH, Maciag T. The heparin-binding (fibroblast) growth factor family of proteins. *Annu Rev Biochem* 1989; 58: 575–606.

Carpenter G, Wahl MI. Epidermal growth factor family in *Peptide Growth Factors and Their Receptors* (Sporn MB and Roberts AB, eds.), Springer-Verlag, Berlin, 1990; 69–171.

Chen RH, Moses HL, Maruoka EM, Derynck R, Kawabata M. Phosphorylation-dependent interaction of the cytoplasmic domain of the type I and II TGFβ receptors. *J Biol Chem* 1995; 270: 12235–12241.

Chowdhury A, Fukuda R, Fukumoto S. Growth factor mRNA expression in normal colorectal mucosa and in uninvolved mucosa from ulcerative colitis patients. *J Gastroenterol* 1996; 31: 353–360.

Claesson-Welsh L. Signal trasduction by the PDGF receptors. *Prog Growth Factor Res* 1994; 5: 37–54.

Coerper S, Sigloch E, Cox D, Starlinger M, Köveker G, Becker HD. Recombinant human transforming growth factor beta 3 accelerates gastric ulcer healing in rats. *Scand J Gastroenterol* 1997; 32: 985–990.

Cohen S. Purification of a nerve-growth promoting protein from the mouse salivary gland and its neuro-cytotoxic antiserum. *Proc Natl Acad Sci USA* 1960; 46: 302–311.

Cohen S. Isolation of a mouse submaxillary gland protein accelerating incisor eruption and eyelid opening in the new-born animal. *J Biol Chem* 1962; 237: 1555–1562.

De Larco J.E. & Todaro G.J. Growth factors from murine sarcoma virus-transformed cells. *Proc Natl Acad Sci USA* 1978; 75: 4001–4005.

Derynck R. TGF-β-receptor mediated signaling. *Trends Biochem Sci* 1994; 19: 548–553.

Drumm B, Cutz E, Tomkins KB, Cook D, Hamilton JR, Sherman P. Urogastrone/epidermal growth factor in treatment of congenital microvillus atrophy. *Lancet* 1988; i: 111–112.

Elder JB, Gillespie IE, Canguli PC, Delamore WI, Gregory H. Effect of urogastrone in the Zollinger-Ellison syndrome. *Lancet* 1975; ii: 424–427.

Elder JB, Williams G, Lacey E, Gregory H. Cellular localisation of human urogastrone epidermal growth factor. *Nature* 1978; 271: 466–467.

Ernst H, Konturek P, Hahn EG, Brzozowski T, Konturek SJ. Acceleration of wound healing in gastric ulcers by local injection of neutralizing antibody to transforming growth factor β1. *Gut* 1996; 39: 172–175.

Fantl WJ, Johnson DE, Williams LT. Signalling by receptor tyrosine kinases. *Ann Rev Biochem* 1993; 61: 453–481.

Feldman EJ, Aures D, Grossman MI. Epidermal growth factor stimulates ornithine decarboxylase activity in the digestive tract of the mouse. *Proc Soc Exp Biol Med* 1978; 159: 400–402.

Fiocchi, C. Inflammatory bowel disease: etiology and pathogenesis. *Gastroenterology* 1998; 115: 182–205.

Galzie Z, Kinsella AR, Smith J.A. Fibroblast growth factors and their receptors. *Biochem Cell Biol* 1997; 75: 669–685.

Ganderton D, Hider RC, Barlow D. *Polypeptide and Protein Drugs: Production, Characterization and Formulations.* Ellis Horwood, New York, 1991.

Gangwar S, Pauletti GM, Wang B, Siahaan TJ, Stella VJ, Borchardt RT. Prodrug strategies to enhance the intestinal absorption of peptides. *DDT* 1997; 2: 148–155.

Giladi E, Raz E, Karmeli F, Okon E, Rachmilewitz D. Transforming growth factor-beta gene therapy ameliorates experimental colitis in rats. *Eur J Gastroenterol Hepatol* 1995; 7: 341–347.

Gospodarowitz D, Bialecki H, Greenburg GM. Purification of the fibroblast growth factor activity factor from bovine brain. *J Biol Chem* 1978; 253: 3736–3734.

Gregory H. Isolation and structure of urogastrone and its relationship to epidermal growth factor. *Nature* 1975; 257: 325–327.

Gresik EW, Noen H, Barka H. Epidermal growth factor-like material in rat submandibular gland. *Am J Anat* 1979; 156: 83–89.

Groenen LC, Nice EC, Burgess AW. Structure-function relationships for the RGF/TGF-α family of mitogens. *Growth Factors* 1994; 11: 235–257.

Guglietta A, Hervada T, Nardi RV, Lesch CA. Effect of PDGF-BB on gastric lesions and acid secretion in rats. *Scand J Gastroenterol* 1992; 27: 673–676.

Guglietta A, Lesch CA. Effect of h-EGF and h-EGF 1-48 on histamine stimulated gastric acid secretion in rats and monkeys. *J Physiol* (Paris) 1993; 87: 343–347.

Guglietta A, Lesch CA, Sanchez B. Protective and healing effect of hEGF

1-48 on TNBS-induced colonic damage in rats: a morphometric evaluation. *Gut* 1993; 34: S38.

Guglietta, A. Possible clinical use of peptide growth factors in the GI tract: perspectives and obstacles. *Exp Clin Gastroenterol* 1993; 3: 1–6.

Guglietta A, Lesch CA, Romano M, McClure RW, Coffey RJ. Effect of transforming growth factor α on gastric acid secretion in rats and monkeys. *Dig Dis Sci* 1994; 39: 177–182.

Guglietta A, Sullivan PB. Clinical applications of epidermal growth factor. *Eur J Gastroenterol Hepatol* 1995; 7: 945–950.

Guglietta A, Kraus ER, Sanchez B, Lesch CA. Protective effect of EGF on iodoacetamide model of colitis. *Gastroenterology* 1996; 110: A919.

Guglietta A, Lesch CA, Kraus ER, Sanchez B. Effect of EGF receptor ligands on TNBS colitis in rats. *Gastroenterology* 1997; 112: A379.

Haedo W, Gonzalez T, Mas JA, Franco S, Gra B, Soto G, Alonso A, Lopez-Saura P. Oral human recombinant epidermal growth factor in the treatment of patients with duodenal ulcer. *Rev Esp Enferm Dig* 1996; 88: 409–413.

Hansson HA, Hong L, Helander HF. Changes in gastric EGF, EGF receptors and acidity during healing of gastric ulcer in rats. *Acta Physiol Scand* 1990; 138: 241–242.

Hart CE, Forstrom JW, Kelly JD, Seifert RA, Smith RA, Ross R, Murray MJ, Bowen-Pope DF. Two classes of PDGF receptor recognize different isoforms of PDGF. *Science* 1988; 240: 1529–1531.

Heitz PUV, Kasper M, Noordenn SV, Polak JM, Gregory H, Pearse AGE. Immunohistochemical localization of urogastrone to human duodenal and submandibular glands. *Gut* 1978; 19: 408–413.

Heldin CH, Backstrom G, Östman A, Hammacher A, Rönnstrand L, Rubin K, Nister M, Westermark B. Binding of different forms of PDGF to human fibroblasts: evidence for two separate receptor types. *EMBO J* 1988; 7: 1387–1293.

Hoffmann P, Zeeh JM, Lakshmmanan J, Wu VS, Procaccino F, Reinshagen M, McRoberts JA, Eysselein VE. Increased expression of transforming growth factor alpha precursors in acute experimental colitis in rats. *Gut* 1997; 41: 195–202.

Hull MA, Cullen DJE, Hudson N, Hawkey CJ. Basic fibroblast growth factor treatment for non-steroidal anti-inflammatory drug associated gastric ulceration. *Gut* 1995; 37: 610–612.

Itoh M, Matsuo Y. Gastric ulcer treatment with intravenous human epidermal growth factor: a double-blind controlled clinical study. *J Gastroenterol Hepatol* 1994; 9: S78–S83.

Jankowski J, Hopwood D, Wormsley KG. Expression of epidermal growth factor, transforming growth factor alpha and their receptor in gastro-oesophageal diseases. *Dig Dis* 1993; 11: 1–11.

Keck PJ, Hauser SD, Krivi G, Sanzo K, Warren T, Feder J, Connolly DT. Vascular permeability factor, an endothelial cell nitogen related to PDGF. *Science* 1989; 246: 1309–1312.

Kjellen G, Fransson SG, Lindstrom F, Sokjer H, Tibbling L. Esophageal function, radiography and dysphagia in Sjögren's syndrome. *Dig Dis Sci* 1986; 31: 225–229.

Koffman CG, Elder JB, Ganguli PC. Effect of urogastrone on gastric secretion and serum gastrin concentration in patients with duodenal ulceration. *Gut* 1982; 23: 951–956.

Konturek SJ, Dembinski A, Warzecha Z, Brzozowski TM, Gregory H. Role of epidermal growth factor in healing of chronic gastroduodenal ulcers in rats. *Gastroenterology* 1988; 94: 1300–1307.

Konturek PC, Brzozowski T, Konturek SJ, Ernst H, Drozdowicz D, Pajdo R, Hahn, EG. Expression of epidermal growth factor and transforming growth factor alpha during ulcer healing. Time sequence study. *Scand J Gastroenterol* 1997a; 32: 6–15.

Lawrence DA. Transforming growth factor-β: a general review. *Eur Cytokine Netw* 1996; 7: 363–374.

Lesch CA, Guglietta A. PD153035, an EGF receptor (EGFr) tyrosine-kinase specific inhibitor, reverses the effect of EGF on gastric acid secretion and TNBS colitis in rats. *Gastroenterology* 1995; 108: A735.

Levi-Montalcini R, Cohen S. Effects of the extract of the mouse submaxillary salivary glands on the sympathetic system of mammals. *Ann NY Acad Sci* 1960; 85: 324–341.

Luck MS, Bass P. Effect of epidermal growth factor on experimental colitis in the rat. *J Pharmacol Exp Therap* 1994; 264: 984–990.

Maccini DM, Veit BC. Salivary epidermal growth factor in patients with and without acid peptic disease. *Am J Gastroenterol* 1990; 85: 1102–1104.

Meyer-Ingold W, Eichner W. Platelet-derived growth factor. *Cell Biol Intl* 1995; 19: 389–398.

Miyazono K, Hellman U, Wernstedt C, Heldin CH. Transforming growth factor-β: latent forms, binding proteins and receptors. *Growth Factors* 1993; 8: 11–22.

Mustoe TA, Landes A, Cromack DT, Mistry D, Griffin A, Deuel TF, Pierce GF. Differential acceleration of healing of surgical incisions in the rabbit gastrointestinal tract by platelet derived growth factor and transforming growth factor beta 1. *Surgery* 1990; 198: 324–330.

Neurath MF, Fuss I, Kelsall BL, Presky DH, Waegell W, Strober W. Experimental granulomatous colitis in mice is abrogated by induction of TGF beta mediated oral tolerance. *J Exp Med* 1996; 183: 2605–2616.

Ohmura E, Emoto N, Tsushima T, Watanabe S, Takeuchi T, Kawamura M, Shigemoto M, Shizume K. Salivary immunoreactive human epidermal growth factor (IR-hEGF) in patients with peptic ulcer disease. *Hepatogas-troenterology* 1987; 34: 160–163.

Otto W, Wright N. Trefoil peptides: coming up clover. *Curr Biol* 1994; 4: 835–838.

Partanen J, Vainikka S, Korhonen J, Armstrong E, Alitalo K. Diverse receptors for fibroblast growth factors. *Prog Growth Factor Res* 1992; 4: 69–83.

Pimentel E. *Handbook of Growth Factors.* CRC, Boca Raton, FL, 1994.

Piotrowski J, Majka J, Sano S, Nowak P, Murty VL, Slomiany A, Slomiany BL. Enhancement in gastric mucosal EGF and PDGF receptor expression with ulcer healing sulglycotide. *Gen Pharmacol* 1995; 26: 749–753.

Playford RJ. Recombinant peptides for gastrointestinal ulceration: still early days. *Gut* 1997; 40: 286–287.

Pringent SA, Lemoine NR. Type 1 (EGFR-related) family of growth factor receptors and their ligands. *Prog Growth Factor Res* 1992; 4: 1–24.

Procaccino F, Reinshagen M, Hoffmann P, Zeeh JM, Lakshmanan J, McRoberts JA, et al. Protective effect of epidermal growth factor in an experimental model of colitis in rats. *Gastroenterology* 1994; 107: 12–17.

Proper JA, Bjornson CL, Moses HL. Mouse embryos contain polypetide growth factors capable of inducing a reversible neoplastic phenotype in non-transformed cells in culture. *J Cell Physiol* 1982; 110: 169–174.

Rohrer SP, Birzin ET, Mosley RT, Berk SC, Hutchins SM, Shen DM, et al. Rapid identification of subtype-selective agonists of the somatostatin receptor through combinatorial chemisty. *Science* 1998; 282: 737–740.

Romano M, Polk WH, Awad JA, Arteaga CL, Nanney LB, Wargovich MJ, et al. Transforming growth factor alpha protection against drug-induced injury of the rat gastric mucosa in-vivo. *J Clin Invest* 1992; 90: 2409–2421.

Romano M, Kraus ER, Boland CR, Coffey RJ. Comparison between transforming growth factor alpha and epidermal growth factor in the protection of rat gastric mucosa against drug-induced injury. *Ital J Gastroenterol* 1994; 26: 223–28.

Romano M, Lesch CA, Meise KS, Veljaca M, Sanchez B, Kraus ER, et al. Increased gastroduodenal concentration of transforming growth factor α in adaptation to aspirin in monkeys and rats. *Gastroenterology* 1996; 110: 1446–1455.

Ross R, Glomset J, Kariya B, Harker L. Platelet-dependent serum factor that stimulates the proliferation of arterial smooth muscle cells in vitro. *Proc Natl Acad Sci USA* 1974; 71: 1207–1210.

Salcedo JA, Al-Kawas F. Treatment of *Helicobacter* infection. *Arch Intern Med* 1998; 158: 842–851.

Sandor Z, Szali D, Charette M, Szabo S. Platelet-derived growth factor (PDGF) accelerate the healing of experimental ulcerative colitis in rats. *Gastroenterology* 1995; 108: A208.

Sands BA, Podolsky DK. Trefoil peptide family. *Ann Rev Physiol* 1996; 58: 253–273.

Sandor ZS, Singh G, Szabo S. Effect of vascular endothelial growth factor (VEGF) on experimental ulcerative colitis in rats. *Gastroenterology* 1998; 114: G4403.

Satoh H, Shino A, Inatomi N, Nagaya H, Sato F, Szabo S, Folkman, J. Effect of rhbFGF-mutein Cs23 (TGP-580) on the healing of gastric ulcers induced by acetic acid in rats. *Gastroenterology* 1991; 100: A155.

Savage CR Jr, Inagami T, Cohen S. Primary structure of epidermal growth factor. *J Biol Chem* 1972; 247: 7612–7621.

Seno W, Sasada R, Iwane M, Sudo K, Kurokawa T, Ito K, Igarashi K. Stabilizing basic fibroblast growth factor using protein engineering. *Biochem Biophys Res Commun* 1988; 151: 701–708.

Sheikh SH, Shaw-Stiffel TA. Gastrointestinal manifestation of Sjögren's syndrome. *Am J Gastroenterol* 1995; 90: 9–14.

Shing Y, Folkman J, Sullivan R. Heparin affinity: a purification of a tumor-derived capillary endothelial cell growth factor. *Science* 1984; 223: 1296–1299.

Skov-Olsen P, Poulsen SS, Therkelsen K, Nexo E. Oral administration of synthetic human urogastrone promotes healing of chronic duodenal ulcers in rats. *Gastroenterology* 1986; 90: 911–917.

Slomiany BL, Liu J, Keogh JP, Piotrowski J, Slomiany A. Enhancement of gastric mucos epidermal growth factor and platelet-derived growth factor receptor expression by sucralfate. *Gen Pharmacol* 1992; 23: 715–718.

Sullivan PB, Brueton MJ, Tabara ZB, Goodlad RA, Lee CY, Wright NA. Epidermal growth factor in necrotising enteritis. *Lancet* 1991; 338: 53–54.

Szabo S, Folkman J, Vattay P, Morales RE, Kato K. Duodenal ulcerogens: the effect of FGF on cysteamine-induced duodenal ulcer, in *Mechanism of Peptic Ulcer Healing* (Halter F, Garner A, Tytgat GNJ, eds.) Kluwer, London, 1991, pp. 139–150.

Szabo S, Folkaman J, Vattay P, Morales RE, Pinkus GE, Kato K. Accelerated healing of duodenal ulcers by oral administration of a mutein of fibroblast growth factor in rats. *Gastroenterology* 1994; 106: 1106–1111.

Szabo S, Kusstatscher S, Sandor Z, Sakoulas G. Molecular and cellular basis of ulcer healing. *Scand J Gastroenterol* 1995a; 30(Suppl 208): 3–8.

Szabo S, Kusstatscher S, Sakoulas G, Sandor Z, Vincze A, Jadus, M. Growth factors: New "endogenous drugs" for ulcer healing. *Scand J Gastroenterol* 1995b; 30(Suppl 210): 15–18.

Szabo S, Sandor Z. Basic fibroblast growth factor and PDGF in GI diseases. *Baill Clin Gastroenterol* 1996; 10: 97–112.

Szabo S, Vincze A, Sandor Z, Jadus M, Gombos Z, Pedram A, et al. Vascular approach to gastroduodenal ulceration. New studies with endothelins and VEGF. *Dig Dis Sci* 1998; 43: 40S–45S.

Takasugi M, Hayakawa A, Khakata H. Gastric involvement in Sjögren's syndrome simulating early gastric cancer. *Endoscopy* 1979; 4: 263–266.

Tarnawski A, Stachura J, Krause WJ, Douglass TJ, Gergely H. Quality of gastric ulcer healing: a new emerging concept. *J Clin Gastroenterol* 1991; 13(Suppl 1): S42–S47.

Tarnawski A, Stachura J, Durbin T, Sarfeh IJ, Gergely H. Increased expression of epidermal growth factor receptor during gastric ulcer healing in rats. *Gastroenterology* 1992a; 102: 695–698.

Tarnawski A, Stachura J, Durbin T, Gergely H, Douglas TG. Sucralfate treatment induced increased expression of EGF and TGFα and their common receptor in the gastric mucosa. A key to the ulcer healing and trophic action? Gastroenterology, 1992b; 102: A175.

Tarnawski A, Arakawa T, Wang H, Kobayashi K. Rebamipide treatment accelerates healing of experimental gastric ulcers. Action mediated by activation of EGF and its receptor expression in ulcerated gastric mucosa. *Arch Pharmacol* 1998; 358(Suppl 2): A508.

Ullrich A, Schlessinger J. Signal transduction by receptors with tyrosine kinase activity. *Cell* 1990; 61: 203–212.

Vattay P, Gyömber E, Morales RE, Kato, K. Effect of orally administered platelet-derived growth factor (PDGF) on healing of chronic duodenal ulcers and gastric secretion in rats. *Gastroenterology* 1991; 100: A180.

Walker-Smith JA, Phillips AD, Walford N, Gregory H, Fitzgerald JD. Intravenous epidermal growth factor/urogastrone increases small-intestinal cell proliferation in congenital microvillus atrophy. *Lancet* 1985; ii: 1239–1240.

Wolfe MM, Bynum TE, Parson WG, Malone KM, Szabo S. Safety and efficacy of an angiogenic peptide, basic fibroblast growth factor (bFGF), in treatment of gastroduodenal ulcers: a preliminary report. *Gastroenterology* 1994; 106: A212.

Wright NA, Pike C, Elia G. Induction of a novel epidermal growth factor-secreting cell lineage by mucosal ulceration in human gastrointestinal stem cells. *Nature* 1990a; 343: 82–85.

Wright NA, Pike CM, Elia G. Ulceration induces a novel epidermal growth factor-secreting cell lineage in human gastrointestinal mucosa. *Digestion* 1990b; 46: 125–133.

Zhu X, Hsu BT, Rees DC. Structural studies of the binding of the anti-ulcer drug sucrose octasulfate to acidic fibroblast growth factor. *Structure* 1993; 15: 27–34.

5   Tachykinins

From Basic Concepts to Therapeutic Implications

Peter Holzer

CONTENTS

1. INTRODUCTION

A Short History of Substance P and Tachykinins

In 1931, von Euler and Gaddum reported that both gut and brain contained a substance that caused contraction of intestinal smooth muscle, and that was different from any of the endogenous compounds known at that time. Quantitative estimations of the novel principle were made by comparing the activity of extracts with the effect of a standard preparation referred to as "P" on the tracings and in the

From: *Drug Development: Molecular Targets for GI Diseases*
Edited by: T. S. Gaginella and A. Guglietta © Humana Press Inc., Totowa, NJ

Table 1
Amino Acid Sequence of Mammalian Tachykinins

Tachykinin	Amino acid sequence
Substance P	H-Arg-Pro-Lys-Pro-Gln-Gln-**Phe**-Phe-**Gly-Leu-Met.NH**$_2$
Neurokinin A	H-His-Lys-Thr-Asp-Ser-**Phe**-Val-**Gly-Leu-Met.NH**$_2$
Neurokinin B	H-Asp-Met-His-Asp-Phe-**Phe**-Val-**Gly-Leu-Met.NH**$_2$

Amino acids common to all three tachykinins are set in bold.

protocols, so that, since 1934, the term "substance P" (SP) has been used in the literature. SP resisted chemical identification for 40 yr, until its isolation was inadvertently accomplished by Chang and Leeman (1970) in an attempt to isolate corticotrophin-releasing factor from the hypothalamus. The peptide nature of SP, however, had been inferred before that, when a close similarity was noted between its pharmacological properties and those of peptides isolated from amphibian skin (e.g., physalaemin, kassinin) and mollusc salivary glands (e.g., eledoisin). By referring to the fast contraction of intestinal smooth muscle produced by these peptides, Erspamer (1981) called them "tachykinins" (TKs) to distinguish them from "bradykinin," which causes a comparatively slow response.

The term "tachykinins" now names a large family of small peptides of nonmammalian and mammalian origin. They share many pharmacological properties, because they contain the C-terminal amino acid sequence Phe-X-Gly-Leu-Met-NH$_2$ as their common structural feature (Table 1), which is important for their affinity to TK receptors. SP, as well as the related neurokinin A (NKA) and neurokinin B (NKB), which were discovered in the 1980s (Nakanishi, 1987), are the principal mammalian TKs (Table 1), whose sequence of 10–11 amino acids is conserved within this class of animals. Along with the cloning of the TK and TK receptor genes by Nakanishi (1987, 1991), exceptional progress has been made in TK pharmacology, culminating in the development of potent and selective antagonists for all three TK receptors (Regoli et al., 1994; Maggi, 1995). Based on Lembeck's (1953) and Otsuka and Yoshioka's (1993) proposal that SP is a transmitter of nociceptive afferent neurons involved in neurogenic inflammatory processes, TK antagonists were modeled to yield novel drugs with anti-inflammatory and antinociceptive properties. As the pathophysiological implications of TKs in the gut were uncovered, it has been learned that TK antagonists also hold particular potential in the treatment of inflammatory bowel disease (IBD), irritable bowel syndrome (IBS), and other gastrointestinal (GI) disorders of considerable socioeconomic impact.

2. MOLECULAR BIOLOGY
OF THE TK SYSTEM

Like other regulatory peptides, the TKs are derived from larger precursor peptides, the preprotachykinins (PPT), which are encoded by two different genes: The *PPT-A* gene contains the sequences for both SP and NKA; the *PPT-B* gene encodes NKB only. The primary RNA transcript of the *PPT-A* gene is alternatively spliced to produce four different forms of PPT-A messenger ribonucleic acid (mRNA), termed α-PPT, β-PPT, γ-PPT, and δ-PPT (Nakanishi, 1987; Holzer and Holzer-Petsche, 1997a). SP can be produced by translation of all four PPT-A mRNAs, but sequences coding for NKA are found in β-PPT and γ-PPT mRNA only. Because *PPT-A* is the TK gene that is primarily expressed in the GI tract, SP and NKA are the TKs that predominate in this organ system; NKB is largely absent (Holzer and Holzer-Petsche, 1997a). In the rat intestine, γ-PPT-A accounts for as much as 80–90% of the TK-encoding mRNA, while β-PPT-A comprises about 10–20% and α-PPT-A less than 1% of the total SP/NKA-encoding mRNA (Sternini et al., 1989).

As predicted by pharmacological and biochemical studies, three TK receptors have been identified by their genomic and molecular structure in a number of mammals, including man (Gerard et al., 1991; Hershey et al., 1991; Nakanishi, 1991). These receptors are currently termed NK_1, NK_2, and NK_3 receptors, although a definite decision on their nomenclature is pending. Unlike the TKs themselves, the TK receptors exhibit small differences in their amino acid sequence and structure among different mammalian species (Fong et al., 1992; Jensen et al., 1994). These variations account for species-related potency differences of nonpeptide TK receptor antagonists, given that nonpeptide antagonists do not bind to the same epitopes of the receptor protein to which the agonists bind (Gether et al., 1993; Fong et al., 1995). In addition, TK receptors can occur in multiple forms, which differ in their affinity for agonists and/or antagonists, as is the case for NK_1 (Maggi and Schwartz, 1997; Ciucci et al., 1998), NK_2 (Maggi et al., 1993b; Croci et al., 1998) and NK_3 (Krause et al., 1997; Johnson et al., 1998) receptors. The cloned TK NK_1, NK_2, and NK_3 receptors belong to the superfamily of guanosine triphosphate (GTP)-binding protein-coupled receptors with seven transmembrane-spanning domains, an extracellular N-terminus, and an intracellular C-terminal segment (Gerard et al., 1991; Hershey et al., 1991; Nakanishi, 1991). In terms of second-messenger systems, it is primarily the phospholipase C/phosphoinositide signaling pathway, which is operated by all three TK receptors (Hershey et al., 1991; Nakanishi, 1991; Regoli et al., 1994; Maggi, 1995; Holzer and Holzer-Petsche, 1997a).

3. TK RECEPTOR PHARMACOLOGY

Pharmacologically, mammalian TK receptors were originally differentiated by the use of certain nonmammalian TKs that exhibit distinct potency rank orders in various assay preparations (Regoli et al., 1994; Maggi, 1995; Holzer and Holzer-Petsche, 1997a). In contrast, SP, NKA, and NKB exhibit little receptor selectivity, and the view that NK_1 receptors are SP-preferring, NK_2 receptors are NKA-preferring, and NK_3 receptors are NKB-preferring is largely erroneous, because SP, NKA, and NKB are full agonists at all three TK receptors, and the differences in their affinity to these receptors can be negligible (Maggi and Schwartz, 1997). There are, however, synthetic and metabolically stable analogs that display considerable receptor selectivity as agonists (Table 2), and hence can be used for the pharmacological, biochemical, and autoradiographic characterization of TK receptors (Regoli et al., 1994; Maggi, 1995; Holzer and Holzer-Petsche, 1997a). The activity of SP, NKA, and NKB at their receptors is regulated by agonist-induced receptor internalization and the activity of membrane-bound proteases, such as neutral endopeptidase EC 3.4.24.11 (Bowden et al., 1994; Maggi, 1995; Holzer and Holzer-Petsche, 1997a; Southwell et al., 1998). A few biological actions of TKs are not brought about by interaction of their C-terminal hexapeptide sequence with TK receptors, but depend on other features of the molecule, a typical example

Table 2
Examples of Selective Tachykinin Receptor Agonists and Antagonists

Ligand type	NK_1 receptor	NK_2 receptor	NK_3 receptor
Peptide-derived receptor-selective agonists	SP methyl ester [Sar^9]-SP sulphone GR-73,632	[β-Ala^8]-NKA-(4-10) [Nleu^{10}]-NKA-(4-10) GR-64,349	Senktide [MePhe^7]-NKB
Peptide-derived receptor-selective antagonists	GR-82,334 FK-888	GR-94,800 MEN-10,627 MEN-11,420	PD-161,182
Nonpeptide receptor-selective antagonists	CP-96,345 (human) CP-99,994 (human) RP-67,580 (rat) SR-140,333 (human, rat) GR-205,171 (human) LY-306,740 (human) L-742,694 (human)	SR-48,968 (human, rat) SR-144,190 (human, rat)	SR-142,801 (human) SB-223,412 (human)

Many of the nonpeptide antagonists exhibit high affinity to either the respective human (and guinea pig) or rat (and mouse) tachykinin receptors. Their relative species selectivity is indicated in brackets. For further information, *see* Snider *et al.* (1991) and Lowe (1996) regarding CP-96,345 and CP- 99,994, Catalioto *et al.* (1998) regarding MEN-10,627 and MEN-11,420, Polley *et al.* (1997) regarding GR-205,171, Gitter *et al.* (1995) regarding LY-306,740, Rupniak *et al.* (1997) regarding L-742,694, Emonds-Alt *et al.* (1997) regarding SR-144,190, Sarau *et al.* (1997) regarding SB-223,412, Regoli *et al.* (1994) and Holzer and Holzer-Petsche (1997a) regarding the other compounds.

117

being the activity of SP to degranulate mast cells by direct interaction with GTP-binding proteins in the mast cell membrane (Bueb et al., 1990).

The heterogeneity of TK receptors has been confirmed by the discovery and development of potent and selective NK_1, NK_2, and NK_3 receptor antagonists of peptide and nonpeptide structure (Maggi et al., 1993b; Regoli et al., 1994; Maggi, 1995; Lowe, 1996; Holzer and Holzer-Petsche, 1997a). The available TK antagonists can be roughly grouped into three categories, the first group of which was discovered when certain L-amino acids in the sequence of SP were replaced by D-amino acids (Maggi et al., 1993b). Further modification and conformational constraining of TK molecules gave way to antagonists characterized by improved potency, selectivity towards NK_1, NK_2, and NK_3 receptors (Table 2), metabolic stability, and lack of nonspecific effects (Maggi et al., 1993b). A typical example of this class of peptide-based antagonists is the cyclic compound nepadutant (MEN-11,420), a water-soluble NK_2 receptor antagonist, which displays high receptor selectivity, high potency, oral bioavailability, and a long duration of action (Catalioto et al., 1998).

A new era began with the introduction of highly active nonpeptide antagonists for all three TK receptor types (Table 2). Although the first compounds, such as the quinuclidine NK_1 receptor antagonist, CP-96,345 (Snider et al., 1991), displayed nonspecific effects on L-type calcium and other membrane channels (Regoli et al., 1994; Maggi, 1995; Holzer and Holzer-Petsche, 1997a), the specificity of many subsequently developed compounds, derived from different lead structures, has been greatly improved. Unlike SR-140,333, most nonpeptide NK_1 receptor antagonists exhibit marked species differences in their activity (Table 2), in that they possess high affinity to either the human and guinea pig or the rat and mouse NK_1 receptor (Snider et al., 1991; Fong et al., 1992; Maggi et al., 1993b; Jensen et al., 1994; Gitter et al., 1995; Lowe, 1996; Holzer and Holzer-Petsche, 1997a; Polley et al., 1997; Rupniak et al., 1997). Potent and selective nonpeptide antagonists of NK_2 and NK_3 receptors were also developed (Lowe, 1996; Emonds-Alt et al., 1997; Holzer and Holzer-Petsche, 1997a; Sarau et al., 1997), and the pharamacokinetic properties of all antagonists expanded in terms of oral bioavailability and blood–brain barrier penetrability.

3.1. SP and NKA: Neuropeptides of the Gut

Although some TKs may be expressed by enterochromaffin and immune cells of the GI mucosa (Castagliuolo et al., 1997; Holzer and Holzer-Petsche, 1997b), most of the SP and NKA present in the gut is derived from two groups of neurons: intrinsic enteric neurons and extrinsic primary afferent nerve fibers (Holzer and Holzer-Petsche, 1997b). The predominant source of TKs is the enteric nervous system (Holzer and Holzer-Petsche, 1997b), which has its cell bodies in the myenteric and submucosal (submucous) plexuses (Fig. 1), and supplies all GI effector systems (Furness et al., 1992; Costa et al., 1996; Holzer and Holzer-Petsche, 1997b). Most enteric SP-positive neurons in the guinea pig small intestine, which have been extensively studied, co-express choline acetyltransferase (Fig. 1), which means that TKs are cotransmitters of cholinergic neurons (Furness et al., 1992; Costa et al., 1996). Neuroanatomical tracing studies have identified several classes of enteric SP neurons (Fig. 1) that differ regarding morphology, chemical coding, and projection (Furness et al., 1992; Costa et al., 1996).

The other important source of SP and NKA in the gut is extrinsic afferent neurons (Fig. 1), most of which originate from dorsal root ganglia, reach the gut via sympathetic (splanchnic, colonic and hypogastric) and sacral parasympathetic (pelvic) nerves, and pass through prevertebral ganglia where they form collateral synapses with sympathetic ganglion cells (Green and Dockray, 1988; Holzer and Holzer-Petsche, 1997a, 1997b). In contrast, vagal afferents emanating from the nodose ganglia make a relatively small contribution to the GI SP content (Green and Dockray, 1988; Bäck et al., 1994; Holzer and Holzer-Petsche, 1997a, 1997b; Suzuki et al., 1997). The spinal afferents project primarily to submucosal arteries and arterioles, where they form a para- and perivascular network of axons (Fig. 1), although some axons also supply mucosa, enteric nerve plexuses, and muscle layers (Furness et al., 1982; Green and Dockray, 1988; Holzer and Holzer-Petsche, 1997a, 1997b). Characteristically, many spinal afferents containing SP co-express calcitonin gene-related peptide, a combination of peptides that is not found in enteric neurons of the rodent and canine gut (Gibbins et al., 1987; Green and Dockray, 1988; Sternini, 1992).

As is expected for transmitters with a vesicular co-localization, depolarization of enteric neurons leads to an even co-release of acetylcholine

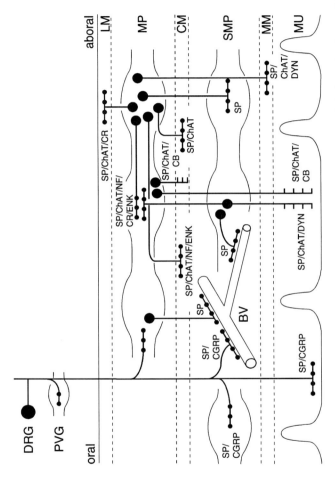

Fig. 1. Schematic summary of the various classes of SP-immunoreactive neurons and their projections within the guinea pig small intestine, with information on the coexistence with other neuropeptides or neuronal markers. BV, blood vessel; CB, calbindin; CGRP, calcitonin gene-related peptide; ChAT, choline acetyltransferase; CM, circular muscle; CR, calretinin; DRG, dorsal root ganglion; DYN, dynorphin; ENK, enkephalin; LM, longitudinal muscle; MM, muscularis mucosae; MP, myenteric plexus; MU, mucosa; NF, neurofilament protein; PVG, prevertebral ganglion; SMP, submucosal plexus.

120

(ACh), SP, and NKA by an exocytotic process that involves influx of extracellular Ca^{2+} via N-type calcium channels (Maggi et al., 1994a; Holzer and Holzer-Petsche, 1997a; Lippi et al., 1998). TK release from extrinsic afferents can specifically be elicited by the excitotoxin capsaicin (Holzer and Holzer-Petsche, 1997a, 1997b), because receptors for this drug (vanilloid receptors) are exclusively expressed on spinal, trigeminal (Caterina et al., 1997), and vagal (Helliwell et al., 1998) afferent neurons.

4. PHYSIOLOGICAL AND PHARMACOLOGICAL ACTIONS OF TKs IN THE GUT

4.1. Actions of TKs on GI Motility

Although SP was discovered as a gut-contracting peptide, it is now evident that TKs can both stimulate and inhibit GI motility, the net response depending on the type and site of TK receptors that are activated (Fig. 2). Nerve-independent facilitation of GI motor activity is brought about by NK_1 receptors on interstitial cells of Cajal (Sternini et al., 1995; Grady et al., 1996; Portbury et al., 1996b; Vannuchi et al., 1997; Lavin et al., 1998) and NK_2 as well as NK_1 receptors on muscle cells (Grady et al., 1996; Portbury et al., 1996a), as is also true for the human intestine (Maggi et al., 1990; Giuliani et al., 1991; Croci et al., 1998; Smith et al., 1998). NK_3 receptors are largely confined to enteric neurons (Grady et al., 1996; Mann et al., 1997), and predominantly mediate cholinergic contraction of the intestinal musculature (Holzer and Holzer-Petsche, 1997a). However, some NK_3 receptors and, in particular, NK_1 receptors (Sternini et al., 1995; Grady et al., 1996; Portbury et al., 1996b; Mann et al., 1997; Vannuchi et al., 1997; Johnson et al., 1998) are also present on inhibitory motor pathways within the enteric nervous system (Fig. 2), and thus enable SP and NKA to depress motor activity (Jin et al., 1993; Maggi et al., 1993a) and peristalsis (Holzer, 1997) via release of the inhibitory transmitters nitric oxide and vasoactive intestinal polypeptide. In vivo, all three TK receptors participate in the ability of SP and NKA to stimulate intestinal motility in the rat, and to replace the regular pattern of interdigestive motor activity by a pattern of irregular activity reminiscent of postprandial motility (Lördal et al., 1998). The motor effects of TKs on the human gut are very similar (Lördal et al., 1997).

oral   aboral

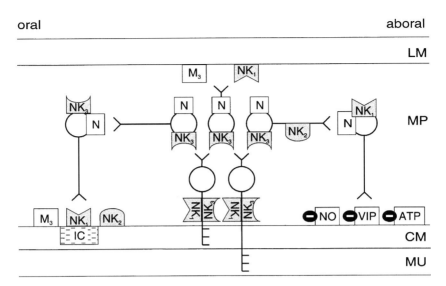

Fig. 2. Schematic summary of the implications of tachykinins and tachykinin NK_1, NK_2, and NK_3 receptors in ascending and descending motor pathways of the guinea pig small intestine. Circles depict neuronal somata. ATP, adenosine triphosphate; CM, circular muscle; IC, interstitial cells; LM, longitudinal muscle; M_3, muscarinic type 3 acetylcholine receptor; MP, myenteric plexus; MU, mucosa; N, nicotinic acetylcholine receptor; NO, nitric oxide; VIP, vasoactive intestinal polypeptide.

The motor actions of TKs have a bearing on the neural control of GI motility (Fig. 2). Enteric motor pathways can be activated by two different populations of myenteric sensory neurons: neurons that are connected to the circular muscle and monitor distention, and neurons that project into the mucosa and are sensitive to mechanical or chemical stimulation of the villi (Furness et al., 1998). TKs are released from either type of intrinsic sensory neuron (Fig. 1), and, via activation of NK_3 receptors, lead to activation of ascending excitatory and descending inhibitory motor pathways (Johnson et al., 1996, 1998). In addition, intrinsic sensory neurons form self-reinforcing networks (Furness et al., 1998), in which they communicate via NK_3 and, to some extent, NK_1 receptors (Fig. 2). Further on, TKs, acting via NK_3 receptors, contribute to transmission from ascending interneurons to excitatory motor neurons; transmission to inhibitory motor neurons involves NK_1, but not NK_3 receptors (Johnson et al., 1998). In many instances, particularly in the ascending excitation of the circular muscle, TKs synergize with ACh in the transmission process (Grider, 1989; Holzer et al., 1993,1998; Holzer and Maggi, 1994; Maggi et al., 1994b; Johnson et al., 1996, 1998; Lecci et al., 1998). This synergistic action, with ACh overriding the action of SP and NKA under physiological conditions, needs to be borne in mind when the implications of TKs in GI regulation are considered as a potential target for therapeutic intervention.

4.2. Actions of TKs on GI Ion and Fluid Transport

TKs can influence the gastric secretion of acid, bicarbonate, and pepsinogen in certain mammalian species, but it is not known whether these pharmacologically ill-defined effects play a role in the physiological control of gastric secretory processes (Holzer and Holzer-Petsche, 1997b). In contrast, there is considerable evidence for TKs participating in the neural control of secretory activity in the small and large intestine, although the identity of the involved TK receptors is subject to regional and species differences (Holzer and Holzer-Petsche, 1997b). TKs can act directly on enterocytes to stimulate chloride and bicarbonate secretion, an action that is mediated by NK_1 receptors in the guinea pig colon (Cooke et al., 1997a), but by NK_2 receptors in the rat small intestine (Portbury et al., 1996a; Hällgren et al., 1997). A major part of the secretory response to SP and NKA, however, is brought about by NK_1 and NK_3 receptors on enteric neurons (Grady et al., 1996; Portbury et al., 1996b; Cooke et al., 1997b; Holzer and Holzer-Petsche, 1997b; Mann et al., 1997; Moore et al., 1997; MacNaughton et al., 1997). NK_1 receptors have likewise been localized to enteric neurons and mucosal cells in the human antrum and duodenum (Smith et al., 1998).

The neurogenic action of SP and NKA to elicit electrolyte and fluid secretion is consistent with the emerging concept that TKs are transmitters of enteric secretory reflex pathways (Fig. 3). Some of the secretory reflexes are initiated by activation of enterochromaffin cells, which function as sensory transducers of luminal stimuli, and activate enteric sensory neurons via 5-hydroxytryptamine (5-HT) acting on 5-HT_{1P} receptors (Cooke et al., 1997b, 1997c). The release of 5-HT from enterochromaffin cells is under the inhibitory control of TKs acting

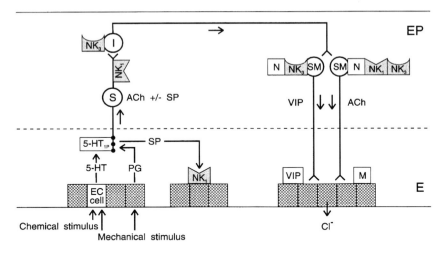

Fig. 3. Schematic summary of the implications of tachykinins and tachykinin NK_1, NK_2 and NK_3 receptors in secretomotor reflexes of the guinea pig colon. Chemical stimuli from the lumen may act on enterochromaffin (EC) cells to release 5-HT, which stimulates enteric sensory neurons (S) of a secretomotor reflex. Circles depict neuronal somata. ACh, acetylcholine; E, epithelium; EP, enteric nerve plexuses; I, interneurons; M, muscarinic acetylcholine receptor; N, nicotinic acetylcholine receptor; PG, prostaglandins; SM, secretomotor neurons; TK, tachykinin; VIP, vasoactive intestinal polypeptide.

via NK_1 and, indirectly, NK_3 receptors (Ginap and Kilbinger, 1997). Activation of intrinsic sensory neurons via 5-HT and/or prostaglandins (Cooke et al., 1997b) can induce secretory activity via two different mechanisms (Fig. 3). On the one hand, sensory neurons activate secretory reflex pathways involving interneurons and both cholinergic and noncholinergic secretomotor neurons (Cooke et al., 1997b, 1997c; Holzer and Holzer-Petsche, 1997b). TKs acting via NK_1 and NK_3 receptors participate in the transmission to secretomotor neurons, which cause ion secretion through release of ACh and/or vasoactive intestinal polypeptide (Cooke et al., 1997b; Holzer and Holzer-Petsche, 1997b; MacNaughton et al., 1997). On the other hand, SP (and other transmitters, such as ACh) can be released from axon collaterals of intrinsic sensory neurons close to the epithelial effector cells, and elicit chloride secretion via an axon reflex type of mechanism (Cooke et al., 1997a). Finally, TKs released from extrinsic afferent neurons in response to capsaicin or *Clostridium difficile* toxin A can also stimulate enteric secretomotor neurons through activation of NK_1 receptors (Mantyh et al., 1996b; MacNaughton et al., 1997).

4.3. Vascular and Immunological Actions of TKs in the Gut

SP and NKA are vasoactive peptides, and may induce vasodilatation or vasoconstriction in the digestive tract, the type of action depending on the vascular bed and species under study. Dilatation of vessels is typically mediated by NK_1 receptors, whereas TK-induced vasoconstriction may be brought about by all three TK receptor types (Holzer and Holzer-Petsche, 1997b). It is, however, uncertain whether the effects of TKs on GI blood flow are of pathophysiological relevance. The expression of NK_1 receptors by endothelial cells (Smith et al., 1998) may have a bearing on the NK_1 receptor-mediated increase in venular permeability, which is consistently seen in the mouse gut only (Figini et al., 1997). This reaction facilitates the extravasation of proteins, fluid, and leukocytes, whose activity, like that of mast cells, may also be directly stimulated by SP (Holzer, 1992). It remains to be examined whether TKs are responsible for the ability of afferent neuron stimulation to increase myeloperoxidase activity and to release interleukin-1 and prostaglandin E_2 in the guinea pig gallbladder (Prystowsky and Rege, 1997).

5. PATHOPHYSIOLOGICAL IMPLICATIONS OF TKs IN THE GUT

5.1. Pathological Changes in Expression of TKs and TK Receptors

GI infection and inflammation can be associated with changes in the tachykininergic innervation of the gut (Table 3), but the alterations are often variable and ill-defined as to whether they are primary or secondary to the disease (Holzer and Holzer-Petsche, 1997b). For instance, the intestinal tissue levels of SP are increased in ulcerative colitis, but decreased in Crohn's disease (Table 3). To shed more light on this issue, several experimental studies have attempted to reproduce disease-related changes in the GI TK system (Table 3), and thus to

Table 3
Tachykinin Changes in Gastrointestinal Disease

Species and region	Insult or disease	Peptide	Change
Human stomach	Gastroesophageal reflux	SP	Decrease (Wattchow et al., 1992)
	Nonulcer dyspepsia	SP	Increase (Kaneko et al., 1993)
Human ileum	Pouchitis	SP	Increase (Keranen et al., 1996)
Rat small intestine	Trichinella spiralis	SP	Increase (Swain et al., 1992)
	γ-Irradiation	SP	Decrease (Esposito et al., 1996)
	Escherichia coli endotoxin	SP, NKA	Decrease (Hellström et al., 1997)
	Clostridium difficile toxin A	SP	Increase (Castagliuolo et al., 1997)
	Nippostrongylus brasiliensis	SP	Increase (Masson et al., 1996)
Mouse small intestine	T. spiralis	SP	Increase (Agro and Stanisz, 1993)
	Schistosoma mansoni	SP	Decrease (Varilek et al., 1991)
Guinea pig small intestine	T. spiralis	SP	Decrease (Palmer and Koch, 1995)
	TNBSA ileitis	SP	Decrease (Miller et al., 1993)
Ferret small intestine	T. spiralis	SP	Decrease (Palmer and Greenwood, 1993)
Human colon	Crohn's disease	SP	Decrease (Kimura et al., 1994)
	Ulcerative colitis	SP	Increase (Koch et al., 1987; Bernstein et al., 1993; Keranen et al., 1995)
		SP	Decrease (Kimura et al., 1994)
Rat colon	TNBSA colitis	SP	Decrease (Renzi et al., 1992; Reinshagen et al., 1996)
	Dextran sulfate colitis	SP	Increase (Kishimoto et al., 1994; Björck et al., 1997)
Rabbit colon	Immune complex colitis	SP	Decrease (Eysselein et al., 1991; Reinshagen et al., 1995)

establish experimental models with which to study the pathophysiological mechanisms behind the observed TK perturbations.

Although some of the experimentally induced alterations mirror those seen in IBD (Table 3), the results are conclusive only when changes in the TK tissue levels have been related to changes in gene transcription or peptide release. Thus, colitis evoked by trinitrobenzene sulfonic acid (TNBSA) in the rat leads to increased transcription of β-PPT mRNA (Renzi et al., 1994), but the tissue level of SP is reduced, which points to enhanced release of the TK during the initial phase of the inflammatory reaction (Renzi et al., 1992; Reinshagen et al., 1996). SP is likewise depleted from the rabbit colon affected by immune-complex-induced inflammation (Eysselein et al., 1991), although, in this case, the expression of β-PPT mRNA remains unaltered (Reinshagen et al., 1995). Inflammation-induced release of SP is indicated by the elevated concentrations of SP in rat blood plasma, which accompany the increase of SP synthesis in dextran-sulfate-induced colitis (Kishimoto et al., 1994) and the decrease in intestinal SP levels caused by γ-irradiation (Esposito et al., 1996). Infection with *Salmonella dublin* enhances PPT mRNA in macrophages of various lymphoid organs within the gut (Bost et al., 1992; Bost, 1995), and macrophages in the rat ileum treated with *Clostridium difficile* toxin A release greater amounts of SP than macrophages from normal ileum (Castagliuolo et al., 1997).

A finding of considerable potential is the observation that IBD (Mantyh et al., 1995) and pseudomembranous colitis caused by infection with *C. difficile* (Mantyh et al., 1996a) are associated with upregulation and ectopic expression of NK_1 receptors on intestinal blood vessels and lymphoid structures (Mantyh et al., 1996a). Although NK_1 receptor upregulation in ulcerative colitis is confined to active, pathologically positive specimens of the colon, the ectopic expression of NK_1 receptors in Crohn's disease is seen in pathologically positive and negative samples alike (Mantyh et al., 1995). Experimental enteritis evoked by *C. difficile* toxin A in the rat is associated with a rapid expression of NK_1 receptors on epithelial cells (Pothoulakis et al., 1998), which normally possess NK_2 receptors only (Portbury et al., 1996a). Mononuclear cells in the human colonic mucosa represent another target system that contains NK_1 receptors (Goode et al., 1998), and *S. dublin* infection enhances the expression of NK_1 receptor mRNA in macrophages of lymphoid organs in the rat (Bost et al., 1992). The functional significance of the upregulated and ectopically expressed NK_1 receptors remains unclear, however, because the upregulation of TK receptors seen in IBD has not yet been observed in experimentally induced inflammation of the gut. To the contrary, TNBSA-induced colitis in the rat decreases NK_1 and NK_2 receptor mRNA expression in vasculature, muscle, and nerve (Renzi et al., 1996), a change that is thought to reflect a consequence, not cause, of the inflammatory reaction (Evangelista et al., 1996).

5.2. Implications of TKs in GI Motor Disturbances

There is pharmacological evidence to indicate that the derangement of GI motility caused by anaphylaxis, inflammation, trauma, and stress may involve SP and NKA (Table 4), and it is tempting to infer that some perturbations of GI motility in both IBS and IBD depend on TKs alike. It seems that extrinsic afferents releasing TKs are of particular importance, given that they are sensitive to tissue irritation and injury (Holzer and Holzer-Petsche, 1997a). On the one hand, tachykininergic afferent neurons probably participate in autonomic intestino-intestinal reflexes, in which SP and NKA released from the central endings of afferent neurons in the spinal cord or brainstem mediate transmission to the efferent reflex arc. Such a central role is reflected by the contribution that TKs make to emesis, the peritoneogastric reflex, the rectocolonic reflex, and postoperative ileus (Table 4). TKs may also participate in short-loop sympathetic reflexes, which are relayed by prevertebral ganglia (Fig. 1), because the sympathetic neurons in these ganglia receive not only preganglionic, but also primary afferent input (Otsuka and Yoshioka, 1993; Holzer and Holzer-Petsche, 1997a).

On the other hand, TKs released from the peripheral terminals of afferent neurons in the gut are expected to interfere with GI motility (Barthó and Holzer, 1995), and the motor dysfunctions caused by esophageal acidification, anaphylaxis, and local inflammation are indeed ameliorated by TK receptor antagonists (Table 4). In addition, experimental inflammation alters the motor effects of TKs in the intestine. Thus, ricin-evoked ileitis in the rabbit causes upregulation of neurogenic contractions that are mediated by TKs (Goldhill et al., 1997), and inflammation induced by γ-irradiation enhances the sensitivity of the rat jejunum to contract in response to SP (Esposito et al., 1996). Furthermore, TKs can stimulate migrating giant contractions of the colon (Tsukamoto et al., 1997), an action that is of pathophysiological significance, because the giant

Table 4
Tachykinin Implications in Pathological Disturbances of Gastrointestinal Motility

Stimulus or insult	Motor dysfunction	Tachykinin receptor implication
Cancer chemotherapy, motion sickness	Emesis (various species)	NK$_1$ receptors (Holzer and Holzer-Petsche, 1997a)
Luminal acidification	Relaxation of lower esophageal sphincter (ferret)	NK$_1$ receptors (Blackshaw and Dent, 1997)
Intraperitoneal irritation	Inhibition of gastric motility or emptying (peritoneogastric reflex in rat)	NK$_1$ receptors (Holzer-Petsche and Rordorf-Nikolić, 1995; Julia and Buéno, 1997)
Abdominal surgery	Inhibition of gastrointestinal transit (intestinointestinal reflex in rat)	NK$_1$ receptors (Espat et al., 1995)
Ovalbumin anaphylaxis	Disruption of migrating motor complex in small intestine (rat)	NK$_1$ receptors (Fargeas et al., 1993)
Castor oil-induced diarrhea	Giant colonic contractions (rat)	NK$_2$ and, partly, NK$_1$ receptors (Croci et al., 1997)
Rectal distention	Inhibition of colonic motility (rectocolonic reflex in rat)	NK$_1$ receptors (Julia et al., 1994)
Restraint stress	Increased defecation (rat)	NK$_1$ receptors (Ikeda et al., 1995; Castagliuolo et al., 1996)

contractions associated with castor-oil-evoked inflammation and diarrhea are prevented by a NK_2 receptor antagonist, and reduced by a NK_1
receptor antagonist (Croci et al., 1997). It would seem that NK_2 receptor
antagonists are beneficial in depressing exaggerated motility caused by
infection and inflammation, particularly because they are spasmolytic in
the rat colon, without having constipating activity (Croci et al., 1997).
Conversely, NK_1 receptor antagonists may be used to interrupt the pathological downregulation of motility associated with gastroesophageal
reflux of acid, abdominal surgery, and peritonitis (Table 4).

5.3. Implications of TKs in Diarrhea and GI Inflammation

Pathological changes in GI fluid and electrolyte secretion are frequent
manifestations of infection and inflammation, and there is reasonable
evidence to assume that SP and NKA participate in a variety of hypersecretory and inflammatory reactions of the gut (Table 5). For instance,
C. difficile toxin A causes capsaicin-sensitive extrinsic afferents in the
rat and mouse ileum to release SP, which, via activation of NK_1 receptors, excites enteric secretomotor neurons, and leads to degranulation
of mast cells, macrophage and granulocyte activation, hypersecretion,
inflammation, and necrosis (Pothoulakis et al., 1994; Mantyh et al.,
1996a, 1996b; Castagliuolo et al., 1997; Wershil et al., 1998). This
concept is corroborated by the observation that genetic deletion of the
NK_1 receptor protects from the secretory and inflammatory responses
to *C. difficile* toxin A in the mouse ileum (Castagliuolo et al., 1998).
Experimental pancreatitis evoked by ceruletide is likewise ameliorated
in NK_1 receptor knock-out mice (Bhatia et al., 1998).

Experiments with TK receptor antagonists indicate that SP and NKA
take part in the hypersecretory and inflammatory responses associated
with delayed-type hypersensitivity and *Trichinella spiralis* infection
(Table 5), but not in the diarrhea caused by cholera toxin (Pothoulakis
et al., 1994). The action of castor oil, TNBSA, and rectal distention
to stimulate secretion and cause inflammation in the gut, involves
activation of multiple TK receptors (Table 5), whose interrelationship
has not yet been fully delineated. SP is particularly important for the
initiation of TNBSA-evoked colitis in the rat and guinea pig, because
NK_1 receptor antagonists inhibit granulocyte infiltration during the first
12 h after TNBSA administration but are of inconsistent effectiveness
during later stages of the inflammatory response (McCafferty et al.,

Table 5
Tachykinin Implications in Intestinal Hypersecretion and Inflammation

Stimulus or insult	Dysfunction	Tachykinin receptor implication
Ceruletide	Pancreatitis (mouse)	NK$_1$ receptors (Bhatia et al., 1998)
Trichinella spiralis	Inflammation and lymphocyte proliferation in small intestine (mouse)	NK$_1$ receptors (Kataeva et al., 1994)
Clostridium difficile toxin A	Granulocyte infiltration, mast cell and macrophage activation, hypersecretion and inflammation in small intestine (rat and mouse)	NK$_1$ receptors (Pothoulakis et al., 1994; Mantyh et al., 1996a, 1996b; Castagliuolo et al., 1997, 1998; Wershil et al., 1998)
Delayed-type hypersensitivity to DNBSA (after DNFB exposure)	Mast cell degranulation and plasma leakage in small intestine (mouse)	NK$_1$ receptors (Kraneveld et al., 1995)
TNBSA	Granulocyte infiltration and damage in ileum (guinea pig)	NK$_2$ and NK$_1$ receptors (Mazelin et al., 1998)
	Granulocyte infiltration in colon (guinea pig)	NK$_1$ receptors (Wallace et al., 1998)
	Granulocyte infiltration and damage in colon (rat)	NK$_1$ receptors and NK$_2$ receptors (McCafferty et al., 1994; Mazelin et al., 1998; Wallace et al., 1998)
Castor oil	Diarrhea (rat)	NK$_2$ and, partly, NK$_1$ receptors (Croci et al., 1997)
Rectal distention	Hypersecretion in colon (rat)	NK$_1$, NK$_2$, and NK$_3$ receptors (Eutamene et al., 1997)

DNBSA, dinitrobenzene sulfonic acid; DNFB, dinitrofluorobenzene.

1994; Reinshagen et al., 1996; Mazelin et al., 1998; Wallace et al., 1998), possibly because of NK_1 receptor downregulation (Evangelista et al., 1996). It must not be overlooked, however, that some proinflammatory actions of TKs in TNBSA-evoked ileitis and colitis (Table 5) are mediated by NK_2 and NK_3 receptors (Mazelin et al., 1998).

TKs are messengers at the interface between the nervous and immune system, and it seems that mast cells, lymphocytes, granulocytes, and macrophages are under the influence of tachykininergic neurons in the gut (Maggi, 1997a). SP-positive nerve fibers lie in close proximity to mucosal mast cells (Stead et al., 1987), from which histamine and other factors are released by the peptide (Shanahan et al., 1985; Lowman et al., 1988). Indeed, the mucosal inflammation elicited by *C. difficile* toxin A in the rat and mouse ileum (Pothoulakis et al., 1994; Wershil et al., 1998), and the plasma protein leakage caused by a delayed-type hypersensitivity reaction in the mouse small intestine (Kraneveld et al., 1995), involve both TKs and mast-cell-derived factors. Analogously, SP acting via NK_1 receptors can aggravate experimental injury of the rat gastric mucosa through mast cell degranulation (Karmeli et al., 1991); TKs acting via NK_2 receptors enhance gastric mucosal resistance to injury (Stroff et al., 1996; Improta et al., 1997).

Other SP-reactive immune cells in the gut include lymphocytes (Stanisz et al., 1987), which coincides with the ability of a NK_1 receptor antagonist to attenuate lymphocyte proliferation in the small intestine of *T. spiralis*-infected mice (Kataeva et al., 1994). A regulatory influence of TKs on granulocytes is suggested by the finding that the granulocyte infiltration caused by *C. difficile* toxin A and TNBSA in the rat intestine is attenuated by a NK_1 receptor antagonist (Pothoulakis et al., 1994; McCafferty et al., 1994). The interrelationship between the TK and immune system is of a bidirectional nature, because the hypersecretory reaction of the rat colon to interleukin-1β depends on TKs (Eutamene et al., 1995). In addition, immune cells are not only targets, at which SP acts to modify immune responses, but, under pathological conditions, can themselves be induced to synthesize and release TKs. This is true for rat peritoneal macrophages exposed to bacterial endotoxin (Bost et al., 1992), macrophages in the mucosa of the rat ileum exposed to *C. difficile* toxin A (Castagliuolo et al., 1997), eosinophils from intestinal granulomas of *Schistosoma*-infected mice (Weinstock and Blum, 1990), and eosinophils from the mucosa of the inflamed human colon (Metwali et al., 1994).

5.4. Implications of TKs
in Visceral Hypersensitivity and Pain

Because SP and NKA are transmitters of nociceptive afferents innervating the gut, it is logical to think of an implication of these peptides
in visceral nociception. TKs may facilitate the excitation of extrinsic
afferents in the gut, and also participate in the central transmission of
nociceptive traffic in the spinal cord and brainstem. Irritant chemicals
as well as immunological and inflammatory mediators release SP and
NKA within the intestinal wall, where these peptides may lead to
sensitization or even excitation of extrinsic afferents (Buéno et al.,
1997; Maggi, 1997b). Indeed, pain reactions to intraperitoneal administration of the noxious chemical, acetic acid (Julia and Buéno, 1997),
and rectal distention (Julia et al., 1994) are inhibited by a NK_2, but
not NK_1, receptor antagonist. NK_1 receptors, however, may also come
into play and contribute to the pseudoaffective (cardiovascular)
responses elicited by peritoneal irritation (Holzer-Petsche and Rordorf-
Nikolić, 1995). Both NK_1 and NK_2 receptors are likewise involved in
the pseudoaffective (hypotensive) response to jejunal distention in the
rat (McLean et al., 1998).

Which transmission relays in the visceral pain pathways depend on
NK_2 receptors is not known. The available data point to a peripheral site
of action, because NK_2 receptors are absent from the spinal cord of adult
mammals (Urban et al., 1994), and TKs are unlikely to penetrate the
blood–brain barrier. This argument is supported by the ability of intraperitoneally injected SP and NK_2 receptor agonists to elicit abdominal writh-
ing reactions, which are indicative of pain (Julia et al., 1994; Kishimoto
et al., 1994; Julia and Buéno, 1997). The peripheral algesic effect of TKs
could be of pathophysiological significance, given that the rise of SP
tissue levels in dextran-sulfate-induced colitis (Kishimoto et al., 1994),
and in nonulcer dyspepsia (Kaneko et al., 1993), is associated with pain.
Because extrinsic afferents in the gut do not seem to possess receptors
for TKs, it is inferred that TK-evoked sensitization or excitation of afferents is indirect and a sequel of changes in muscle tone, which excites
mechanosensitive afferents, or other TK-induced processes that ultimately sensitize or excite nociceptive afferents (Maggi, 1997b). Notably,
the NK_2-receptor-mediated hypersensitivity to intestinal distention,
which is observed in rats infected with *Nippostrongylus brasiliensis*, is
confined to areas of hypermastocytosis (McLean et al., 1997).

Physiology   Pathology

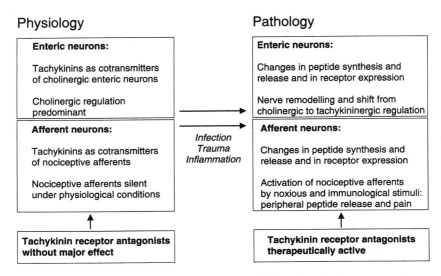

Fig. 4. Chart diagram of some neuronal and functional changes associated with intestinal inflammation, which highlight tachykinins as possible targets for novel therapeutic strategies.

6. CONCLUSIONS

The TKs, SP and NKA, participate in the physiological regulation of various digestive functions, an implication that is portrayed by the cell-specific expression of these peptides and their receptors in the gut. SP and NKA are cotransmitters of enteric cholinergic neurons, which control GI motor activity, secretion of electrolytes and fluid, and vascular and immune functions. In addition, TKs are expressed in extrinsic afferent nerve fibers, from which they can be released in response to irritant or noxious stimulation of the digestive tract. Gut disorders of various etiology, particularly those caused by infection and inflammation, are related to changes in the GI expression of TKs and their receptors (Fig. 4). It is hypothesized, therefore, that the contribution of tachykininergic neurons to normal GI physiology is out of balance in the diseased gut (Fig. 4). Nerve remodeling, and a shift in the enteric nervous system away from cholinergic toward tachykininergic regulation, takes place in experimental infection and inflammation of the intestine (Masson et al., 1996). In accordance with this scheme

(Fig. 4), it has been observed that TK receptor antagonists are not very active in the normal gut, but are able to correct disturbed motility, hypersecretion, tissue homeostasis, and pain associated with certain forms of intestinal anaphylaxis, infection, and inflammation. Extrapolation of these experimental findings to disorders of the human digestive system identifies TK receptors as novel targets for gastroenterological therapy. However, TKs are messengers within a multifactorial control system, and manipulation of a particular TK receptor alone may not be therapeutically sufficient.

ACKNOWLEDGMENTS

The author is grateful to Ulrike Holzer-Petsche for her help with the graphs. Work in the author's laboratory was supported by the Austrian Science Foundation (grants P9473-MED and P11834-MED) and the Jubilee Foundation of the Austrian National Bank (grants 4905 and 6237).

REFERENCES

Agro A, Stanisz AM. Inhibition of murine intestinal inflammation by anti-substance P antibody. *Reg Immunol* 1993; 5: 120–126.

Bäck N, Ahonen M, Häppölä O, Kivilaakso E, Kiviluoto T. Effect of vagotomy on expression of neuropeptides and histamine in rat oxyntic mucosa. *Digest Dis Sci* 1994; 39: 353–361.

Barthó L, Holzer P. Inhibitory modulation of guinea pig intestinal peristalsis caused by capsaicin involves calcitonin gene-related peptide and nitric oxide. *Naunyn Schmiedeberg's Arch Pharmacol* 1995; 353: 102–109.

Bernstein CN, Robert ME, Eysselein VE. Rectal substance P concentrations are increased in ulcerative colitis but not in Crohn's disease. *Am J Gastroenterol* 1993; 88: 908–913.

Bhatia M, Saluja AK, Hofbauer B, Frossard JL, Lee HS, Castagliuolo I, et al. Role of substance P and the neurokinin 1 receptor in acute pancreatitis and pancreatitis-associated lung injury. *Proc Natl Acad Sci USA* 1998; 95: 4760–4765.

Björck S, Jennische E, Dahlström A, Ahlman H. Influence of topical rectal application of drugs on dextran sulfate-induced colitis in rats. *Digest Dis Sci* 1997; 42: 824–832.

Blackshaw LA, and Dent J. Lower oesophageal sphincter responses to noxious oesophageal chemical stimuli in the ferret: involvement of tachykinin receptors. *J Auton Nerv Syst* 1997; 66: 189–200.

Bost KL. Inducible preprotachykinin mRNA expression in mucosal lymphoid organs following oral immunization with *Salmonella. J Neuroimmunol* 1995; 62: 59–67.

Bost KL, Breeding SA, Pascual DW. Modulation of the mRNAs encoding substance P and its receptor in rat macrophages by LPS. *Reg Immunol* 1992; 4: 105–112.

Bowden JJ, Garland AM, Baluk P, Lefevre P, Grady EF, Vigna SR, Bunnett NW, McDonald DM. Direct observation of substance P-induced internalization of neurokinin 1 (NK$_1$) receptors at sites of inflammation. *Proc Natl Acad Sci USA* 1994; 91: 8964–8968.

Bueb JL, Mousli M, Bronner C, Rouot B, Landry Y. Activation of G$_i$-like proteins, a receptor-independent effect of kinins in mast cells. *Mol Pharmacol* 1990; 38: 816–822.

Buéno L, Fioramonti J, Delvaux M, Frexinos J. Mediators and pharmacology of visceral sensitivity: from basic to clinical investigations. *Gastroenterology* 1997; 112: 1714–1743.

Castagliuolo I, Keates AC, Qiu BS, Kelly CP, Nikulasson S, Leeman SE, Pothoulakis C. Increased substance P responses in dorsal root ganglia and intestinal macrophages during *Clostridium difficile* toxin A enteritis in rats. *Proc Natl Acad Sci USA* 1997; 94: 4788–4793.

Castagliuolo I, LaMont JT, Qiu BS, Fleming SM, Bhaskar KR, Nikulasson ST, Kornetsky C, Pothoulakis C. Acute stress causes mucin release from rat colon: role of corticotropin releasing factor and mast cells. *Am J Physiol* 1996; 271: G884–G892.

Castagliuolo I, Riegler M, Pasha A, Nikulasson S, Lu B, Gerard C, Gerard NP, Pothoulakis C. Neurokinin–1 (NK–1) receptor is required in *Clostridium difficile*-induced enteritis. *J Clin Invest* 1998; 101: 1547–1550.

Catalioto R-M, Criscuoli M, Cucchi P, Giachetti A, Giannotti D, Giuliani S, et al. MEN 11420 (Nepadutant), a novel glycosylated bicyclic peptide tachykinin NK$_2$ receptor antagonist. *Br J Pharmacol* 1998; 123: 81–91.

Caterina MJ, Schumacher MA, Tominaga M, Rosen TA, Levine JD, Julius D. Capsaicin receptor: a heat-activated ion channel in the pain pathway. *Nature* 1997; 389: 816–824.

Chang MM, Leeman SE. Isolation of a sialogogic peptide from bovine hypothalamic tissue and its characterization as substance P. *J Biol Chem* 1970; 245: 4784–4790.

Ciucci A, Palma C, Manzini S, Werge TM. Point mutation increases a form of the NK$_1$ receptor with high affinity for neurokinin A and B and septide. *Br J Pharmacol* 1998; 125: 393–401.

Cooke HJ, Sidhu M, Fox P, Wang YZ, Zimmermann EM. Substance P as a mediator of colonic secretory reflexes. *Am J Physiol* 1997a; 272: G238–G245.

Cooke HJ, Sidhu M, Wang YZ. 5-HT activates neural reflexes regulating secretion in the guinea-pig colon. *Neurogastroenterol Motil* 1997b; 9: 181–186.

Cooke HJ, Sidhu M, Wang YZ. Activation of 5-HT$_{1P}$ receptors on submucosal afferents subsequently triggers VIP neurons and chloride secretion in the guinea-pig colon. *J Auton Nerv Syst* 1997c; 66: 105–110.

Costa M, Brookes SJ,H, Steele PA, Gibbins I, Burcher E, Kandiak CJ. Neurochemical classification of myenteric neurons in the guinea-pig ileum. *Neuroscience* 1996; 75: 949–967.

Croci T, Aureggi G, Manara L, Emonds-Alt X, Le Fur G, Maffrand, J-P, Mukenge S, Ferla G. *In vitro* characterization of tachykinin NK$_2$-receptors modulating motor responses of human colonic muscle strips. *Br J Pharmacol* 1998; 124: 1321–1327.

Croci T, Landi M, Emonds-Alt X, Le Fur G, Maffrand, J-P, Manara L. Role of tachykinins in castor oil diarrhoea in rats. *Br J Pharmacol* 1997; 121: 375–380.

Emonds-Alt X, Advenier C, Cognon C, Croci T, Daoui S, Ducoux JP, et al. Biochemical and pharmacological activities of SR 144190, a new nonpeptide tachykinin NK$_2$ receptor antagonist. *Neuropeptides* 1997; 31: 449–458.

Erspamer V. Tachykinin peptide family. *Trends Neurosci* 1981; 4: 267–269.

Espat NJ, Cheng G, Kelley MC, Vogel SB, Sninsky CA, Hocking MP. Vasoactive intestinal peptide and substance P receptor antagonists improve postoperative ileus. *J Surg Res* 1995; 58: 719–723.

Esposito V, Linard C, Maubert C, Aigueperse J, Gourmelon P. Modulation of gut substance P after whole-body irradiation: a new pathological feature. *Digest Dis Sci* 1996; 41: 2070–2077.

Euler US, von, Gaddum JH. An unidentified depressor substance in certain tissue extracts. *J Physiol (London)* 1931; 72: 74–87.

Eutamene H, Theodorou V, Fioramonti J, Buéno L. Implication of NK$_1$ and NK$_2$ receptors in rat colonic hypersecretion induced by interleukin$_1$: role of nitric oxide. *Gastroenterology* 1995; 109: 483–489.

Eutamene H, Theodorou V, Fioramonti J, Buéno L. Rectal distention-induced colonic net water secretion in rats involves tachykinins, capsaicin sensory, and vagus nerves. *Gastroenterology* 1997; 112: 1595–1602.

Evangelista S, Maggi M, Renzetti AR. Down-regulation of substance P receptors during colitis induced by trinitrobenzene sulfonic acid in rats. *Neuropeptides* 1996; 30: 425–428.

Eysselein VE, Reinshagen M, Cominelli F, Sternini C, Davis W, Patel A, et al. Calcitonin gene-related peptide and substance P decrease in the rabbit colon during colitis. A time study. *Gastroenterology* 1991; 101: 1211–1219.

Fargeas MJ, Fioramonti J, Buéno L. Involvement of capsaicin-sensitive afferent nerves in the intestinal motor alterations induced by intestinal anaphylaxis in rats. *Int Arch Allergy Immunol* 1993; 101: 190–195.

Figini M, Emanueli C, Grady EF, Kirkwood K, Payan DG, Ansel J, et al. Substance P and bradykinin stimulate plasma extravasation in the mouse gastrointestinal tract and pancreas. *Am J Physiol* 1997; 272: G785–G793.

Fong TM, Huang RC, Yu H, Swain CJ, Underwood D, Cascieri MA, Strader CD. Mutational analysis of neurokinin receptor function. *Can J Physio Pharmacol* 1995; 73: 860–865.

Fong TM, Yu H, Strader CD. Molecular basis for the species selectivity of the neurokinin–1 receptor antagonists CP–96,345 and RP67580. *J Biol Chem* 1992; 267: 25,668–25,671.

Furness JB, Bornstein JC, Murphy R, Pompolo S. Roles of peptides in transmission in the enteric nervous system. *Trends Neurosci* 1992; 15: 66–71.

Furness JB, Kunze WAA, Bertrand PP, Clerc N, Bornstein JC. Intrinsic primary afferent neurons of the intestine. *Prog Neurobiol* 1998; 54: 1–18.

Furness JB, Papka RE, Della NG, Costa M, Eskay RL. Substance P-like immunoreactivity in nerves associated with the vascular system of guinea-pigs. *Neuroscience* 1982; 7: 447–459.

Gerard NP, Garraway LA, Eddy RL, Shows TB, Iijima H, Paquet JL, Gerard C. Human substance P receptor (NK–1): organization of the gene, chromosome localization, and functional expression of cDNA clones. *Biochemistry* 1991; 30: 10,640–10,646.

Gether U, Johansen TE, Snider RM, Lowe JA, Nakanishi S, Schwartz TW. Different binding epitopes on the NK_1 receptor for substance P and nonpeptide antagonist. *Nature* 1993; 362: 345–348.

Gibbins IL, Furness JB, Costa M. Pathway-specific patterns of the co-existence of substance P, calcitonin gene-related peptide, cholecystokinin and dynorphin in neurons of the dorsal root ganglia of the guinea-pig. *Cell Tissue Res* 1987; 248: 417–437.

Ginap T, Kilbinger H. NK_1- and NK_3-receptor mediated inhibition of 5-hydroxytryptamine release from the vascularly perfused small intestine of the guinea-pig. *Naunyn Schmiedeberg's Arch Pharmacol* 1997; 356: 689–693.

Gitter BD, Bruns RF, Howbert JJ, Waters DC, Threlkeld PG, Cox LM, et al. Pharmacological characterization of LY303870: a novel, potent and selective nonpeptide substance P (neurokinin–1) receptor antagonist. *J Pharmacol Exp Ther* 1995; 275: 737–744.

Giuliani S, Barbanti G, Turini D, Quartara L, Rovero P, Giachetti A, Maggi CA. NK$_2$ tachykinin receptors and contraction of circular muscle of the human colon: characterization of the NK$_2$ receptor subtype. *Eur J Pharmacol* 1991; 203: 365–370.

Goldhill JM, Shea-Donohue T, Ali N, Pineiro-Carrero VM. Tachykininergic neurotransmission is enhanced in small intestinal circular muscle in a rabbit model of inflammation. *J Pharmacol Exp Ther* 1997; 282: 1373–1378.

Goode T, O'Connell J, Sternini C, Anton P, Wong H, O'Sullivan GC, Collins JK, Shanahan F. Substance P (neurokinin–1) receptor is a marker of human mucosal but not peripheral mononuclear cells: molecular quantitation and localization. *J Immunol* 1998; 161: 2232–2240.

Grady EF, Baluk P, Böhm S, Gamp PD, Wong H, Payan DG, et al. Characterization of antisera specific to NK$_1$, NK$_2$ and NK$_3$ neurokinin receptors and their utilization to localize receptors in the rat gastrointestinal tract. *J Neurosci* 1996; 16: 6975–6986.

Green T, Dockray GJ. Characterization of the peptidergic afferent innervation of the stomach in the rat, mouse and guinea-pig. *Neuroscience* 1988; 25: 181–193.

Grider JR. Identification of neurotransmitters regulating intestinal peristaltic reflex in humans. *Gastroenterology* 1989; 97: 1414–1419.

Hällgren A, Flemström G, Hellström PM, Lördal M, Hellgren S, Nylander O. Neurokinin A increases duodenal mucosal permeability, bicarbonate secretion, and fluid output in the rat. *Am J Physiol* 1997; 273: G1077-G1086.

Helliwell RJA, McLatchie LM, Clarke M, Winter J, Bevan S, McIntyre P. Capsaicin sensitivity is associated with the expression of the vanilloid (capsaicin) receptor (VR1) mRNA in adult rat sensory ganglia. *Neurosci Lett* 1998; 250: 177–180.

Hellström PM, Al Saffar A, Ljung T, Theodorsson E. Endotoxin actions on myoelectric activity, transit, and neuropeptides in the gut: role of nitric oxide. *Digest Dis Sci* 1997; 42: 1640–1651.

Hershey AD, Polenzani L, Woodward RM, Miledi R, Krause JE. Molecular and genetic characterization, functional expression, and mRNA expression patterns of a rat substance P receptor. *Ann New York Acad Sci* 1991; 632: 63–78.

Holzer P. Peptidergic sensory neurons in the control of vascular functions: mechanisms and significance in the cutaneous and splanchnic vascular beds. *Rev Physiol Biochem Pharmacol* 1992; 121: 49–146.

Holzer P. Involvement of nitric oxide in the substance P-induced inhibition of intestinal peristalsis. *NeuroReport* 1997; 8: 2857–2860.

Holzer P, Holzer-Petsche U. Tachykinins in the gut. Part I. Expression, release and motor function. *Pharmacol Ther* 1997a; 73: 173–217.

Holzer P, Holzer-Petsche U. Tachykinins in the gut. Part II. Roles in neural excitation, secretion and inflammation. *Pharmacol Ther* 1997b; 73: 219–263.

Holzer P, Lippe IT, Heinemann A, Barthó L. Tachykinin NK$_1$ and NK$_2$ receptor-mediated control of peristaltic propulsion in the guinea-pig small intestine *in vitro*. *Neuropharmacology* 1998; 37: 131–138.

Holzer P, Maggi CA. Synergistic role of muscarinic acetylcholine and tachykinin NK–2 receptors in intestinal peristalsis. *Naunyn Schmiedeberg's Arch Pharmacol* 1994; 349: 194–201.

Holzer P, Schluet W, Maggi CA. Ascending enteric reflex contraction: roles of acetylcholine and tachykinins in relation to distension and propagation of excitation. *J Pharmacol Exp Ther* 1993; 264: 391–396.

Holzer-Petsche U, Rordorf-Nikolić T. Central versus peripheral site of action of the tachykinin NK$_1$-antagonist RP 67580 in inhibiting chemonociception. *Br J Pharmacol* 1995; 115: 486–490.

Ikeda K, Miyata K, Orita A, Kubota H, Yamada T, Tomioka K. RP67580, a neurokinin$_1$ receptor antagonist, decreased restraint stress-induced defecation in rat. *Neurosci Lett* 1995; 198: 103–106.

Improta G, Broccardo M, Tabacco A, Evangelista S. Central and peripheral antiulcer and antisecretory effects of Ala^5-NKA-(4–10), a tachykinin NK$_2$ receptor agonist, in rats. *Neuropeptides* 1997; 31: 399–402.

Jensen CJ, Gerard NP, Schwartz TW, Gether U. Species selectivity of chemically distinct tachykinin nonpeptide antagonists is dependent on common divergent residues of the rat and human neurokinin–1 receptors. *Mol Pharmacol* 1994; 45: 294–299.

Jin JG, Misra S, Grider JR, Makhlouf GM. Functional difference between SP and NKA: relaxation of gastric muscle by SP is mediated by VIP and NO. *Am J Physiol* 1993; 264: G678–G685.

Johnson PJ, Bornstein JC, Burcher E. Roles of neuronal NK$_1$ and NK$_3$ receptors in synaptic transmission during motility reflexes in the guinea pig ileum. *Br J Pharmacol* 1998; 124: 1375–1384.

Johnson PJ, Bornstein JC, Yuan SY, Furness JB. Analysis of contributions of acetylcholine and tachykinins to neuro-neuronal transmission in motility reflexes in the guinea pig ileum. *Br J Pharmacol* 1996; 118: 973–983.

Julia V, Buéno L. Tachykininergic mediation of viscerosensitive responses to acute inflammation in rats: role of CGRP. *Am J Physiol* 1997; 272: G141–G146.

Julia V, Morteau O, Buéno L. Involvement of neurokinin 1 and 2 receptors in viscerosensitive response to rectal distension in rats. *Gastroenterology* 1994; 107: 94–102.

Kaneko H, Mitsuma T, Uchida K, Furusawa A, Morise K. Immunoreactive somatostatin, substance P, and calcitonin gene-related peptide concentrations of the human gastric mucosa in patients with nonulcer dyspepsia and peptic ulcer disease. *Am J Gastroenterol* 1993; 88: 898–904.

Karmeli F, Eliakim R, Okon E, Rachmilewitz D. Gastric mucosal damage by ethanol is mediated by substance P and prevented by ketotifen, a mast cell stabilizer. *Gastroenterology* 1991; 100: 1206–1216.

Kataeva G, Agro A, Stanisz AM. Substance P-mediated intestinal inflammation: inhibitory effects of CP 96,345 and SMS 201–995. *Neuroimmunomodulation* 1994; 1: 350–356.

Keranen U, Järvinen H, Kiviluoto T, Kivilaakso E, Soinila S. Substance P- and vasoactive intestinal polypeptide-immunoreactive innervation in normal and inflamed pouches after restorative proctocolectomy for ulcerative colitis. *Digest Dis Sci* 1996; 41: 1658–1664.

Keranen U, Kiviluoto T, Järvinen H, Bäck N, Kivilaakso E, Soinila S. Changes in substance P-immunoreactive innervation of human colon associated with ulcerative colitis. *Digest Dis Sci* 1995; 40: 2250–2258.

Kimura M, Masuda,T, Hiwatashi N, Toyota T, Nagura H. Changes in neuropeptide-containing nerves in human colonic mucosa with inflammatory bowel disease. *Pathol Int* 1994; 44: 624–634.

Kishimoto S, Kobayashi H, Machino H, Tari A, Kajiyama G, Miyoshi A. High concentrations of substance P as a possible transmission of abdominal pain in rats with chemical induced ulcerative colitis. *Biomed Res* 1994; 15(Suppl 2): 133–140.

Koch TR, Carney JA, Go VL. Distribution and quantitation of gut neuropeptides in normal intestine and inflammatory bowel diseases. *Digest Dis Sci* 1987; 32: 369–376.

Kraneveld AD, Buckley TL, van Heuven-Nolsen D, van Schaik Y, Koster AS, Nijkamp FP. Delayed-type hypersensitivity-induced increase in vascular permeability in the mouse small intestine: inhibition by depletion of sensory neuropeptides and NK_1 receptor blockade. *Br J Pharmacol* 1995; 114: 1483–1489.

Krause JE, Staveteig PT, Mentzer JN, Schmidt SK, Tucker JB, Brodbeck RM, Bu JY, Karpitskiy VV. Functional expression of a novel human neurokinin–3 receptor homolog that binds [^{3}H]senktide and [^{125}I-MePhe^7]-neurokinin B, and is responsive to tachykinin peptide agonists. *Proc Natl Acad Sci USA* 1997; 94: 310–315.

Lavin ST, Southwell BR, Murphy R, Jenkinson KM, Furness JB. Activation of neurokinin–1 receptors on interstitial cells of Cajal of the guinea-pig small intestine by substance P. *Histochem Cell Biol* 1998; 110: 263–271.

Lecci A, Giuliani S, Tramontana M, De Giorgio R, Maggi CA. The role of tachykinin NK_1 and NK_2 receptors in atropine-resistant colonic propulsion in anaesthetized guinea-pigs. *Br J Pharmacol* 1998; 124: 27–34.

Lembeck F. Zur Frage der zentralen Übertragung afferenter Impulse—III. Mitteilung. Das Vorkommen und die Bedeutung der Substanz P in den dorsalen Wurzeln des Rückenmarks. *Arch Exp Pathol Pharmakol* 1953; 219: 197–213.

Lippi A, Santicioli P, Criscuoli M, Maggi CA. Depolarization evoked co-release of tachykinins from enteric nerves in the guinea-pig proximal colon. *Naunyn Schmiedeberg's Arch Pharmacol* 1998; 357: 245–251.

Lördal M, Bränström R, Hellström PM. Mediation of irregular spiking activity by multiple neurokinin-receptors in the small intestine of the rat. *Br J Pharmacol* 1998; 123: 63–70.

Lördal M, Theodorsson E, Hellström PM. Tachykinins influence interdigestive rhythm and contractile strength of human small intestine. *Digest Dis Sci* 1997; 42: 1940–1949.

Lowe JA. Nonpeptide tachykinin antagonists: medicinal chemistry and molecular biology. *Medicinal Res Rev* 1996; 16: 527–545.

Lowman MA, Rees PH, Benyon RC, Church MK. Human mast cell heterogeneity: histamine release from mast cells dispersed from skin, lung, adenoids, tonsils, and colon in response to IgE-dependent and nonimmunologic stimuli. *J Allergy Clin Immunol* 1988;81: 590–597.

MacNaughton W, Moore B, Vanner S. Cellular pathways mediating tachykinin-evoked secretomotor responses in guinea pig ileum. *Am J Physiol* 1997; 273: G1127–G1134.

Maggi CA. Mammalian tachykinin receptors. *Gen Pharmacol* 1995; 26: 911–944.

Maggi CA. Effects of tachykinins on inflammatory and immune cells. *Regul Pept* 1997a; 70: 75–90.

Maggi CA. Tachykinins as peripheral modulators of primary afferent nerves and visceral sensitivity. *Pharmacol Res* 1997b; 36: 153–169.

Maggi CA, Holzer P, Giuliani S. Effect of ω-conotoxin on cholinergic and tachykininergic excitatory neurotransmission to the circular muscle of the guinea-pig colon. *Naunyn Schmiedeberg's Arch Pharmacol* 1994a; 350: 529–536.

Maggi CA, Patacchini R, Barthó L, Holzer P, Santicioli P. Tachykinin NK_1 and NK_2 receptor antagonists and atropine-resistant ascending excitatory reflex to the circular muscle of the guinea pig ileum. *Br J Pharmacol* 1994b; 112: 161–168.

Maggi CA, Patacchini R, Giachetti A, Meli A. Tachykinin receptors in the circular muscle of the guinea pig ileum. *Br J Pharmacol* 1990; 101: 996–1000.

Maggi CA, Patacchini R, Meini S, Giuliani S. Nitric oxide is the mediator of tachykinin NK_3 receptor-induced relaxation in the circular muscle of the guinea pig ileum. *Eur J Pharmacol* 1993a; 240: 45–50.

Maggi CA, Patacchini R, Rovero P, Giachetti A. Tachykinin receptors and tachykinin receptor antagonists. *J Auton Pharmacol* 1993b; 13: 23–93.

Maggi CA, Schwartz TW. Dual nature of the tachykinin NK_1 receptor. *Trends Pharmacol Sci* 1997;18: 351–354.

Mann PT, Southwell BR, Ding Y-Q, Shigemoto R, Mizuno N, Furness JB. Localisation of neurokinin 3 (NK_3) receptor immunoreactivity in the rat gastrointestinal tract. *Cell Tissue Res* 1997; 289: 1–9.

Mantyh CR, Maggio JE, Mantyh PW, Vigna SR, Pappas TN. Increased substance P receptor expression by blood vessels and lymphoid aggregates in *Clostridium difficile*-induced pseudomembranous colitis. *Digest Dis Sci* 1996a; 41: 614–620.

Mantyh CR, Pappas TN, Lapp JA, Washington MK, Neville LM, Ghilardi JR, et al. Substance P activation of enteric neurons in response to intraluminal *Clostridium difficile* toxin A in the rat ileum. *Gastroenterology* 1996b; 111: 1272–1280.

Mantyh CR, Vigna SR, Bollinger RR, Mantyh PW, Maggio JE, Pappas TN. Differential expression of substance P receptors in patients with Crohn's disease and ulcerative colitis. *Gastroenterology* 1995; 109: 850–860.

Masson SD, McKay DM, Stead RH, Agro A, Stanisz A, Perdue MH. *Nippostrongylus brasiliensis* infection evokes neuronal abnormalities and alterations in neurally regulated electrolyte transport in rat jejunum. *Parasitology* 1996; 113: 173–182.

Mazelin L, Theodorou V, Moré J, Emonds-Alt X, Fioramonti J, Buéno L. Comparative effects of nonpeptide tachykinin receptor antagonists on experimental gut inflammation in rats and guinea-pigs. *Life Sci* 1998; 63: 293–304.

McCafferty D-M, Sharkey KA, Wallace JL. Beneficial effects of local or systemic lidocaine in experimental colitis. *Am J Physiol* 1994; 266: G560–G567.

McLean PG, Garcia-Villar R, Fioramonti J, Buéno L. Effects of tachykinin receptor antagonists on the rat jejunal distension pain response. *Eur J Pharmacol* 1998; 345: 247–252.

McLean PG, Picard C, Garcia-Villar R, Moré J, Fioramonti J, Buéno L. Effects of nematode infection on sensitivity to intestinal distension: role of tachykinin NK_2 receptors. *Eur J Pharmacol* 1997; 337: 279–282.

Metwali A, Blum AM, Ferraris L, Klein JS, Fiocchi C, Weinstock JV. Eosinophils within the healthy or inflamed human intestine produce substance P and vasoactive intestinal peptide. *J Neuroimmunol* 1994; 52: 69–78.

Miller MJ, Sadowska-Krowicka H, Jeng AY, Chotinaruemol S, Wong M, Clark DA, Ho W, Sharkey KA. Substance P levels in experimental ileitis in guinea pigs: effects of misoprostol. *Am J Physiol* 1993; 265: G321–G330.

Moore BA, Vanner S, Bunnett NW, Sharkey KA. Characterization of neurokinin–1 receptors in the submucosal plexus of guinea pig ileum. *Am J Physiol* 1997; 273: G670–G678.

Nakanishi S. Substance P precursor and kininogen: their structures, gene organizations, and regulation. *Physiol Rev* 1987; 67: 1117–1142.

Nakanishi S. Mammalian tachykinin receptors. *Annu Rev Neurosci* 1991; 14: 123–136.

Otsuka M, Yoshioka K. Neurotransmitter functions of mammalian tachykinins. *Physiol Rev* 1993; 73: 229–308.

Palmer JM, Greenwood B. Regional content of enteric substance P and vaso-active intestinal peptide during intestinal inflammation in the parasitized ferret. *Neuropeptides* 1993; 25: 95–103.

Palmer JM, Koch TR. Altered neuropeptide content and cholinergic enzymatic activity in the inflamed guinea pig jejunum during parasitism. *Neuropeptides* 1995; 28: 287–297.

Polley JS, Gaskin PJ, Perren MJ, Connor HE, Ward P, Beattie DT. Activity of GR205171, a potent non-peptide tachykinin NK_1 receptor antagonist, in the trigeminovascular system. *Regul Pept* 1997; 68: 23–29.

Portbury AL, Furness JB, Southwell BR, Wong H, Walsh JH, and Bunnett NW. Distribution of neurokinin–2 receptors in the guinea-pig gastrointestinal tract. *Cell Tissue Res* 1996a; 286: 281–292.

Portbury AL, Furness JB, Young HM, Southwell BR, Vigna SR. Localisation of NK_1 receptor immunoreactivity to neurons and interstitial cells of the guinea-pig gastrointestinal tract. *J Comp Neurol* 1996b; 367: 342–351.

Pothoulakis C, Castagliuolo I, LaMont JT, Jaffer A, O'Keane JC, Snider RM, Leeman SE. CP–96,345, a substance P antagonist, inhibits rat intestinal responses to *Clostridium difficile* toxin A but not cholera toxin. *Proc Natl Acad Sci USA* 1994; 91: 947–951.

Pothoulakis C, Castagliuolo I, Leeman SE, Wang C-C, Li H, Hoffman BJ, Mezey E. Substance P receptor expression in intestinal epithelium in *Clostridium difficile* toxin A enteritis in rats. *Am J Physiol* 275, G68–G75.

Prystowsky JB, Rege RV. Neurogenic inflammation in cholecystitis. *Digest Dis Sci* 1997; 42: 1489–1494.

Regoli D, Boudon A, Fauchère JL. Receptors and antagonists for substance P and related peptides. *Pharmacol Rev* 1994; 46: 551–599.

Reinshagen M, Adler G, Eysselein VE. Substance P gene expression in acute experimental colitis. *Regul Pept* 1995; 59: 53–58.

Reinshagen M, Patel A, Sottili M, French S, Sternini C, Eysselein VE. Action of sensory neurons in an experimental rat colitis model of injury and repair. *Am J Physiol* 1996; 270: G79–G86.

Renzi D, Calabró A, Panerai C, Tramontana M, Evangelista S, Milani S, Surrenti C. Preprotachykinin mRNA expression in the colonic tissue during experimental colitis in rats. *Digestion* 1994; 55 (Suppl 2): 36.

Renzi D, Calabró A, Panerai C, Tramontana M, Evangelista S, Surrenti C. NK1- and NK2-receptor gene expression during TNB-induced colitis in rats. *Gut* 1996; 39(Suppl 3): A137.

Renzi D, Tramontana M, Panerai C, Surrenti C, Evangelista S. Decrease of calcitonin gene-related peptide, but not vasoactive intestinal polypeptide and substance P, in the TNB-induced experimental colitis in rats. *Neuropeptides* 1992; 22: 56–57.

Rupniak NMJ, Tattersall FD, Williams AR, Rycroft W, Carlson EJ, Cascieri MA, et al. In vitro and in vivo predictors of the anti-emetic activity of tachykinin NK$_1$ receptor antagonists. *Eur J Pharmacol* 1997; 326: 201–209.

Sarau HM, Griswold DE, Potts W, Foley JJ, Schmidt DB, Webb EF, et al. Nonpeptide tachykinin receptor antagonists. 1. Pharmacological and pharmacokinetic characterization of SB 223412, a novel, potent and selective neurokinin–3 receptor antagonist. *J Pharmacol Exp Ther* 1997; 281: 1303–1311.

Shanahan F, Denburg JA, Fox J, Bienenstock J, Befus D. Mast cell heterogeneity: effects of neuroenteric peptides on histamine release. *J Immunol* 1985; 135: 1331–1337.

Smith VC, Sagot MA, Couraud JY, Buchan AMJ. Localization of the neurokinin 1 (NK–1) receptor in the human antrum and duodenum. *Neurosci Lett* 1998; 253: 49–52.

Snider RM, Constantine JW, Lowe JAI, Longo KP, Lebel WS, Woody HA, et al. A potent nonpeptide antagonist of the substance P (NK$_1$) receptor. *Science* 1991; 251: 435–437.

Southwell BR, Seybold VS, Woodman HL, Jenkinson KM, Furness JB. Quantitation of neurokinin 1 receptor internalization and recycling in guinea-pig myenteric neurons. *Neuroscience* 1998; 87: 925–931.

Stanisz AM, Scicchitano R, Dazin P, Bienenstock J, Payan DG. Distribution of substance P receptors on murine spleen and Peyer's patch T and B cells. *J Immunol* 1987; 139: 749–754.

Stead RH, Tomioka M, Quinonez G, Simon GT, Felten SY, Bienenstock J. Intestinal mucosal mast cells in normal and nematode-infected rat intestines are in intimate contact with peptidergic nerves. *Proc Natl Acad Sci USA* 1987; 84: 2975–2979.

Sternini C. Enteric and visceral afferent CGRP neurons. Targets of innervation and differential expression patterns. *Ann NY Acad Sci* 1992; 657: 170–186.

Sternini C, Anderson K, Frantz G, Krause JE, Brecha N. Expression of substance P/neurokinin A-encoding preprotachykinin messenger ribonucleic acids in the rat enteric nervous system. *Gastroenterology* 1989; 97: 348–356.

Sternini C, Su D, Gamp PD, Bunnett NW. Cellular sites of expression of the neurokinin–1 receptor in the rat gastrointestinal tract. *J Comp Neurol* 1995; 358: 531–540.

Stroff T, Plate S, Seyed Ebrahim J, Ehrlich K-H, Respondek M, Peskar BM. Tachykinin-induced increase in gastric mucosal resistance: role of primary afferent neurons, CGRP, and NO. *Am J Physiol* 1996; 271: G1017–G1027.

Suzuki T, Kagoshima M, Shibata M, Inaba N, Onodera S, Yamaura T, Shimada H. Effects of several denervation procedures on distribution of calcitonin gene-related peptide and substance P immunoreactive fibers in rat stomach. *Dig Dis Sci* 1997; 42: 1242–1254.

Tsukamoto M, Sarna SK, Condon RE. A novel motility effect of tachykinins in normal and inflamed colon. *Am J Physiol* 1997; 35: G1607–G1614.

Urban L, Thompson SWN, Dray A. Modulation of spinal excitability: co-operation between neurokinin and excitatory amino acid neurotransmitters. *Trends Neurosci* 1994; 17: 432–438.

Vannucchi MG, De Giorgio R, Faussone-Pellegrini MS. NK_1 receptor expression in the interstitial cells of Cajal and neurons and tachykinin distribution in rat ileum during development. *J Comp Neurol* 1997; 383: 153–162.

Varilek GW, Weinstock JV, Williams TH, Jew J. Alterations of the intestinal innervation in mice infected with *Schistosoma mansoni*. *J Parasitol* 1991; 77: 472–478.

Wallace JL, McCafferty D-M, Sharkey KA. Lack of beneficial effect of a tachykinin receptor antagonist in experimental colitis. *Regul Pept* 1998; 73: 95–101.

Wattchow DA, Jamieson GG, Maddern GJ, Furness JB, Costa M. Distribution of peptide-containing nerve fibers in the gastric musculature of patients undergoing surgery for gastroesophageal reflux. *Ann Surg* 1992; 216: 153–160.

Weinstock JV, Blum AM. Release of substance P by granuloma eosinophils in response to secretagogues in murine schistosomiasis Mansoni. *Cell Immunol* 1990; 125: 380–385.

Wershil BK, Castagliuolo I, Pothoulakis C. Direct evidence of mast cell involvement in *Clostridium difficile* toxin A-induced enteritis in mice. *Gastroenterology* 1998; 114: 956–964.

6 CCK_A Receptors in Gastrointestinal Disorders

New Therapeutic Implications

Massimo D'Amato, Francesco Makovec, and Lucio C. Rovati

Contents

1. INTRODUCTION

Knowledge of the pathophysiological roles of gastrointestinal (GI) peptides has progressed with the advances in peptide chemistry. However, a decisive step has been the development of potent and specific peptide receptor antagonists, which not only became important experimental tools for elucidating the physiological roles of peptide hormones, but also in defining the contribution of peptide hormones to disease states, but they may even ultimately prove to be important as therapeutic agents. Among all GI peptides, nonpeptidic molecules with potent and

From: *Drug Development: Molecular Targets for GI Diseases*
Edited by: T. S. Gaginella and A. Guglietta © Humana Press Inc., Totowa, NJ

selective antagonistic properties have been made available for gastrin and cholecystokinin (CCK). Comprehensive reviews on the biological actions of CCK (Mutt, 1980; Morley, 1982; Crawley and Vanderhaeghen, 1985; Albus, 1988; Brawley 1991; Hökfelt et al., 1991; Moran and McHugh, 1991; Smith and Gibbs, 1992; Crawley and Corvin 1994; Walsh, 1994a, 1994b) and on CCK receptors (Dourish and Hill, 1987; Jensen et al., 1990; Woodruff and Hughes, 1991; Silvente-Poirot et al., 1993; Williams and Blevins, 1993; D'Amato et al., 1994; Rasmussen, 1995; Wang, 1995) are available. Moreover, Adler and Beglinger (1991), provide comprehensive coverage of the role of CCK in the control of GI functions with the use of CCK antagonists. In addition, an international conference on CCK, sponsored by the New York Academy of Science, took place in 1993 (Reeve et al., 1994).

This chapter focuses on the available clinical data concerning the effect of CCK_A-antagonists on GI functions, and discusses the potential therapeutic application of CCK_A-antagonists in GI disorders.

2. CCK, CCK RECEPTORS, AND CCK RECEPTOR ANTAGONISTS

When it was first discovered, the function of CCK was considered to be simple and straightforward: CCK has long been recognized as the major regulator of gallbladder contraction (Ivy and Oldberg 1928) and pancreatic secretion (Harper and Raper, 1943). Considerable evidence, however, now supports the regulation of the motor and sensory functions at various levels of the alimentary tract as the major physiological role of CCK.

The biological actions of CCK are mediated by receptors located on the target organ. High-affinity CCK binding sites were initially demonstrated in rat pancreatic acini (Sankaran et al., 1980) and rat cerebral cortex (Hay et al., 1980). These sites showed distinct differences in their specificity for various CCK-related peptides (Innis and Snyder, 1980; Makovec et al., 1986). These CCK receptors have been pharmacologically classified on the basis of their affinity for the peptide agonists, CCK and gastrin, which share the same COOH-terminal peptide sequence, but differ in the sulfation at the sixth (gastrin) and seventh (CCK) tyrosyl residues. Given their anatomical location, they were classified as CCK receptors type A (alimentary) and B (brain) (Moran et al., 1986). Extensive evidence now indicates that CCK$_A$ receptors are also present in the brain and CCK$_B$ receptors in the periphery (Woodruff and Hughes, 1991), but the original nomenclature still holds. A third receptor subtype was initially believed to exist, and was named gastrin receptor, because it was characterized on isolated canine parietal cells (Soll et al., 1984); this receptor has subsequently been shown to be identical to the CCK$_B$ receptor (Song et al., 1993), and therefore this receptor is also referred to as CCK$_B$/gastrin receptor. Recently, human gallbladder (CCK$_A$) (Ulrich et al., 1993), as well as brain and gastric (CCK$_B$/gastrin), receptors (Pisegna et al., 1992) have been cloned, and show discrete proportion of homology. Furthermore, it has also been shown that a single amino acid of the CCK$_B$/gastrin receptors determines the specificity for nonpeptide antagonists (Beiborn et al., 1993).

The CCK$_A$ receptor mediates most of the activities of CCK in the GI system. It has relative affinities for CCK$_8$ (i.e., the sulphated COOH-terminal octapeptide of CCK), which are about 100× those for desulfated CCK$_8$, and 1000× those for CCK$_4$ or gastrin. CCK$_A$ receptors are present on the pancreatic acinar cells and gallbladder, as well as on alimentary tract muscle, neurons in the myenteric plexus, vagal afferents from the GI tract, and also in certain brain nuclei, including the interpeduncular nucleus, the area postrema, and the nucleus tractus solitarius. The CCK$_B$/gastrin receptor mediates gastrin-induced effects in the GI tract, and the actions of CCK in the central nervous system (CNS). Its affinity for CCK$_8$ is only 10× more than that for desulfated CCK$_8$, gastrin, and CCK$_4$, and it is therefore much less selective than the CCK$_A$ receptor. Some general and major characteristics of the CCK$_A$ and CCK$_B$/gastrin receptors are shown in Table 1, examples of different chemical classes of CCK-receptor antagonists are shown in Table 2, and some distinctive pharmacological properties of the CCK receptors are shown in Table 3.

In the GI tract, the CCK$_B$/gastrin receptor (Beinfeld, 1983) chiefly mediates the stimulation of gastric acid secretion by gastrin from parietal cells (Soll et al., 1984), the release of histamine (a more potent stimulus than gastrin for acid secretion from the parietal cells) from enterochromaffin-like cells (Nakata et al., 1992), and contraction of smooth muscle cells (Grider and Makhlouf, 1990). A thorough review of the CCK$_B$/gastrin receptor, its physiological and possibly therapeutical significance at GI and CNS levels, is beyond the scope of this chapter.

Table 1
Cholecystokinin and Gastrin Receptors

Nomenclature	CCK_A	CCK_B/gastrin
Gene	CCK_AR	CCK_BR
Chromosomal localization	4p16.2-15.1	11p15.4
Structural information (human)	428 aa 7TM P32238	447 aa 7TM P32239
G-protein effector	$G_{q/11}$	$G_{q/11}$
Predominant effectors	IP_3/DG	IP_3/DG
Predominant anatomical distribution	GI tract > CNS	CNS > GI tract
Potency order of endogenous ligands	CCK_8 >>>> gastrin = des-CCK_8 = CCK_4	CCK_8 > gastrin = CCK_4

7TM, seven transmembrane domains; IP_3, inositol triphosphate; DG, diacylglycerol; GI, gastrointestinal; CNS, central nervous system. Each > symbol stands for ×10.

However, CCK has been proposed as a significant neurotransmitter/neuromodulator in the CNS, and a possible involvement of CCK in the pathogenesis of anxiety and panic disorders has been hypothesized (Harro et al., 1993). Therefore, specific CCK_B/gastrin receptor antagonists, in addition to the more classical GI indication (peptic ulcer [Makovec and D'Amato, 1997]), have then been proposed, based on results of preliminary animal experiments (Hughes et al., 1990), as new potential anxiolytics. Some of these CCK_B/gastrin receptor antagonists have also been tested in humans: CI-988 (Singh et al., 1991) (formerly PD134308 [38]), L-365,260 (Lotti and Chang, 1989), and spiroglumide (formerly CR 2194 [Makovec et al., 1992]).

3. THERAPEUTIC POTENTIAL OF CCK_A RECEPTOR IN GI DISORDERS

Six CCK_A-receptor antagonists have been tested in humans, at least to the authors' present knowledge. Among these, loxiglumide and its active enantiomer, dexloxiglumide, are now the CCK_A antagonists at the

Table 2
Chemical Classes of CCK-Receptor Antagonists

Class	Example
Cyclic nucleotide	Dibutyryl cGMP
Partial sequences	COOH-terminal fragments of CCK; CCK-JMV-180
Natural products	Asperlicin; virginiamycin; tetronothiodin
Substituted benzodiazepines derivatives	Devazepide; L-365,260; FK-480; L-740,093; YM022
Amino acid derivatives	
Aspartic acid	2-NAP
Glutamic acid	Proglumide; lorglumide; loxiglumide (and its D-enantiomer dexloxiglumide); spiroglumide
Serine	TP-680
Tryptophan	Benzotrip
Dipeptoids	CI-988
Pyrazolidones	LY-206,890; LY-262,291
Ureidoacetamides	RP69758
Ureidobenzapines	CP-212454
Indolyl derivatives	SR-27,897B; T0632
Anthranilic acid derivatives	CR 2945

most advanced stage of clinical research in gastroenterology. Although some of the results obtained by using one antagonist could be confirmed by using another one, care must be taken in extrapolating the results obtained with one compound to the whole class, especially from the toxicological point of view. The human studies with CCK$_A$-receptors antagonists have been of fundamental importance because they provided compelling evidence for the physiological role(s) of CCK, but, more importantly, these studies provided the rationale for the use of CCK$_A$-receptors antagonists in GI disorders, as outlined hereafter. The potential clinical application of CCK$_A$ antagonists will be presented according to an anatomical subdivision whose order has been chosen according to the chronological order by which the concepts of the pathophysiological roles of CCK were developed.

Table 3
Pharmacological Properties of CCK-Receptor Subtypes

	CCK_A	CCK_B/gastrin
Selective agonists	A71623	[N-methyl-Nle[28,31]] desulfated CCK_8
Selective antagonists (pA_2)	Devazepide (9.8)	CI-988 (8.1)
	Loxiglumide (6.3)	L-365,260 (7.5)
	Dexloxiglumide ((K_i vs [125I]BH-CCK$_8$ = 130 nM)	LY-262691 (7.5)
		Spiroglumide (K_i vs [125I]BH-CCK$_8$ =
	PD-140,548 (7.9–8.6)	600 nM)
	SR-27,897 (9.2)	Virginiamycin (K_i vs
	2-NAP (pk$_B$ = 6.5)	[125I]BH-CCK$_8$ =
	T-0632 (9.6)	570 nM)
		YM022 (10.2)
Selective radioligands	[³H]devazepide (0.2 nM)	[³H]L-365,260 (2.0 nM)
		[³H]PD-140,376 (0.2 nM)
		[³H]- or [125I]gastrin

pA$_2$, negative logarithm of the antagonist concentration giving a dose-ratio of 2; K$_i$, antagonist concentration giving half-maximal occupation of the receptor site; pK$_B$, negative logarithm of the equilibrium dissociation constant of a competitive antagonist.

3.1. Gallbladder

Although postulated since its discovery, the exact role of CCK in the regulation of gallbladder physiology in man remained unclear until relatively recently, when the development of sensitive and specific bioassays for plasma CCK measurement (Liddle et al., 1984, 1985) established that feeding produces an increase in plasma CCK, which is correlated with a concomitant decrease in gallbladder volumes (Liddle et al., 1985). In addition, iv infusion of CCK, which produced a CCK plasma level mimicking those obtained after feeding, induced a decrease in gallbladder volumes comparable to those seen after a meal (Liddle et al., 1985). However, the real breakthrough was represented by the availability of potent and selective CCK$_A$ receptor antagonists. Indeed, the administration of devazepide and loxiglumide in a dose-dependent manner, inhibited the decrease in gallbladder volume produced by exogenously administered CCK (Liddle et al., 1989; Malesci et al.,

1990; Konturek et al., 1989), or its analog, cerulein, (Niderau et al., 1989), or by ingestion of food (Liddle et al., 1989; Konturek et al., 1989; Malesci et al., 1992). Taken together, these studies made clear that endogenous CCK is the most important regulating factor of gallbladder contraction in response to feeding, providing a rationale for the application of CCK$_A$ antagonists in biliary colics. Preliminary studies actually suggest that patients with biliary colic, refractory to standard antispasmodic treatments, obtained prompt and efficient relief with loxiglumide by oral or iv route (Beglinger et al., 1989). Moreover, it is conceivable that CCK$_A$ receptor antagonists might be also used in the treatment of disorders associated with the abnormal responses of the sphincter of Oddi to CCK, such as biliary dyskinesia or recurrent pancreatitis (Hildebrand et al., 1990).

3.2. Pancreas

The effect of CCK on pancreatic function and morphology have recently been reviewed (Niederau et al., 1994). This subheading concentrates on exocrine pancreatic secretion, because the experimental evidence of a trophic effect in man is still scarce.

The role of CCK in pancreatic exocrine secretion has been clearly elucidated, because CCK potently stimulates pancreatic enzyme secretion as part of a complex interaction with other hormonal and neural factors that balance stimulation and inhibition of pancreatic secretion. CCK interacts with CCK$_A$ receptors on pancreatic acinar cells from several species, including humans (Gardner and Jensen 1987; Jensen et al., 1980). In humans, exogenous CCK or its analog, cerulein (Jensen et al., 1980; Beglinger et al., 1985; Kerstens et al., 1985; Adler et al., 1991; Schmidt et al., 1991; Scarpignato, 1992), as well as treatments that increase endogenous CCK circulating levels (Walsh et al., 1982; Owyang et al., 1986), determine an increase of pancreatic exocrine secretion (Jensen et al., 1980; Beglinger et al., 1985; Owyang et al., 1986; Schmidt et al., 1991; Cantor et al., 1992; Katschinski et al., 1992). In addition, if the elevated plasma CCK concentration is reduced to basal levels, exocrine pancreatic secretion is also reduced (Owyang et al., 1986). Although atropine can completely block the increase in exocrine pancreatic secretion stimulated by exogenous (Schmidt et al.,

1991; Scarpignato, 1992) or endogenous CCK (Adler et al., 1991), CCK_A receptor antagonists are able to completely block the effect of exogenous CCK (Schmidt et al., 1991; Scarpignato, 1992), but only partially reduced enzyme secretions stimulated by endogenous CCK (Adler et al., 1991; Schmidt et al., 1991; Cantor et al., 1992; Scarpignato, 1992). Taken together, these findings indicate that cholinergic innervation is the major mediator of the pancreatic response to a meal in humans (Beglinger et al., 1992). However, because the CCK_A antagonist loxiglumide can abolish the CCK-induced response, and reduce by up to 70% the response to a meal (Scarpignato, 1992), the cholinergic pathway probably represents the primary target on which CCK interacts to modulate postprandial pancreatic secretion. In addition to neural cholinergic inputs, CCK also interacts with the hormone secretin to amplify pancreatic fluid and electrolyte secretion (Konturek et al., 1995). Therefore, all the studies on exocrine pancreatic secretion seem to indicate that CCK contributes to the maintenance of a normal duodenal pH by amplifying, directly or indirectly, pancreatic bicarbonate secretion.

In addition to the physiological control of pancreatic secretion, CCK is also involved in the regulation of pancreatic enzyme synthesis (Rovati, 1991), which can be inhibited by CCK_A receptor antagonists. The inhibition of both pancreatic secretion and enzyme synthesis by CCK_A antagonists could help in treating acute pancreatitis, as already suggested by different experimental models (Rovati, 1991). Furthermore, another clinical target for CCK_A receptor antagonists is chronic pancreatitis. The rational for this indication is based on the existence of a negative feedback regulation of human pancreatic enzyme synthesis by CCK. The reduction of the enzyme secretion typical of chronic pancreatitis caused by a disturbance of this feedback regulation would result in a pancreatic overstimulation of the pancreas, which may be responsible for the recurrence of abdominal pain episodes in chronic pancreatitis patients. The use of CCK_A antagonists may provide pain relief. However, the results of ongoing clinical studies are needed to provide an adequate support to this hypothesis.

CCK has been also proposed as a candidate in the regulation of endocrine pancreatic function. Results from these studies conflict across different species. However, recent studies with the CCK_A antagonists, devazepide (Liddle et al., 1990) and loxiglumide (Fried et al., 1991; Hildebrand et al., 1991; Schmidt et al., 1991; Baum et al., 1992), in humans indicate that endogenous CCK, acting at CCK$_A$ receptors, may not be a critical factor in insulin or glucagon secretion, but may be critical in the regulation of pancreatic polypeptide secretion (Niderau et al., 1994).

CCK has been reported to exert a trophic effect on pancreatic cellular growth, to potentiate the action of carcinogens, and possibly to be a growth factor for pancreatic cancer (Rovati, 1991; Niderau et al., 1994). Because of these overall findings and of the dissatisfaction with the present treatments for pancreatic cancer, there is a rationale for the CCK$_A$ antagonists to be tested therapeutically in clinical trials. Two clinical trials have been performed to test the therapeutic effect of CCK$_A$ antagonists (Abruzzese et al., 1992; Militello et al., 1997). Although the results of these studies failed to demonstrate any impact of devazepide and loxiglumide, respectively, on tumor progression, only a small number of patients were treated, the trials were too short to show an effect in the presence of a progressive disease such as pancreatic cancer, a wider range of doses might have been tested, and the CCK-receptor status was unknown. This last point, the expression of CCK receptors in pancreatic carcinoma, is the most important issue to be considered. CCK receptors have been demonstrated on cancer tissue in some experiments (Upp et al., 1987; Bell et al., 1992), and it would be useful to know the CCK receptors' status and their functionality whenever possible, because their absence might be responsible for the poor clinical results described.

3.3. Esophagus

The esophagus retains two major functions: it propels the bolus in a caudal direction, and minimizes, if not prevents, reflux of gastric content from the stomach by creating an effective barrier consisting of a 3–5-cm-long high-pressure zone, the lower esophageal sphincter (LES), which effectively separates the esophagus from the stomach. Physiologically, LES pressure falls after swallowing, favoring food progression distally into the stomach. However, even in healthy subjects, physiological reflux of gastric content may occur as a result of a sudden, transient relaxation of the LES (TLESR) unrelated to swallowing, particularly after meals (Dent et al., 1980). These TLESRs are now recognized as the primary underlying mechanism of gastro-esophageal reflux disease (GERD) (Mittal et al., 1995). It is well known that fat is a potent stimulant of CCK secretion (Liddle et al., 1985), and exogenous CCK is able to decrease LES pressure (Resin et al., 1973; Lederboer et al., 1995), suggesting that CCK is involved in the mechanism responsible for LES competence. Several lines of evidence indicate that CCK is involved through a CCK_A-receptor-mediated mechanism. First of all, it has been shown that an effective CCK_A antagonism by loxiglumide is able to antagonize meal-induced decrease in LES pressure (Katschinski et al., 1992, 1994). Furthermore, loxiglumide is also able to reverse the increased occurrence rate of TLESRs induced in a variety of experimental models, as shown in a series of randomized, double-blind, placebo-controlled studies in healthy volunteers (Boulant et al., 1996; Trudgil et al., 1996; Boeckxstaens et al., 1998; Clave et al., 1998; Zerbib et al., 1998), as well as in patients with GERD (Fakhry et al., 1997; Trudgill et al., 1998).

These studies also showed that the CCK_A receptors are probably located in the afferent limbs of the gastroesophageal reflux pathway of a neural reflex, consisting of vagal afferents sending information to the nucleus tractus solitarius in the brain stem. This signal subsequently activates the dorsomotor nucleus of the vagus and the nucleus ambiguous, whose efferent motor output travels down through the vagus nerve, and activates the same inhibitory motor neurons in the LES that are involved with swallow-related relaxation (Mittal et al., 1995).

The location of the CCK_A receptors on the afferent limb is important, because it implies that it is theoretically possible to inhibit the occurrence of TLESRs without interfering with normal LES function, and, therefore, this opens new perspectives for alternative treatment of gastroesophageal reflux disease by using CCK_A receptor antagonists.

Other pathophysiological mechanisms, such as delayed gastric emptying, can play an important role (Pope, 1994) in the pathogenesis of GERD. Gastroparesis occurs in 40% of patients with GERD (Cunningham et al., 1991), but the delay in gastric emptying is not always marked, and its significance is uncertain; however, some authors believe that gastric emptying may be one of the most important gastric factors in GERD (Scarpignato et al., 1993). Although not all patients with reflux have delayed gastric emptying, in those whose emptying is delayed, the acid clearance from the esophagus is also delayed, and the esophagus is then exposed to a pH of less than 4.0 for a longer time, thus furthering the production of lesions.

Although the effectiveness of antisecretory treatment with H$_2$-receptor antagonists or proton pump inhibitors provide valid evidence that GERD is somehow an acid-related disorder, acid hypersecretion is seen only in a minority of patients with GERD (Collen et al., 1994; Dent, 1994). Thus, it appears that the acid is in the wrong place, rather than secreted in a wrong, exaggerated, quantity. Therefore, disordered motility, rather than acid hypersecretion, appears to be the chief cause of GERD. This is further corroborated by the prevalence of symptoms suggestive of dysmotility, such as early satiety, bloating, and regurgitation, in these patients. In addition, prokinetic agents, such as substituted benzamides and cisapride, are drugs commonly and quite successfully used in the treatment of GERD, especially when associated with antisecretive therapy (Titgat et al., 1996).

Loxiglumide has been shown to accelerate gastric emptying in healthy volunteers, as well as in nonulcer dyspepsia patients (NUD), as it will be described in more detail in Subheading 3.4; also, CCK$_A$ antagonists might be of therapeutic value in GERD, not only because they prevent the postprandial decrease in LES pressure and reduce the occurrence of TLESRs, but also because they accelerate gastric emptying.

In addition to their apparent selective capability to reduce the occurrence of TLESRs, to prevent the postprandial fall of LES pressure, and to have a gastrokinetic effect, the use of CCK$_A$ antagonists in the management of GERD might represent a new therapeutic approach, also, because of the most obvious ability of this class of compounds to inhibit postprandial gallbladder contraction in a dose-dependent manner. The inhibition of gallbladder emptying by decreasing the amount of bile in the intestine (Hildebrand et al., 1990), reduces the chance of bile to reflux into the stomach, and then up into the esophagus. Although acid is an important damaging agent (Titgat et al., 1996), the addition of bile produces more mucosal damage than acid or pepsin alone (Sagaie-Shirazi et al., 1975).

3.4. Stomach

The role of endogenous CCK in the regulation of gastric motor functions has been subject to extensive investigation in a variety of species, including man. Several lines of evidence seem to suggest that

CCK plays an important role in the regulation of gastric emptying. In addition, the role of endogenous CCK in the control of gastric acid secretion has recently been better elucidated. Comprehensive reviews on the research in this area, including clinical data on the effect of CCK and CCK_A-antagonists on gastric motility (Scarpignato, 1992; Beglinger, 1994; Scarpignato et al., 1993) and on gastric acid secretion (Soll et al., 1985, 1989; Schubert and Shamburek, 1990), respectively, have been published. In this subheading, all available evidence obtained in human studies will be discussed, focusing on the effect of CCK and CCK_A-antagonists first on the gastric motor function, and then on the gastric secretory function.

Exogenous application of CCK, or of the CCK analog, cerulein, at pharmacological doses, slows the gastric emptying rate in man, by contracting the pyloric sphincter and relaxing the proximal stomach (Chey et al., 1970; Debas et al., 1975; Yamagishi and Debas, 1978; Scarpignato et al., 1981; Valenzuela and Defilippi, 1981; Anika, 1982). It has been suggested that the vagus nerve is involved in mediating these effects, and there is evidence that vagal afferents and an intact gastric branch are critical (Scarpignato et al., 1981; Dockray, 1991; Schwartz et al., 1993). In addition, doses of CCK that produced plasma levels similar to those obtained postprandially, significantly delayed gastric emptying in humans (Liddle et al., 1986; Kleibeuker et al., 1988).

CCK plasma levels promptly increase in response to a meal whose composition has selective effects on the release of endogenous CCK, with proteins and amino acids being potent stimulants of CCK in humans (Liddle et al., 1985). Because digestive products of fat and proteins are potent inhibitors of gastric emptying, this constitutes indirect supporting evidence that CCK has a role in the regulation of gastric motility (Meyer, 1987).

The concept has been elaborated that the slowing effect of CCK on gastric emptying would regulate its own release: whenever food enters the duodenum, CCK is then promptly released; CCK stimulates gallbladder contraction and pancreatic secretion, and at the same time inhibits gastric emptying. As a consequence, less food is delivered into the duodenum, which in turn reduces the stimulus for further CCK release. CCK would then play a role as an integrator of postprandial digestive functions (Sagaie-Shirazi et al., 1975).

CCK_A receptor antagonists have been used as pharmacological tools to investigate the role of endogenous CCK in the regulation of gastric emptying. Several studies have been conducted with somewhat conflicting results, probably caused by methodological problems. A statistically significant acceleration of gastric emptying rate (vs control) of solid–liquid meals has been reported in six studies with loxiglumide (Meyer et al., 1989; Li Bassi et al., 1990; Fried et al., 1991; Chua et al., 1994; Borovicka et al., 1996; Schwizer et al., 1996), in one study with devazepide (Cantor et al., 1992), and in one study with SR27897B (Kreiss et al., 1995); in two other studies with loxiglumide (Corazziari et al., 1990; Niederau et al., 1993), and another with devazepide (Liddle et al., 1989), no significant differences were found.

These apparent conflicting results may be explained in several ways: first, different techniques were used to measure gastric emptying, and, when the same technique was used (e.g., scintigraphy), data were not always provided about the validation of the method, to discriminate between the solid and liquid phase of the emptying (Niederau et al., 1993); second, different authors used different meals, in terms of composition and caloric content; third, different populations were studied, because some studies were performed in healthy volunteers and others in patients with functional dyspepsia. Although there is a wide overlap in terms of gastric emptying rate between these two groups, it is widely accepted that the gastric emptying is more frequently delayed in patients rather than in healthy subjects, in whom it is more difficult to show an acceleration; last, the sample size of these experiments was not always adequate, and therefore they did not have a sufficient statistical power to detect a significant difference.

Taking into account these methodological problems, it is difficult to compare one study with another. However, the body of evidence seems to favor the conclusion that CCK$_A$-antagonists are able to accelerate gastric emptying rate, corroborating further the important role of postprandially released (endogenous) CCK in the regulation of gastric emptying of a mixed meal in humans, even though, because of the aforementioned discrepancies, factors other than CCK might certainly contribute to the regulation of gastric emptying.

Other indirect but important evidence on the role of CCK on gastric motor functions comes also from those experiments in which the ingestion or the duodenal infusion of fat was used as an experimental model to study the influence of endogenous CCK. Dietary fat induces a variety of effects on the upper GI tract, including the abrupt interruption of the cyclic occurrence of the interdigestive migrating motor complex, and the increase of the so called gastric receptive relaxation (which is the relaxation that occurs in the gastric fundus in response to food intake).

The effects of CCK_A-blockade on antroduodenal motility after sham feeding, as well as after fat ingested or perfused into the duodenum, have also been investigated. With sham feeding experiments, it has been shown that antroduodenal motility is primarily under cholinergic control. Cholinergic blockade with atropine completely abolished increase of antroduodenal motility, gastropancreatic secretion, and pancreatic polypeptide and gastrin secretion induced by sham feeding; CCK_A blockade with loxiglumide induced a reduction of the motility, and virtually suppressed the frequency of coordinated antroduodenal contraction, and of pancreatic polypeptide secretion (Katschinski et al., 1992). The effects of duodenal perfusion of a mixed liquid meal on antroduodenal responses were also studied, and it was found that atropine and loxiglumide both reduced the antroduodenal motor response to the meal, with the effect of atropine more pronounced at the antral level; the loxiglumide effect was more pronounced at the duodenal level (Katschinski et al., 1996). This leads to the conclusion that both cholinergic input and endogenous CCK are major stimulatory regulators of antroduodenal motility. Taken together, these results seem also to indicate the existence of a regional heterogeneity of cholinergic and CCK control. Cholinergic input predominates in the antrum, and CCK predominates in the duodenum, and both systems seem to be equipotent in the pylorus.

Further evidence that, at the antroduodenal level, the motor response induced by fat is regulated by a CCK_A-receptor-dependent mechanism comes from another study, which showed that loxiglumide prevented the decrease of the antroduodenal motor response to meal ingestion (De Giorgio et al., 1994).

Another gastric motor effect induced by dietary fat is the increase of the so-called gastric receptive relaxation. Lipid instillation directly into the stomach induces a significant increase in gastric fundus compliance, which was not affected by the presence of an effective CCK_A receptor blockade, which instead prevented the decrease in gastric tone (Mesquita et al., 1994, 1997). The dynamic and tonic properties of the fundus in response to lipids seem therefore regulated by different mechanisms, with endogenous CCK playing a role in the modulation of gastric tone, and other factors being involved in the regulation of gastric accommodation.

The effects obtained with loxiglumide on fundal and antroduodenal motility seem to confirm that endogenous CCK is implicated also in the regulation of fundal and antroduodenal motor response, and may help to explain the gastrokinetic effect of CCK$_A$-antagonists. They also provide a robust rational for the use of this class of drug in motor disorders of the proximal GI tract.

In addition to the gastrokinetic action, CCK$_A$ antagonists may indeed have the added advantage of an interaction with the sensory pathways from the gut. In addition to the aforementioned motor effects, lipids instilled into the duodenum induce meal-like fullness, followed by nausea, in healthy volunteers (Feinle et al., 1996). In the presence of effective CCK$_A$-receptor blockade, a significant reduction of these sensations was observed, indicating that endogenous CCK is probably involved in the modulation of sensation originating in the gut through a CCK$_A$-receptor-dependent mechanism (Feinle et al., 1996).

As mentioned above, CCK$_A$ antagonists can be considered a new class of gastrokinetic drugs because they reduce the CCK-induced delay of gastric emptying, and accelerate gastric emptying of liquid, as well as solid, standard meals. Loxiglumide has been shown to accelerate the pathologically delayed gastric emptying of mixed solid–liquid meals in NUD patients, and to relieve their symptoms (Li Bassi et al., 1990; Chua et al., 1994). In addition, a randomized, double-blind, placebo-controlled clinical study in NUD symptomatic patients (enrolled only if they also had a delayed gastric emptying) showed a symptomatic beneficial effect statistically superior to the effect of placebo also in those subjects in whom gastric emptying was not significantly accelerated (Chua et al., 1994). The results of this preliminary clinical study in functional dyspepsia confirm that no definite correlation between symptomatic improvement and acceleration of gastric emptying occurs. The clinical benefit experienced by patients suggests that CCK$_A$ antagonists may be of therapeutic value in functional dyspepsia. However, further studies in a larger patient population are necessary to confirm this hypothesis, as well as to determine the role of CCK in the pathogenesis of this clinical condition and the mechanism of action of the drug of this class.

The role of CCK in gastric acid secretion is an area of relatively recent investigation, although the effects of the related peptide, gastrin, have been well documented (for reviews, see Soll et al., 1985; Soll, 1989; Schubert and Shamburek 1990). Exogenous administration of

CCK has produced conflicting reports regarding its role in gastric acid secretion. In vitro, CCK and gastrin are equipotent stimulants (Wank et al., 1992). When exogenously infused in different species, including man, CCK is only a weak stimulant of gastric acid secretion, compared to gastrin (Evans et al., 1988). The effects of exogenous CCK on gastric acid secretion in humans have been known for many years: CCK stimulated basal acid secretion, but inhibited gastrin-stimulated acid secretion (Wormsley 1968; Stening et al., 1969; Stening and Grossman 1969; Brooks et al., 1970; Brooks and Grossman 1970; Corazziari et al., 1979). The possibility that CCK could have a dual role, one stimulatory and one inhibitory, was proposed by Soll et al. (1985). These investigators put forward the hypothesis that CCK could act at the parietal cell to stimulate acid secretion, but could also inhibit acid secretion by releasing somatostatin from cells in the gastric mucosa. Recent studies with CCK antagonists support this hypothesis, that the inhibitory effect of CCK depends on somatostatin release mediated by CCK_A receptors. More precisely, CCK has been reported to inhibit gastrin- and peptone-stimulated acid secretion in humans, and this inhibition was blocked by loxiglumide (Jensen et al., 1980; Konturek et al., 1990; Burckhardt et al., 1994). Taken together, these studies provide evidence that endogenous CCK may play a role in the inhibitory regulation of gastric acid secretion, although the inhibition induced by CCK is achieved only when suprapharmacological doses of CCK_A antagonists are used in conditions of stimulation of gastric acid secretion.

3.5. Small and Large Intestine

CCK is thought to stimulate motility patterns of the fed state in the small bowel; in the colon, CCK stimulates electrical spike activity associated with segmenting contractions, and may be involved in the postprandial gastrocolonic reflex (Snape and Cohen, 1979). The ascending colon acts as a storage area for colonic contents, and, in idiopathic chronic constipation, the abnormality is usually located in the ascending colon. The hypothesis could then be put forward that a drug acting at this level of the colon could be expected to accelerate the transit. If it is postulated that endogenous CCK would exert an inhibitory effect on the propulsive motility in the ascending colon, as indicated by preliminary experiments (Fossati-Marchal et al., 1994), this inhibitory action could theoretically be reversed by CCK$_A$-antagonists. This hypothesis has been tested, and is now supported by clinical experimental data. Oral administration of loxiglumide in healthy volunteers accelerates colonic transit (Meyer et al., 1989), and loxiglumide was also effective in significantly accelerating the colonic transit time in chronically and severely constipated elderly nursing home patients (Meier et al., 1993). In both healthy volunteers and constipated patients, the principal site of action of the drug seemed to be located in the ascending colon, as indicated by the observation that segmental colonic transit was markedly accelerated in the ascending colon (Fried et al., 1991; Meier et al., 1993). In addition, the constipated patients also experienced an increase in the number of bowel movements and a reduction in the use of enemas and laxatives, which may have important socioeconomical implications (Meier et al., 1994). Finally, dexloxiglumide, the active enantiomer of loxiglumide, has been shown to accelerate the colonic transit time, in an experimental model of constipation (Meier et al., 1994, 1997).

In addition to constipation, another possible therapeutic application of CCK$_A$ antagonists is irritable bowel syndrome (IBS). Characteristically, IBS patient's symptoms and motor abnormalities are concentrated during the waking state, but both are absent during sleep. Alteration of meal-induced responses might play a major role in the pathophysiology of IBS (Wingate, 1990). Eating a meal can increase the motor activity in the ileum, and this response could be, at least in part, attributed to CCK. Patients with IBS show an exaggerated motor response to food intake (Kellow and Phillips, 1987). Exogenous administration of CCK, at doses in the physiological range, induced a dose-dependent increased in ileal motility. In addition, this CCK-induced increased ileal motility was greater in patients with IBS than in healthy controls (Kellow et al., 1988). The first observation that CCK may be involved in the pathophysiology of IBS comes, however, from earlier studies that showed that CCK administration to IBS patients is able to exacerbate the symptoms of the disease (Harvey and Read, 1973). In addition to symptoms, particularly abdominal pain, CCK can also produce some of the motility disorders of the disease (Roberts-Thomson et al., 1992). A further confirmation of these earlier findings comes from a very recent study, in which an exaggerated and prolonged CCK release in response to a fat meal was elicited in IBS patients (Sjolund et al., 1996).

A pilot therapeutic study using loxiglumide in IBS seems to indicate a therapeutic potential of CCK_A antagonists in IBS, and therefore it would confirm an involvement of CCK in the pathophysiology of IBS (Cann et al., 1994). The mechanism by which loxiglumide might be clinically beneficial is currently under investigation. Preliminary evidence seems to indicate that a CCK_A-mediated mechanism does not play a major role in the regulation of the interdigestive and postprandial motility of the left colon (Niederau et al., 1992). However, loxiglumide, at clinical doses, interferes with the gastrocolonic reflex and ileal motility, and is able to selectively slow proximal colonic transit time in IBS patients (Barrow et al., 1994).

In addition, at the same clinical doses, loxiglumide significantly decreased the postprandial increase of rectal sensations and pain in IBS patients. Preliminary observations show that these changes were not paralleled by relevant motility changes.

The rationale for the use of CCK_A antagonists in IBS is therefore because of their ability to reduce the abnormally increased sensitivity and reactivity in IBS patients, because of the possible involvement of CCK in the transduction of sensory signals originating from the gut. Although the first clinical data are encouraging, further studies are warranted.

4. CONCLUSION

The GI peptide field has recently entered a new era, because of the development of nonpeptide receptor antagonists, which can be used extensively to study peptide physiology and potentially as therapeutic agents. The discovery that chemicals with no apparent structural similarity to peptide hormones can selectively block binding of naturally occurring peptides to their receptors, has allowed us to overcome the lack of agents with good bioactivity after oral administration, which had long hampered therapeutic research in this area. The development of specific, selective, potent, and orally active CCK_A antagonists has allowed a more precise definition of the role(s) of CCK among the major regulators of GI functions. Considerable evidence now supports a physiological role for CCK in the regulation of GI responses. Its effects on esophageal motility, gastric emptying rate, gallbladder and intestinal motility, and pancreatic secretion would suggest that CCK exerts a broad range of regulatory functions in the upper GI tract that would optimize the ratio of nutrients to endogenous secretions, particularly in the proximal small intestine, and elicits a specific pattern of motor responses in the lower GI tract. In addition to the motor effects, CCK seems to be implicated in the modulation of GI tract viscerosensitivity. Taken together, findings provide a rationale for the clinical use of CCK$_A$ receptor antagonists in the treatment of different functional GI disorders, such as IBS, chronic constipation, biliary colics, gastric emptying disorders, nonulcer dyspepsia, GERD, pancreatic disorders, and, possibly, GI cancers.

REFERENCES

Abruzzese JL, Gholson CF, Daugherty K, Larson E, DuBrow R, Berlin R, Levin B. Pilot clinical trial of the cholecystokinin receptor antagonist MK–329 in patients with advanced pancreatic cancer. *Pancreas* 1992; 2: 165–171.

Adler G, Beglinger C. *Cholecystokinin Antagonists in Gastroenterology: Basic and Clinical Status.* Springer-Verlag, Berlin-Heidelberg, 1991.

Adler G, Beglinger C, Braun U, Reinshagen M, Koop I, Schafmayer A, Rovati LC, Arnold R. Interaction of the cholinergic system and cholecystokinin in the regulation of endogenous and exogenous stimulation of pancreatic secretion in humans. *Gastroenterology* 1991; 100: 537–543.

Albus M. Cholecystokinin. *Prog Neuropsychopharmacol Biol Psychiatry* 1988; 12: S5–S21.

Anika MS. Effects of cholecystokinin and caerulein on gastric emptying. *Eur J Pharmacol* 1982; 85: 195–199.

Barrow L, Blackshaw PE, Wilson CG, Rovati L, Spiller RC. Selective slowing of proximal colon transit in irritable bowel syndrome by the cholecystokinin-receptor antagonist, loxiglumide. *Eur J Gastroenterol Hepatol* 1994; 6: 381–387

Baum F, Nauck MA, Ebert R, Cantor P, Hoffmann G, Choudhury AR, Schmidt WE, Creutzfeldt W. Role of endogenously released cholecystokinin in determining postprandial insulin levels in man: effects of loxiglumide, a specific cholecystokinin receptor antagonist. *Digestion* 1992; 53: 189–199.

Beglinger C. Effect of cholecystokinin on gastrin motility in humans. Cholecystokinin. *Ann NY Acad Sci* 1994; 713: 219–225.

Beglinger C, Dill S, Meyer B, Werth B. Treatment of biliary colic with loxiglumide. *Lancet* 1989; 8655: 167.

Beglinger C, Fried M, Whitehouse I, Jansen JBMJ, Lamer CHBW, Gyr K. Pancreatic enzyme response to a liquid meal and to hormonal stimulation. *J Clin Invest* 1985; 75: 1471–1476.

Beglinger C, Hildebrand P, Adler G, Werth B, Luo H, Delco F, Gyr K. Postprandial control of gallbaldder contraction and exocrine pancreatic secretion in man. *Eur J Clin Invest* 1992; 22: 827–834.

Beiborn M, Lee YM, McBride EW, Quinn SM, Kopin AS. Single amino acid of the cholecystokinin-B/gastrin receptors determines specificity for the non-peptide antagonists. *Nature* 1993; 362: 348–350.

Beinfeld MC. Cholecystokinin in the central nervous system. *Neuropeptides* 1983; 3: 411–419.

Bell RH Jr, Kuhlman ET, Jensen RT, Longnecker DS. Overexpression of cholecystokinin receptors in azaserine-induced neoplasms of the rat pancreas. *Cancer Res* 1992; 52: 3295–3299.

Boeckxstaens GE, Fakhry N, D'Amato M, Hollloway RH, Hirsch D, Vrij V, Tytgat GNJ. Involvement of cholecystokinin-A receptors in transient lower esophageal sphincter relaxations triggered by gastric distension. *Am J Gastroenterol* 1998; 93: 1823–1828.

Borovicka J, Kreiss C, Asal K, Remy B, Mettraux C, Wells A, et al. Role of cholecystokinin as a regulator of solid and liquid gastric emptying in humans. *Am J Physiol* 1996; 271: G448–G453.

Boulant J, Mathieus S, D'Amato M, Abergel A, Dapoigny M, Bommelaer G. Cholecystokinin in transient lower esophageal sphincter relaxations due to gastric distension in humans. *Gut* 1997; 40: 575–581.

Brooks AM, Grossman MI. Effect of secretion and cholecystokinin on pentagastrin-stimulated gastric acid secretion in man. *Gastroenterology* 1970; 59: 114–119.

Brooks AM, Agosti A, Bertaccini G, Grossman MI. Inhibition of gastric acid secretion in man by peptide analogues of cholecystokinin. *N Engl J Med* 1970; 282: 535–538.

Burckhardt B, Delco F, Ensinck JW, Meier R, Bauerfeind P, Aufderhaar U, et al. Cholecystokinin is a physiological regulator of gastric acid secretion in man. *Eur J Clin Invest* 1994; 24: 370–376.

Cann PA, Rovati LC, Smart H, Spiller RC, Whorwell PJ. Loxiglumide a CCK-A antagonist, in irritable bowel syndrome: a pilot multicentre clinical study. *Ann NY Acad Sci* 1994; 713: 449–450.

Cantor P, Mortensen PE, Myhre J, Gjorup I, Worning H, Stahl E, Survill TT. Effect of the cholecystokinin receptor antagonist MK–329 on meal-stimulated pancreatobiliary output in humans. *Gastroenterology* 1992; 102: 1242–1252.

Chey WY, Hitanant S, Hendricks J, Lorber SH. Effect of secretion and cholecystokinin on gastric emptying and gastric secretion in man. *Gastroenterology* 1970; 58: 820–827.

Chua AS, Bekkering M, Rovati LC, Keeling PW. Clinical efficacy and prokinetic effect of the CCK-A antagonist loxiglumide in nonulcer dyspepsia. *Ann NY Acad Sci* 1994; 713: 451–453.

Clave P, Gonzalez A, Moreno A, Lopez R, Farre A, Cusso X, et al. Endogenous cholecystokinin enhances postprandial gastroesophageal reflux in humans through extrasphincteric receptors. *Gastroenterology* 1998; 115: 597–604.

Collen MJ, Johnson DA, Sheridan MJ. Basal acid output and gastric acid hypersecretion in gastro-oesophageal reflux disease. Correlation with ranitidine therapy. *Dig Dis Sci* 1994; 39: 410–417.

Corazziari E, Ricci R, Biliotti D, Bontempo I, Pallotta N, Torsoli A. Oral administration of CCK antagonist loxiglumide inhibits postprandial gallbladder contraction without affecting gastric emptying. *Dig Dis Sci* 1990; 35: 50–54.

Corazziari E, Solomon TE, Grossman MI. Effect of ninety-five percent pure cholecystokinin on gastrin-stimulated acid secretion in man and dog. *Gastroenterology* 1979; 77: 91–95.

Crawley JN, Corwin RL. Biological actions of cholecystokinin. *Peptides* 1994; 15: 731–755.

Crawley JN, Vanderhaeghen JJ. Neuronal cholecystokinin. *Ann NY Acad Sci* 1985; 448: 1–697.

Crawley JN. Cholecystokinin-dopamine interactions. *Trends Pharmacol Sci* 1991; 12: 232–235.

Cunningham KM, Horowitz M, Riddell PS, Maddern GJ, Myers JC, Holloway RH, Wishart JM, Jamieson GG. Relations among autonomic nerve dysfunction oesophageal motility and gastric emptying in gastro-oesophageal reflux disease. *Gut* 1991; 32: 1436–1440.

D'Amato M, Makovec F, Rovati LC. Potential clinical applications of CCK$_A$ receptor antagonists in gastroenterology. *Drug News Perspec* 1994; 7: 87–95.

De Giorgio R, Stanghellini V, Ricci-Maccarini M, Morselli-Labate AM, Barbara G, Franzoso L, et al. Effects of dietary fat on postprandial gastrointestinal motility are inhibited by a cholecystokinin type A receptor antagonist. *Ann NY Acad Sci* 1994; 703: 226–231.

Debas HT, Farroq O, Grossman MI. Inhibition of gastric emptying is a physiological action of cholecystokinin. *Gastroenterology* 1975; 68: 1211–1217.

Dent J. Roles of gastric acid and pH in the pathogenesis of gastro-oesophageal reflux disease. *Scand J Gastroenterol* 1994; 29(Suppl 201) 55–61.

Dent J, Dodds WJ, Friedman RH, Sekiguchi T, Hogan WJ, Arndorfer RC, Petrie DJ. Mechanism of gastroesophageal reflux in recumbent asymptomatic human subjects. *J Clin Invest* 1980; 65: 256–259.

Dockray GJ. Mediation and modulation of gastric afferent functions by regulatory peptides, in *Brain-Gut Interactions,* Tache Y, Wingate D, ed., Boston, CRC, pp. 124–130, 1991.

Dourish CT, Hill DR. Classification and function of CCK receptors. *Trends Pharmacol Sci* 1987; 8: 207–208.

Evans BE, Rittle KE, Bock ME, Di Pardo RM, Freidinger RM, Whitter WL, et al. Methods for drug discovery: development of potent, selective, orally effective cholecystokinin antagonist. *J Med Chem* 1988; 31: 2235–2246.

Fakhry N, D'Amato M, Hirsch D, Holloway RH, Vrij V, Mathus-Liegen EMH, Tytgat GNJ, Boeckxstaens GE. Loxiglumide inhibits meal-induced transient LES relaxations in obese patients. *Gastroenterology* 1997; 112: A730.

Feinle C, D'Amato M, Read NW. Cholecystokinin-A receptors modulate gastric sensory and motor responses to gastric distension and duodenal lipid. *Gastroenterology* 1996; 110: 1379–1385.

Fossati-Marchal S, Coffin B, Flourié B, Lémann M, Franchisseur C, Jian R, Rambaud JC. Effects of cholecystokinin octapeptide (CCK-OP) on the tonic and phasic motor activity of the human colon. *Gastroenterology* 1994; 106: A499.

Fried M, Erlacher U, Schwizer W, Löchner C, Koerfer J, Beglinger C, et al. Role of cholecystokinin in the regulation of gastric emptying and pancreatic enzyme secretion in humans. *Gastroenterology* 1991; 101: 503–511.

Fried M, Schwizer W, Beglinger C, Keller U, Jansen JBMJ, Lamers CHBW. Physiological role of cholecystokinin on postprandial insulin secretion and gastric meal emptying in man. Studies with the cholecystokinin receptor antagonist loxiglumide. *Diabetologia* 1991; 34: 721–726.

Gardner JD, Jensen RT. Secretagogue receptors on pancreatic acinar cells. In *Physiology of the Gastrointestinal Tract* (Johnson LR, ed.), Raven, New York, pp. 1109–1126, 1987.

Grider JR, Makhlouf GM. Distinct receptors for cholecystokinin and gastrin on muscle cells of stomach and gallbladder. *Am J Physiol* 1990; 259: G184–G190.

Harper AA, Raper HS. Pancreozymin, a stimulant of the secretion of pancreatic enzymes in extracts of the small intestine. *J Physiol* (London) 1943; 102: 115–125.

Harro J, Vasar E, Bradwejn J. CCK in animal and human research on anxiety. *TIPS* 1993; 14: 244–249.

Harvey RF, Read AE. Effect of cholecystokinin on colonic motility and symptoms in patients with the irritable bowel syndrome. *Lancet* 1973; I: 1–13.

Hay SE, Beinfeld MC, Jensen RT, Goodwin FK, Paul SM. Demonstration of a putative receptor site for cholecystokinin in rat brain. *Neuropeptides* 1980; 1: 53–62.

Hildebrand P, Beglinger C, Gyr K, Jansen JBMJ, Rovati LC, Zuercher M, et al. Effects of a cholecystokinin receptor antagonist on intestinal phase of pancreatic and biliary response in man. *J Clin Invest* 1990; 85: 640–646.

Hildebrand P, Ensinck JW, Ketterer S, Delco S, Mossi S, Bangerter U, Beglinger C. Effect of cholecystokinin antagonist on meal-stimulated insulin and pancreatic polypeptide release in humans. *J Clin Endocrinol Metab* 1991; 72: 1123–1129.

Hökfelt T, Cortes R, Schalling M, Ceccatelli S, Pelto-Huikko M, Persson H, Villar MJ. Distribution patterns of CCK and CCK mRNA in some neuronal and nonneuronal tissues. *Neuropeptides* 1991; 19(Suppl.), 31–34.

Hughes J, Boden P, Costall B, Domeney A, Kelly E, Horwell DC, et al. Development of a class of selective cholecystokinin type B receptor antagonists having potent anxiolytic activity. *Proc Natl Acad Sci USA* 1990; 87: 6728–32.

Innis RB, Snyder SH. Distinct cholecystokinin receptors in brain and pancreas. *Proc Natl Acad Sci USA* 1980; 77: 6917–6921.

Ivy AC, Oldberg E. Hormone mechanism for gallbladder contraction and evacuation. *Am J Physiol* 1928; 86: 599–613.

Jensen RT, Huang SC, Schrenk T, Wank SA, Gardener JD. Cholecystokinin receptor antagonists: ability to distinguish various classes of cholecystokinin receptors, in *Gastrointestinal Endocrinology: Receptors and Post-Receptor Mechanisms* (Thompson JC, ed.) Academic, San Diego, CA, 1990, pp. 95–111.

Jensen RT, Lemp GF, Gardner JD. Interaction of cholecystokinin with specific membrane receptors on pancreatic acinar cells. *Proc Natl Acad Sci USA* 1980; 77: 2079–2083.

Katschinski M, Dahmen G, Reinshagen M, Beglinger C, Koop H, Nustede R, Adler G. Cephalic stimulation of gastrointestinal secretory and motor responses in humans. *Gastroenterology* 1992; 103: 383–391.

Katschinski M, Dippel C, Reinshagen M, Schirra J, Arnold R, Nustede R, Beglinger C, Adler G. Induction of the fed patter of human exocrine pancreatic secretion by nutrients: role of cholecystokinin and neurotensin. *Clin Invest* 1992; 70: 902–908.

Katschinski M, Schirra J, Beglinger C, Langbein S, Wank U, D'Amato M, Arnold R. Intestinal phase of human antro-pyloro-duodenal motility: cholinergic and CCK-mediated regulation. *Eur J Clin Invest* 1996; 26: 574–583.

Katschinski M, Schirra J, Koppelberg T, Arnold R, Beglinger C, Rovati LC, Adler G. Effect of CCK-A receptor blockade on esophageal motility. *Eur J Gastroenterol Hepatol* 1994; 6: 983–986.

Katschinski M, Schirra J, Koppelberg T, Roder M, Arnold R, Beglinger C, Rovati LC, Adler G. Role of CCK as a physiological regulator of esophageal motility in man. *Hell J Gastroneterol* 1992; 5(Suppl.), 158 (Abstract).

Kellow JE, Phillips SF. Altered small bowel motility in the irritable bowel syndrome is correlated with symptoms. *Gastroenterology* 1987; 92: 1885–1893.

Kellow JE, Millar LJ, Phillips SF. Dysmotility of the small intestine is provoked by stimuli in the irritable bowel syndrome. *Gut* 1988; 29: 1236–1243.

Kerstens PJSM, Laners CBHW, Jansen JBMJ, Delong AJL, Hessels M, Hafkenscheid JCM. Physiological plasma concentrations of cholecystokinin stimulate pancreatic enzyme secretion and gallbladder contraction in man. *Life Sci* 1985; 36: 565–569.

Kleibeuker JH, Beekhuis H, Jansen JBMJ, Peirs DA, Lamers CHBW. Cholecystokinin is a physiological hormonal mediator or fat-inhibition of gastric emptying in man. *Eur J Clin Invest* 1988; 18: 173–177.

Konturek JW, Gabryelewicz A, Kulesza E, Konturek SJ, Domschke W. Cholecystokinin (CCK) in the amino acid uptake and enzyme protein secretion by the pancreas in humans. *Int J Pancreatol* 1995; 17: 55–61.

Konturek JW, Konturek SJ, Kurek A, Bogdal J, Olesky J, Rovati L. CCK receptor antagonism by loxiglumide and gall bladder contractions response to cholecystokinin, sham feeding and ordinary feeding in man. *Gut* 1989; 30: 1136–1142.

Konturek SJ, Kwiecien N, Obtulowicz W, Kopp B, Olesky J, Rovati L. Cholecystokinin in the inhibition of gastric secretion and gastric emptying in humans. *Digestion* 1990; 45: 1–8.

Kreiss C, Schwizer W, Borovicka J, Jansen JBMJ, Bouloux C, Pignol R, Bischof-Delaloye A, Fried M. Effect of SR 27897B, a new CCK-A receptor antagonist, on gastric emptying of a solid-liquid meal in humans. *Gastroenterology* 1995; 108: A632.

Lederboer M, Masclee AAM, Batstra MR, Jansen JBMJ, Lamers CBHW. Effect of cholecystokinin on lower oesophageal sphincter pressure and transient lower oesophageal sphincter relaxations in humans. *Gut* 1995; 36: 39–44.

Li Bassi S, Rovati LC, Giacovelli G, Bolondi L, Barbara L. Effects of loxiglumide, a cholecystokinin antagonist in non-ulcer dyspepsia. *Gastroenterology* 1990; 98: A77.

Liddle RA, Gertz BJ, Kanayama S, Beccaria L, Gettys TW, Taylor IL, et al. Regulation of pancreatic endocrine function by cholecystokinin: studies with MK–329, a nonpeptide cholecystokinin receptor antagonist. *J Clin Endocrinol Metab* 1990; 70: 1312–1318.

Liddle RA, Goldfine ID, Williams JA. Bioassays of plasma cholecystokinin in rats: effects of food, trypsin inhibitor, and alcohol. *Gastroenterology* 1984; 87: 542–549.

Liddle RA, Goldfine ID, Rosen MS, Taplitz RA, Williams JA. Cholecystokinin bioactivity in human plasma: molecular forms, responses to feeding, and relationship to gallbladder contractions. *J Clin Invest* 1985; 75: 1144–1152.

Liddle RA, Morita ET, Conrad CK, Williams JA. Regulation of gastric emptying in humans by cholecystokinin. *J Clin Invest* 1986; 77: 992–996.

Liddle RA, Gertz BJ, Kanayama S, Beccaria L, Coker LD, Turnbull TA, Morita ET. Effects of a novel cholecystokinin (CCK) receptor antagonist, MK–329, on gallbladder contraction and gastric emptying in humans. Implications for the physiology of CCK. *J Clin Invest* 1989; 84: 1220–1225.

Lotti VJ, Chang RSL. New and selective non-peptide gastrin antagonist and brain cholecystokinin receptor (CCK-B) ligand: L-365,260. *Eur. J. Pharmacol.* 1989; 162: 273–80.

Makovec F, D'Amato M. CCK$_B$/gastrin receptor antagonists as potential drugs for peptic ulcer therapy. *Drug Dis Today* 1997; 2: 283–293.

Makovec F, Bani M, Chisté R, Revel L, Rovat ILC, Rovati LA. Differentiation of central and peripheral cholecystokinin-antagonistic activity. *Arzeneim-Forsch* 1986; 36: 98–102.

Makovec F, Peris W, Revel L, Giovanetti R, Mennuni L, Rovati LC. Structure–antigastrin activity relationships of new (R)-4-benzamido-5-oxopentanoic acid derivatives. *J Med Chem* 1992; 35: 28–38.

Malesci A, Defazio C, Festorazzi S, Bonato C, Valentini A, Tacconi, M, Rovati LC, Setnikar I. Effect of loxiglumide on gallbladder contractile response to caerulein and food in humans. *Gastroenterology* 1990; 98: 1307–1310.

Malesci A, Defazio C, Festorazzi S, Bonato C, Valentini A, Tacconi M, et al. Dose-response effects of oral loxiglumide on postprandial gall-bladder emptying in man. *Arzeneim-Forsch* 1992; 42: 1359–1362.

Meier R, Beglinger C, Giacovelli G, D'Amato M. Effect of the CCK-A receptor antagonist dexloxiglumide on postprandial gallbladder emptying and colonic transit time in healthy volunteers. *Gastroenterology* 1997; 112: A788.

Meier R, Beglinger C, Thurmshirn M, Meyer M, Rovati LC, Giacovelli G, D'Amato M, Gyr R. Therapeutic effects of loxiglumide, a cholecystokinin antagonist, on chronic constipation in elderly patients, a prospective, randomised, double-blinded, controlled trial. *J Gastroenter Mot* 1993; 5: 129–135.

Meier R, D'Amato M, Pullwitt A, Schneider H, Rovati LC, Beglinger C. Effect of a CCK$_A$ receptor antagonist in an experimental model of delayed colonic transit time in man. *Gastroenterology* 1994; 106: A538.

Mesquita MA, Thompson DG, Ahluwalia NK, Troncon LEA, D'Amato M,

Rovati LC. Role of CCK in the regulation of dynamic and tonic mechanical response of the human gastric fundus to lipids. *Cholecystokinin* 1994; 713: 393–394.

Mesquita MA, Thompson DG, Troncon LEA, D'Amato M, Rovati LC. Effect of cholecystokinin-A receptor blockade on lipid induced gastric relaxation in humans. *Am J Physiol* 1997; 273: G118–G123.

Meyer BM, Werth BA, Beglinger C, Hildebrand P, Jansen JBMJ, Zach D, Rovati LC, Stalder GA. Role of cholecystokinin in regulation of gastrointestinal motor functions. *Lancet* 1989; II: 12–15.

Meyer JH. Motility of the stomach and gastroduodenal junction, in *Physiology of the Gastrointestinal Tract,* (Johnson LR, ed.), Raven, New York, 1987, pp. 613–629.

Militello C, Sperti C, Di Prima F, Pedrazzoli S. Clinical evaluation and safety of loxiglumide (CCK-A receptor antagonist) in nonresectable pancreatic cancer patients. *Pancreas* 1997; 14: 222–228.

Mittal K, Holloway RH, Panagini R, Blackshaw LA, Dent J. Transient lower esophageal sphincter relaxation. *Gastroenterology* 1995; 109: 601–610.

Moran TH, McHugh PR. Gastric mechanisms in CCK satiety, in *Multiple Cholecystokinin Receptors in the CNS* (Dourish CT, et al., eds.), Oxford University Press, Oxford, 1991, pp. 183–205.

Moran TH, Robinson PH, Goldbrich MS. Two brain cholecystokinin receptors: implications for behavioural actions. *Brain Res* 1986; 362: 175–179.

Morley JE. Ascent of cholecystokinin (CCK) from gut to brain. *Life Sci* 1982; 30: 479–493.

Mutt V. Cholecystokinin: Isolation, structure and function, in *Gastrointestinal Hormones* (Glass GBJ, ed), Raven, New York, 1980, pp. 169–203.

Nakata H, Matsui T, Ito M, Taniguchi T, Naribayashi Y, Arima N, et al. Cloning and characterisation of gastrin receptor from ECL carcinoid tumor of Mastomys natalensis. *Biochem Biophys Res Commun* 1992; 187: 1151–1157.

Niederau C, Faber S, Karaus M. Cholecystokinin's role in regulation of colon motility in health and in irritable bowel syndrome. *Gastroenterology* 1992; 102: 1889–1898.

Niederau C, Heintges T, Rovati LC, Strohmeyer G. Effects of loxiglumide on gallbladder emptying in healthy volunteers. *Gastroenterology* 1989; 97: 1331–1336.

Niederau C, Lüthen R, Heintges T. Effects of CCK on pancreatic function and morphology. *Cholecystokinin* 1994; 713: 180–198.

Niederau C, Mecklenbeck W, Heindges T. Cholecystokinin does not delay gastric emptying of regular meals in healthy humans. *Hepatogastroenterology* 1993; 40: 380–383.

Orlando RC. Pathophysiology of gastroesophageal reflux. Oesophageal epithelial resistance, in *Oesophagus*. (Castell DO, ed.) Little Brown, New York, 1992, pp. 463–478.

Owyang C, Louie DS, Tatum D. Feedback regulation of pancreatic enzyme secretion-suppression of cholecystokinin release by trypsin. *J Clin Invest* 1986; 77: 2042–2047.

Pisegna JR, De Weerth A, Huppi K, Wank SA. Molecular cloning of the human brain and gastric cholecystokinin receptor: structure, functional expression and chromosomal localisation. *Biochem Biophys Res Commun* 1992; 189: 296–303.

Pope CE. Acid reflux disorders. *N Engl J Med* 1994; 331: 656–660.

Rasmussen K. Therapeutic potential of cholecystokinin-B antagonists. *Exp Opin Invest Drugs* 1995; 4: 313–322.

Reeve R, Eysselein V, Salomon TE, Go VLW. Cholecystokinin. *Ann NY Acad Sci* 1994; 713: 1–467.

Resin H, Stern DH, Sturdevant RAL, Isenberg JI. Effect of the C-terminal octapeptide of cholecystokinin on lower esophageal sphincter pressure in man. *Gastroenterology* 1973; 64: 946–949.

Roberts-Thomson IC, Fettman MJ, Jonsson JR, Frewin DB. Responses to cholecystokinin octapeptide in patients with functional abdominal pain syndromes. *J Gastroenterol Hepatol* 1992; 7: 293–297.

Rovati LC. Perspectives of CCK antagonists in pancreatic research and clinical use. *Int J Pancreatol* 1991; 8: 215–226.

Sagaie-Shirazi S, Denbesten L, Zike WL. Effect of bile salts on the ionic permeability of the oesophageal mucosa and their role in the production of esophagitis. *Gastroenterology* 1975; 68: 728–733.

Sankaran H, Goldfine I, Deveney CW, Wong KY, Williams JA. Bindings of cholecystokinin to high affinity receptors on isolated rat pancreatic acini. *J Biol Chem* 1980; 255: 1849–53.

Scarpignato C. Cholecystokinin antagonists and motilides: pharmacology and potential in the treatment of gastroesophageal reflux disease and other digestive motor disorders. *Front Gastrointest Res* 1992; 20: 90–128.

Scarpignato C, Varga G, Corradi C. Effect of CCK and its antagonists on gastric emptying. *J Physiol* (Paris) 1993; 87: 291–301.

Scarpignato C, Zimbaro G, Vitulo F, Bertaccini G. Caerulein delays gastric emtying of solids in man. *Arch Int Pharmacodyn Ther* 1981; 249: 98–105.

Schmidt WE, Creutzfeldt W, Hocker M, Nustede R, Choudhury AR, Schelser A, Rovati LC, Olsch UR. Cholecystokinin in receptor antagonist loxiglumide modulates plasma levels of gastro-entero-pancreatic hormones in man. Feedback control of cholecystokinin and gastrin secretion. *Eur J Clin Invest* 1991; 21: 501–511.

Schmidt WE, Creutzfeldt W, Schleser A, Choudhury AR, Nustede R, Hocker M, et al. Role of CCK in regulation of pancreaticobiliary functions and GI motility in humans: Effects of loxiglumide. *Am J Physiol* 1991; 260: G197–G206.

Schubert ML, Shamburek RD. Control of acid secretion. *Gastroenterol Clin North Am* 1990; 19: 1–25.

Schwartz GJ, Berkow G, McHugh PR, Moran TH. Gastric branch vagotomy blocks nutrient and cholecystokinin-induced suppression of gastric emptying. *Am J Physiol Regul Integr Comp Physiol* 1993; 264: R630–R637.

Schwizer W, Borovicka J, Kunz P, Fraser R, Kreiss C, D'Amato M, et al. Role of CCK in the regulation of liquid gastric emptying and gastric motility in humans. Studies with the CCK antagonist loxiglumide. *Gut* 1996; 9: 500–504.

Silvente-Poirot S, Dufresne M, Vaysse N, Fourmy D. Peripheral cholecystokinin receptors. *Eur J Biochem* 1993; 215: 513–529.

Singh L, Field MJ, Huges J, Menzies R, Oles RJ, Vass CA, Woodruff GN. Behavioural properties of CI–988, a selective cholecystokinin-B receptor antagonist. *Br J Pharmacol* 1991; 104: 239–245.

Sjolund K, Ekman R, Lindgren S, Rehfeld JF. Disturbed motilin and cholecystokinin release in the irritable bowel syndrome. *Scand J Gastroenterol* 1996; 31: 1110–1114.

Smith GP, Gibbs J. Development and proof of the CCK hypothesis of satiety, in *Multiple Cholecystokinin Receptors in the CNS* (Dourish CT, et al., eds.) Oxford University Press, Oxford, 1992, pp. 183–205.

Snape WJ JR, Cohen S. Effect of bethanechol, gastrin I, or cholecystokinin on myoelectrical activity. *Am J Physiol* 1979; 236: E458–E463.

Soll AH, Anirian DA, Park J, Elashoff JD, Yamada T. Cholecystokinin potently releases somatostatin from canine fundic mucosal cells in short-term culture. *Am J Physiol* 1985; 248: G569–573.

Soll AH, Amiran DA, Thomas LP, Reedy TJ, Elashoff JD. Gastrin receptors on isolated canine parietal cells. *J Clin Invest* 1984; 73: 1434–1447.

Soll AH. Gastric mucosal receptors, in *Handbook of Physiology, Section 6: The Gastrointestinal System* (Schults SG, Makhlouf GM, Rauner BB, eds.) American Physiological Society, Bethesda, MD, 1989, pp. 193–214.

Song ID, Brown RN, Wiltshire RN, Gantz I, Trent JM, Yamada T. Human gastrin/cholecystokinin type B receptor gene: alternative splice donor site in exon 4 generates two variant mRNAs. *Proc Natl Acad Sci USA* 1993; 90: 9085–9086.

Stening GF, Grossman MI. Gastrin-related peptides as stimulants of pancreatic and gastric secretion. *Am J Physiol* 1969; 217: 252–266.

Stening GF, Johnson LR, Grossman MI. Effect of cholecystokinin and caerulein on gastrin and histamine-evoked gastric secretion. *Gastroenterology* 1969; 57: 44–50.

Trudgill N, D'Amato M, Riley S. Effects of loxiglumide on lower oesophageal sphincter function following a fat meal in healthy volunteers. *Gastroenterology* 1996; 110: A771.

Trudgill N, D'Amato M, Riley S. Loxiglumide inhibits post-prandial transient lower oesophageal sphincter relaxations in patients with gastro-oesophageal reflux disease. *Gastroenterology* 1997; 112: A315.

Tytgat GNJ, Janssens J, Reynolds JC, Wienbeck M. Update on the pathophysiology and management of gastro-oesophageal reflux disease: the role of prokinetic therapy. *Eur J Gastroenterol Hepatol* 1996; 8: 603–611.

Ulrich CD, Ferber I, Holicky E, Hadac E, Buell G, Miller LJ. Molecular cloning and functional expression of the human gallbladder cholecystokinin A receptor. *Biochem Biophys Res Commun* 1993; 193: 204–11.

Upp JR, Singh P, Townsend CM JR, Thompson JC. Predicting response to endocrine therapy in humans pancreatic cancer with cholecystokinin receptors [abstract]. *Gastroenterology* 1987; 92: 1677.

Valenzuela JE, Defilippi C. Inhibition of gastric emptying in humans by secretin, the octapeptide of cholecystokinin, and intraduodenal fat. *Gastroenterology* 1981; 81: 898–902.

Walsh JH. Gastrointestinal hormones: gastrin and cholecystokinin, in *Physiology of the Gastrointestinal Tract* (Johnson LR, et al., eds.), Raven, New York, 1994a, pp. 3–31.

Walsh JH. Gastrointestinal hormones: gastrin and cholecystokinin, in *Physiology of the Gastrointestinal Tract* (Johnson LR, et al., eds.), Raven, New York, 1994b, pp. 49–67.

Walsh JH, Lamers CB, Valenzuela JE. Cholecystokinin-octapeptide like immunoreactivity in human plasma. *Gastroenterology* 1982; 82: 438–444.

Wank SA. Cholecystokinin receptors. *Am J Physiol* 1995; 269: G628–G646.

Wank SA, Pisegna JR, De Weerth A. Brain and gastrointestinal cholecystokinin receptor family: structure and functional expression. *Proc Natl Acad Sc USA* 1992; 89: 8691–8695.

Williams JA, Blevins GT. Cholecystokinin and regulation of pancreatic acinar cell function. *Physiol Rev* 1993; 73: 701–723.

Wingate DL. Functional disorders of the small intestine. *Semin Gastrointest Dis* 1990; 1: 37.

Woodruff GN, Hughes J. Cholecystokinin antagonists. *Ann Rev Pharmacol Toxicol* 1991; 31: 469–501.

Wormsley KG. Gastric response to secretion and pancreozymin in man. *Scand J Gastroenterol* 1968; 3: 632–636.

Yamagishi T, Debas HT. Cholecystokinin inhibits gastric emptying by acting on both proximal stomach and pylorus. *Am J Physiol* 1978; 234: E375–E378.

Zerbib F, Bruley Des Varannes SM, Scarpignato C, Leray V, D'Amato M, Roze C, Galmiche JP. Simultaneous assessment of lower esophageal sphincter function and fundic tone after a mixed meal in healthy humans: role of endogenous cholecystokinin. *Am J Physiol* 1998; 275: G1266–G1273.

7

5-HT$_3$/5-HT$_4$ Receptors in Motility Disorders

New Therapeutic Agents

Sushil K. Sarna, Michel R. Briejer, and Jan A. J. Schuurkes

CONTENTS

1. INTRODUCTION

5-hydroxytryptamine (5-HT) is one of the gut neurotransmitters that have been the focus of drug development in the past few years. One of the reasons for the focus on 5-HT is its strategic location in entero-chromaffin cells (Erspamer, 1996) which are in close proximity to the

From: *Drug Development: Molecular Targets for GI Diseases*
Edited by: T. S. Gaginella and A. Guglietta © Humana Press Inc., Totowa, NJ

mucosal sensory nerve endings, and in interganglionic neurons, which synapse on motor excitatory and motor inhibitory neurons (Gershon and Ross, 1966; Gershon, 1977; Furness and Costa, 1982). Because of this, extensive investigations, ranging from the molecular to clinical levels, have been performed to determine the role of 5-HT in the regulation of gastrointestinal (GI) motility. However, despite all the information currently available regarding 5-HT, its precise role in the regulation of various motility patterns in fasting and fed states, its involvement in the pathophysiology of GI motility disorders, or as a road map to propose specific agonists or antagonists of 5-HT receptors to normalize motility function in disease, are not fully understood. This is partly because of organ-specific multiple levels of control of motility in the intact state, and partly because of the large number of 5-HT receptor subtypes and their diverse locations. Locations and subtypes of receptors vary among species, which makes it more difficult to extrapolate findings from animal models to human disease. This chapter provides a brief analysis of information regarding 5-HT, with special reference to 5-HT$_3$/5-HT$_4$ receptors, which may be relevant to drug development in the treatment of motility disorders. The discussion is focused on stomach, small intestine, and colon only.

2. REGULATION OF GI MOTILITY FUNCTION

The following are some aspects of motility that are important in relation to drug development.

2.1. Motility Targets for Drug Development

The gut smooth muscle exhibits three distinct types of contractions (Fig. 1): rhythmic phasic contractions, ultrapropulsive contractions, and tone (Sarna and Otterson, 1993). The motility function of each type of contraction, and the neurohormonal, electrophysiologic, and cellular mechanisms that regulate them, are very different. The rhythmic phasic contractions produce mixing and slow, orderly distal propulsion of luminal contents in the fasting and the postprandial states. The maximum frequency and direction of propagation of these contractions are

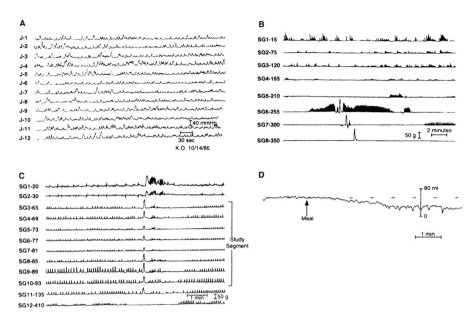

Fig. 1 (A) Postprandial human jejunal phasic contractions recorded with mano-metric catheters. The side-openings (J-1 to J-12) were 2 cm apart. No descend-ing inhibition is seen with phasic contractions. (**B**) GMC started at SG6 and propagated to SG8 strain gage transducer. The GMC at SG6 occurred during an MMC. The MMC would normally take 40–50 min. to propagate from SG6 to SG8, but the GMC propagated the same distance in about 2 min. Note, also, the large amplitude and long duration of the GMC as compared with those of the phasic contractions. SG1 to SG8 indicate the strain gage transduc-ers surgically implanted on the small intestine. The numbers after these sym-bols indicate their distances from the pylorus. (Reproduced with permission from Sarna et al., (1989) *Gastroenterology Clinics of North America*, V. 18. (**C**) An RGC originated at SG11 and rapidly propagated towards the duodenum. The amplitude and duration of the RGC are much greater than those of phasic contractions. (Reproduced with permission from Cowles and Sarna (1990), Am. J. Physiol., 259 (Gastrointest. Liver Physiol., 22), G693–G701. (**D**) Human ileal tone recorded by a barostat. Ingestion of a meal decreased the barostat volume indicating an increase in tone that lasted for several min. (Reproduced with permission from Coffin et al. (1994) Am. J. Physiol., 267 (Gastrointest and Liver Section, 30), G569–G574.

regulated by slow waves generated by smooth muscle cells and interstitial cells of Cajal (Sarna, 1989; Sarna and Otterson, 1993). Release of excitatory and inhibitory neurotransmitters from the motor neurons determines whether the smooth muscle will contract or not. In the presence of an excitatory neurotransmitter, such as acetylcholine (ACh), the smooth muscle contracts only during a slow wave. Therefore, the distance of propagation of individual phasic contractions depends on the length of the segment over which the excitatory neurotransmitter is released concurrently, and the distance over which the slow waves are synchronized (Sarna, 1989; Sarna and Otterson, 1993). In the intact organ, the propagation of contractions is of major importance in propulsion (Cowles and Sarna, 1990).

The above point is important in the development of prokinetic drugs. Potential prokinetic drugs should not only stimulate contractions, but should ensure that they propagate in the caudad direction. Therefore, the effect of potential prokinetics on the organization of slow waves, as well as on neurotransmitter release, must be considered.

The phasic contractions also occur in groups, such as migrating motor complexes (MMCs) and migrating clustered contractions (Szurszewski, 1969; Sarna, 1985; Summers et al., 1983; Kellow et al., 1986). In nonruminants, spontaneous MMCs occur primarily during the fasting state. The MMC cycling in the stomach and the small intestine is disrupted soon after the ingestion of a meal (Bueno and Ruckebusch, 1978), therefore, MMCs normally have no role in postprandial propulsion. In the fasting state, there are no nutrients to propel. This means that the ability of a drug to stimulate MMCs in the fasting state is usually not an indication that it can accelerate small intestinal transit or the rate of gastric emptying. Studies with MMCs in the fasting state may, however, be used to determine the subtypes of receptors involved in the action of drugs and, to a limited extent, their in vivo locus of action.

The ultrapropulsive contractions (Sarna, 1987; Lang and Sarna, 1986; Karaus and Sarna, 1987) are of two types, giant migrating contractions (GMCs; Fig. 1B) and retrograde giant contractions (RGCs; Fig. 1C). The GMCs propagate uninterruptedly and rapidly ($\approx$1 cm/s) over long distances in the caudad direction in the small intestine and colon. The RGCs propagate rapidly in the orad direction ($\approx$10 cm/s) in the upper small intestine, and up to the antrum only. These contractions are much larger in amplitude (2–3× the maximum amplitude of rhythmic phasic contractions) and longer in duration (4–6×) than the phasic contractions (Sarna, 1987; Quigley, 1984). Because of their large amplitude, they strongly occlude the lumen. Strong occlusion of the lumen and long distances of propagation make these contractions highly effective in propulsion. The GMCs and RGCs are not regulated by slow waves (Sarna, 1987; Lang and Sarna, 1986; Lang et al., 1986). The cellular and enteric neural mechanisms of regulation of these contractions are not understood yet. In the canine colon, it seems that substance P, acting directly on smooth muscle cells, may stimulate GMCs (Tsukamoto et al., 1997).

GMCs also produce descending inhibition of ongoing phasic contractions (Otterson and Sarna, 1994), which may help in accommodating the large bolus of luminal contents being propelled ahead of a GMC. The GMCs correspond to the peristaltic contractions originally described by Bayliss and Starling (1899). It is important to note that rhythmic phasic contractions do not produce descending inhibition, even when they propagate in the distal direction (Fig. 1A). The phasic contractions, therefore, do not fit the classic definition of peristalsis.

In animals and in humans (Sarna, 1987; Kellow and Phillips, 1987), under certain conditions, the GMCs may produce the sensation of abdominal discomfort and cramping. Several factors, such as strong contraction of the gut wall beyond nociceptive threshold, or excessive distention of the descending segment because of a large bolus being propelled ahead of a GMC, may contribute to this sensation. A defect in the mechanisms that produce descending inhibition may also contribute to the sensation of pain. In the case of a defect in descending inhibition, the ongoing phasic contractions may not be inhibited, and thus may provide resistance to rapid propulsion by GMCs. Normally, GMCs occur once or twice a day in the terminal ileum and proximal colon (Karaus and Sarna, 1987), but, in certain conditions, such as inflammation, their frequency may be increased to as much as 1/h (Sethi and Sarna, 1991a, 1991b; Jouët et al., 1995). By contrast, the frequency of GMCs is significantly reduced, or they are totally absent, in idiopathic chronic constipation (Bassotti et al., 1988). GMCs in the distal colon also precede defecation (Karaus and Sarna, 1987) or tenesmus. By contrast, MMCs or phasic contractions are not associated with mass movements or abdominal cramping. The RGCs produce ascending inhibition of contractions (Lang and Sarna, 1986), which rapidly regurgitate the contents of the upper small intestine into the antrum, in preparation for vomitus expulsion.

The precise role of increase in tone (Fig. 1D) in propulsion is not known. It is thought, however, that an increase in tone may enhance the propulsive effectiveness of phasic contractions. The reduction in luminal diameter because of increase in tone would cause even smaller amplitude phasic contractions to occlude the lumen, and thus to be more effective in propulsion.

Another important point in drug development is the distinction between longitudinal and circular muscle contractions. There are differences in the innervation of the two muscle layers (Karaus et al., 1987; Wattchow et al., 1995), and there are also differences in the postreceptor signal transduction pathways between the two muscle layers (Kuemmerle et al., 1994; Murthy et al., 1991). In addition, the role of longitudinal muscle contractions that reduce the length of the organ, rather than occlude the lumen, is not known. For this reason, the data from studies in longitudinal muscle cannot be readily related to the effectiveness of a potential drug in modulating motility function.

The importance of the above points is that, in drug development, specific contractions may have to be targeted to achieve a desired goal. For example, in inflammation, a several-fold increase in the frequency of GMCs, and a suppression of phasic contractions, make a major contribution to the symptoms of diarrhea, abdominal cramping, and urgency of defecation (Jouët et al., 1995; Sethi and Sarna, 1991a, 1991b). To minimize these symptoms, the target of drug development should be to inhibit the GMCs, and to stimulate phasic contractions and increase tone. Such opposing goals can be achieved concurrently, if drugs are targeted at the cellular and molecular levels, where the regulating mechanisms may differ for the three types of contractions. Likewise, if slow transit in constipation is to be overcome, the target may be to stimulate colonic GMCs, to cause mass movements, but also to increase tone or stimulate phasic contractions, so that adequate turning over and mixing of fecal contents can be maintained for adequate colonic absorption. In this case, colonic GMCs may have to be stimulated selectively without stimulating small intestinal GMCs. Once again, this can be achieved by choosing molecular targets that differ for the stimulation of GMCs in the two organs. In brief, the aim of stimulating or inhibiting nonspecific contractions by a drug in order to modify motility function in disease, may not be sufficient. The stimulation or inhibition of specific types of contractions that are the cause of motility disturbance, and the effects of drugs on slow waves that regulate the maximum frequency, duration, and distance of propagation of phasic contractions must be considered.

3. CLASSIFICATION

Based on the criteria of pharmacology, molecular structure, and intracellular signal transduction pathways, the subtypes of 5-HT receptors are grouped into seven classes currently recognized by the International Union of Pharmacology (Hoyer, 1994). Of these, the roles of four classes of receptors (5-HT$_1$, 5-HT$_2$, 5-HT$_3$, and 5-HT$_4$) in the regulation of gut motility have been studied extensively. A great deal of work also has been done on 5-HT$_{1P}$ receptors, and reported by Gershon (1995) and others. However, the remainder of this chapter will focus primarily on the potential utilization of 5-HT$_3$/5-HT$_4$ receptors as targets for drug development. Some reports indicate that 5-HT$_{1P}$ receptors may be similar or close to 5-HT$_4$ receptors.

4. PHARMACOLOGY AND LOCALIZATION

Numerous agonists and antagonists of 5-HT$_3$/5-HT$_4$ receptors have been employed for the pharmacological characterization of 5-HT$_3$/5-HT$_4$ receptors. The agonists of 5-HT$_3$ receptors are 2-methyl-5-HT, phenylbiguanide, and m-chloro-analog of phenylbiguanide, but they may also stimulate other receptor subtypes. Substituted benzamides (e.g., zacopride, cisapride, metoclopramide, and renzapride) are selective agonists of 5-HT$_4$ receptors, but they also act as antagonists at other 5-HT receptors, such as 5-HT$_3$ and 5-HT$_{2A}$ (Richardson et al., 1985; Fortune et al., 1983; Kilpatrick et al., 19990; Linnik et al., 1991; Schiavone et al., 1990; Middlefell and Price, 1991; Flynn et al., 1992; Hasler et al., 1991). Highly selective antagonists of 5-HT$_3$ receptor are granisetron, MDL-72222, and ondansetron. Zacopride and tropisetron are relatively selective antagonists of these receptors (Butler et al., 1988, 1990). Zacopride is also a potential agonist at 5-HT$_4$ receptors, and, at higher concentrations, tropisetron acts as a potent antagonist of 5-HT$_4$ receptors. Some of the potent and highly selective antagonists of 5-HT$_4$ receptors are SB 204070, GR 125487, and GR 113808 (Buchheit et al., 1992; Gale et al., 1994a, 1994b; Wardle et al., 1994). The potencies of the above agonists and antagonists may be species- and organ-dependent. The reasons for this variation are not understood, but it may indicate variations in subtypes of receptors among species.

A knowledge of the location of the target receptor is important in drug development. The potential of a drug in normalizing motility function may be greater, if the targeted receptor plays a physiological role in the regulation of the type of contraction responsible for pathophysiology of the disease. The chances for a drug to be effective may be greater also, if the defect producing the pathophysiology is upstream from the targeted receptor. For example, if the defect is in the sensory limb of the motility reflex (stimulation of contractions by the activation of chemo- or mechano-receptors in the mucosa), a good location of the targeted receptor might be on the interganglionic neurons or motor neurons, which lack the normal input from the sensory neurons, but can be stimulated by the drug. The prokinetic agents in the gut may be more effective when the targeted receptors are located on the neurons, from which they mediate the release of endogenous neurotransmitters, such as ACh, rather than on smooth muscle cells, where they directly stimulate receptor-mediated contractions. Even though ACh is the physiological neurotransmitter at the neuroreffector junction for most of the contractions in the gut, agonists of the muscarinic receptors on the gut smooth muscle are not effective prokinetic agents. These agonists stimulate phasic contractions and increase tone, but the contractions thus stimulated may not have physiological spatial organization, because of their concurrent stimulation at all sites. Also, the direct stimulation of smooth muscle muscarinic receptors may disrupt the synchronization of slow waves. In choosing specific target receptors in drug development, it is helpful to know whether the defect producing motility disorders is affecting the motor excitatory or motor inhibitory neurons, or both.

5-HT$_3$ and 5-HT$_4$ receptors are localized primarily on the enteric neurons. The exact location, e.g., excitatory and/or inhibitory motor neurons, interganglionic neurons, or sensory neurons, may be species- and organ-dependent. Multiple locations of these receptors in the enteric neurons of the same organ is most likely. Recent studies indicate that 5-HT$_4$ receptors may also be present on human intestinal circular and longitudinal smooth muscle cells (Kuemmerle et al., 1995). However, it seems that, in the intact state, the apparent affinity of the neuronal receptors is much greater than that of smooth muscle receptors (Graf and Sarna, 1996, 1997; Haga et al., 1996; Yoshida et al., 1991; Wilmer et al., 1993). As a result, the effects of systemically administered 5-HT$_3$/5-HT$_4$ agonists and antagonists may be seen primarily as those resulting from the activation of neuronal receptors. However, a concurrent modulatory effect on smooth muscle receptors cannot be ruled out.

Studies on the flat sheet model of ascending contraction and descending inhibition indicate that, in the rat and human colon, 5-HT$_4$ receptors are localized on sensory neurons, where they release calcitonin gene-related peptide as an intermediate neurotransmitter (Foxx-Orenstein et al., 1996; Grider et al., 1996). 5-HT$_4$ receptor antagonist SDZ-205557 blocks the response to mucosal stroking, but 5-HT$_3$ receptor antagonist LY-279584 has no effect. In the guinea pig distal colon, however, 5-HT$_3$ receptors may also be localized on these neurons, because 5-HT$_3$ receptor antagonists in this species block the response to mucosal stroking. Studies in isolated segments of the guinea pig distal colon, which measured the speed of propulsion of artificial fecal pellets, indicated that 5-HT$_3$ and 5-HT$_4$ receptors may be in parallel pathways; concurrent antagonism of both receptors is required to block the propulsion of fecal pellets (Kadowaki et al., 1993, 1994). These studies clearly establish one of the locations of 5-HT$_3$ and 5-HT$_4$ receptors, but these receptors may also be located at other sites on the enteric neurons, which can also be stimulated by drugs.

In the guinea pig ileum, also, the 5-H$_3$/5-HT$_4$ receptors are located on neurons. The activation of these receptors releases ^{3}H ACh from longitudinal muscle–myenteric plexus preparations (Kilbinger and Wolf, 1992). The activation of 5-HT$_4$ receptors also stimulates longitudinal muscle contractions in isolated segments of the ileum (Buchheit and Buhl, 1991; Craig and Clarke, 1991; Eglen et al., 1990; Tonini et al., 1992), and enhances cholinergic contractions induced by electrical field stimulation. One of these studies indicated that, in isolated ileal segments, activation of 5-HT$_4$ receptors does not stimulate circular muscle contractions (Buchheit and Buhl, 1991). These data indicate that the longitudinal and circular muscle layers may be innervated differently. According to these findings, the 5-HT$_4$ agonists should have little or no effect on propulsion in the intact in vivo guinea pig small intestine, because circular muscle contractions are not affected by these receptors.

5. ELECTROPHYSIOLOGY AND SIGNAL TRANSDUCTION PATHWAYS

Electrophysiologically, the two major types of enteric neurons are S/type I and AH/type II (Bornstein et al., 1994a; Hirst et al., 1974; Nishi and North, 1973). The S/type I neurons generate a sodium-channel-sensitive action potential that is blocked by tetrodotoxin. These neurons exhibit both fast and slow excitatory postsynaptic potentials. They generate continuous spike potentials when depolarized with intracellular current injection. Morphological and histological findings suggest that S/type I neurons are likely to be motor neurons (Bornstein, 1994b). In vivo and in vitro studies also indicate that a subset of motor neurons of the myenteric plexus is sensitive to tetrodotoxin (Jouët et al., 1995; Graf and Sarna, 1996, 1997; Briejer and Schuurkes, 1996; Sarna et al., 1981; Shi and Sarna, 1997; Wood et al., 1972). However, concurrent intracellular recordings of enteric neurons and smooth muscle contractions have not yet been made, to precisely correlate electrophysiological characteristics with the effector response.

The AH/type II neurons do not generate repeated spikes when they are depolarized by single current pulses. Spikes are generated only at the onset of depolarization, after which the cell is hyperpolarized, rendering it refractory. However, during a slow excitatory postsynaptic potential, these cells exhibit continuous spikes.

Iontophoretic application of 5-HT on guinea pig ileal enteric neurons produces a fast excitatory postsynaptic potential (fEPSP), followed by a slow depolarization (Hirst and Silinsky, 1975). The fEPSP is similar to that seen with activation of the nicotinic receptors (Hirst and Silinsky, 1975; Neild, 1980), that are directly coupled to cation channels. This suggested that the receptors mediating the fEPSP in response to 5-HT may also be coupled to a cation channel. Patch clamp studies in cell-free membranes indicated that 5-HT opens channels (9 pS and 15 pS) permeable to sodium and potassium (Derkach et al., 1989). These channels are blocked by the $5-HT_3$ receptor antagonists, ondansetron and tropisetron.

The activation of $5-HT_4$ receptor facilitates fEPSP in guinea pig ileum (Pan and Galligan, 1994; Tonini et al., 1989). The $5-HT_4$ receptors are positively coupled to adenylate cyclase in central nervous system (CNS) neurons (Bockaert et al., 1989; Dumuis et al., 1991). An increase in cyclic adenosine monophosphate (cAMP) causes depolarization in these neurons. However, in the myenteric S/type I and AH/type II neurons, 5-HT$_4$ agonists do not induce depolarization. This raises the question whether these receptors on the enteric neurons are coupled to adenylate cyclase (Pan and Galligan, 1994, 1995). However, studies on dispersed longitudinal and circular muscle cells from the human small intestine show that these receptors are coupled to adenylate cyclase through Gs (Kuemmerle et al., 1994). The increase in cAMP on activation of 5-HT$_4$ receptors induces relaxation of the cells contracted with cholecystokinin 8.

The facilitation of fEPSP by both 5-HT$_3$ and 5-HT$_4$ receptors would enhance the release of ACh from these neurons. This makes these receptors potential targets for prokinetic drugs, because ACh is the final neurotransmitter at the neuroeffector junction to stimulate postprandial phasic contractions. However, as will be discussed in subheading 7.2, stimulation of 5-HT$_3$/5-HT$_4$ receptors, or their antagonism, does not seem to affect small bowel transit in humans. This discrepancy may represent a species difference (electrophysiological data are from guinea pig ileum), or that, in the intact state, the drug concentration at the neurons does not reach the levels used in in vitro experiments to stimulate motility.

6. IN VIVO LOCUS OF ACTION AND REGULATION OF MOTILITY

Systemic administration of test substances lacks the specificity of experiments obtainable in reduced models. However, these experiments provide useful preclinical information, because eventually the drugs must work in the intact state. The specificity of in vivo experiments is enhanced significantly by the use of intracerebroventricular and close intra-arterial administration of test substances. In both cases, the amounts of test substances infused are so small that they have only local effects in the CNS or in the gut wall, respectively.

In the fasting state, iv administration of 5-HT stimulates circular muscle contractions during phase I activity in the canine small intestine (Ormsbee et al., 1984). Close intra-arterial administration of 5-HT also stimulates phasic circular muscle contractions, both in the canine jejunum and the colon (Graf and Sarna, 1996, 1997). The response to close intra-arterial infusion of 5-HT in the jejunum is blocked almost completely by atropine and hexamethonium, indicating that, in the intact state, 5-HT stimulates small intestinal contractions almost entirely through cholinergic neurons acting at a presynaptic site, and involving at least one nicotinic synapse (Graf and Sarna, 1996, 1997). Similar data have been reported in muscle strips from the guinea pig small intestine (Costa and Furness, 1979). In vitro studies on guinea pig proximal colon muscle strips suggest that a part of the response to the activation of 5-HT$_3$ and 5-HT$_4$ receptors may be mediated by neurokinin 1 receptors located on smooth muscle cells (Briejer and Schuurkes, 1997). In the colon, the response to close intra-arterial 5-HT is blocked completely by atropine, but only partially by hexamethonium, indicating that the receptors may be localized on presynaptic neurons, as well as on postsynaptic cholinergic motor excitatory neurons (Graf and Sarna, 1997).

The above studies also indicated that, in the intact state, 5-HT$_2$, but not 5-HT$_3$, receptors are involved in the mediation of the 5-HT response in the canine small intestine (Graf and Sarna, 1996). However, 5-HT$_4$ receptors located on nitronergic neurons may partially inhibit the response by releasing nitric oxide (NO). The blockade of 5-HT$_4$ receptors or the blockade of NO synthase enhances the response to 5-HT (Graf and Sarna, 1996). By contrast, the excitatory response to 5-HT in the colon is mediated primarily by 5-HT$_3$ receptors (Graf and Sarna, 1996).

Findings in the intact state reveal several things in relation to drug development:

1. Even though 5-HT receptors are present on smooth muscle cells (Kuemmerle et al., 1994), their apparent affinity (including factors such as number of receptors and receptor reserve) to 5-HT may be much less than of those on enteric neurons. The smooth muscle effects may not be seen in the intact state, unless a very high concentration of 5-HT is present in the vicinity of these cells.
2. The excitatory effects of 5-HT through cholinergic neurons exceed the inhibitory effects through nitronergic neurons in the colon and the small intestine. Unless the receptors on the nitronergic neurons can be targeted specifically, the net effect of 5-HT may be excitatory in these organs.

3. 5-HT's action in the gut wall stimulates phasic contractions, not GMCs. However, as seen in Subheading 7.3., GMCs in the colon may be stimulated if selective agonists of 5-HT$_4$ receptors, such as cisapride or prucalopride, are used.

Recent studies also indicate that endogenous 5-HT is involved in the stimulation of phase III contractions in the canine and human stomach (Haga et al., 1996; Wilmer et al., 1993). This response may be mediated by 5-HT$_3$ receptors. 5-HT depletion by p-chlorophenylalanine, or by blocking of 5-HT$_3$ receptors by iv administration of ondansetron, significantly inhibits the cycling of gastric phase III activity. This role of 5-HT$_3$ receptors may be specific to the stomach, because inhibition of these receptors has no significant effect on fasting motor activity in the small intestine (Yoshida et al., 1991).

7. FUNCTIONAL ROLE

7.1. Gastric Emptying

The interpretation of gastric emptying studies in relation to drug development is often difficult, because of different types of meals used in these studies. In general, studies with nonnutrient meals and meals containing only one nutrient, such as fat, may not be as useful as those using regular mixed meals. The mechanisms of regulation of gastric emptying of nutrient meals are different from those regulating the emptying of nonnutrient meals (Orihata and Sarna, 1996). As a result, enhanced emptying of a nonnutrient meal in response to a drug does not necessarily imply enhanced emptying of a mixed nutrient meal. Another complexity is that the mechanisms for the regulation of gastric emptying may differ among species, particularly among rodents and higher species, such as dogs and humans. In spite of the established role of 5-HT$_3$ receptors in inducing the fasting phase III cycling in humans and dogs, and in spite of studies showing that 5-HT$_3$ antagonists enhance gastric emptying of nonnutrient or single-nutrient meals in rats and guinea pigs, 5-HT$_3$ receptors seem to play little role in the regulation of gastric emptying in humans (Buchheit et al., 1985; Costell et al., 1987; Eglen et al., 1993; Schiavone et al., 1990). 5-HT$_3$ receptor antagonists also have little effect on the emptying of nutrient meals in rats (Cohen et al., 1990). Similarly, 5-HT$_3$ receptor antagonists, granisetron and ondansetron, fail to normalize gastric emptying in patients with gastric stasis syndrome or anorexia nervosa (Nielsen et al., 1990; Rizzi et al., 1994), and in dogs in which gastric emptying is retarded by an α_2-adrenergic agonist (Gullikson et al., 1991). The lack of a prokinetic effect of 5-HT$_3$ antagonists in dogs is consistent with the finding that, in this species, these agents have little effect on area under postprandial antral contractions (Gullilkson et al., 1991).

In contrast to the above, the agonists of 5-HT$_4$ receptors have shown promise as gastroprokinetic agents in humans. In animals and in humans, cisapride, as well as more specific 5-HT$_4$ agonists, accelerate gastric emptying in the normal state, and in some diseases that delay gastric emptying (Camilleri et al., 1986; Emmanuel et al., 1998; Fraser et al., 1993; Gullikson, et al., 1991; Horowitz et al., 1987; Jian et al., 1985; Richards et al., 1993; Stacher et al., 1987; Van Daele et al., 1984). Cisapride also improves gastric emptying in long-term use (Abell et al., 1991; Camilleri et al., 1989; Corinaldesi et al., 1987). However, there does not seem to be a positive correlation between the improvement in gastric emptying and symptoms of dyspepsia. The mechanisms or the locus of action of 5-HT$_4$ agonists in accelerating gastric emptying remain unknown. These agonists stimulate antral contractions that propagate across the pylorus (Fraser et al., 1993). Gastric emptying, however, is a complex phenomenon that involves several factors, including initial relaxation (accommodation), followed by a gradual contraction of the fundus that transfers the meal into the body of the stomach, antral contractions and their distal propagation, pyloric tone and its phasic contractions, antro-pyloro-duodenal coordination, spatial and temporal organization of duodenal contractions, and neurohormonal feedback from the small intestine to the stomach (Haba and Sarna, 1993). 5-HT$_4$ agonists may affect one or more of these regulating factors to accelerate gastric emptying. In dogs, cisapride accelerates gastric emptying of solid meals by stimulating antro-pyloro-duodenal coordination, as well as duodenal contractions (Orihata and Sarna, 1994).

The primary mechanism of acceleration of gastric emptying by 5-HT$_4$ agonists may be the release of ACh. The efficacy of these compounds will, therefore, depend on the nature of the defect that produces gastric stasis. For example, if the defect is in muscarinic receptors on smooth muscle cells, or at a postreceptor smooth muscle level, the release of ACh may be normal. In this case, the improvement in gastric emptying by 5-HT$_4$ agonists may be minimal. Likewise, if the defect is caused by enteric neuropathy, 5-HT$_4$ agonists may not be effective in releasing Ach.

7.2. Small Intestinal Transit

5-HT$_3$, receptors do not seem to be involved in regulating postprandial small intestinal transit in healthy subjects or in patients with diarrhea-predominant irritable bowel syndrome (IBS) (Steadman et al., 1992; Talley et al., 1989). Similar studies in the rat model are inconclusive, because mouth-to-cecal transit, instead of small bowel transit, was measured (Brown et al., 1991, 1993). These findings are in agreement with in vivo and in vitro findings in animal models, which show that 5-HT$_3$ receptors may not mediate the stimulation of circular muscle contractions by 5-HT (Buchheit and Buhl, 1993, 1991; Craig and Clarke, 1991b; Graf and Sarna, 1996; Tonini et al., 1989).

Evidence indicates that 5-HT$_4$ receptor agonists and antagonists also have little effect on small bowel transit of nonnutrient markers in fasting rats (Clayton and Gale, 1996; Costell et al., 1993). Human studies with cisapride have mostly measured mouth-to-cecum transit, making it difficult to assess the role of 5-HT$_4$ receptors on small bowel transit alone (McCallum et al., 1988).

7.3. Colonic Transit and Defecation

The 5-HT$_3$ receptor antagonist, ondansetron, has been reported to retard colonic transit in healthy subjects (Talley et al., 1990). However, it has no effect on colonic transit, stool weight, stool frequency, or clinical symptoms in diarrhea-predominant IBS patients (Steadman et al., 1992). This may be a classic example in which the type of targeted contraction is important. It is possible that ondansetron retards transit in normal subjects by altering phasic contractions. If diarrhea in IBS patients is caused by an increased frequency of GMCs, ondansetron may have little effect.

Von der Ohe et al. (1994) found that ondansetron by itself does not affect colonic tone or phasic contractions recorded by a barostat and manometric catheters, respectively, but antagonism of 5-HT$_3$ receptors blunts the gastrocolonic response (Björnsson et al., 1998; Von der Ohe et al., 1994) induced by meal ingestion or antral distention. These findings are consistent with those in the intact canine colon that 5-HT-induced contractions are mediated by 5-HT$_3$ receptors (Graf and Sarna, 1997).

Various reports indicate that the 5-HT$_4$ agonists, cisapride and prucalopride, increase stool frequency to varying degrees in a subset of patients with idiopathic constipation (Emmanuel et al., 1998; Gomme and Verlinden, 1986; Krevsky et al., 1989; Müller-Lissner et al., 1987; Rajendran et al., 1992; Varheyen et al., 1987). The acceleration of transit occurs primarily in the ascending and transverse colon (Krevsky et al., 1989). The potential of 5-HT$_4$ agonists in accelerating colonic transit is supported by in vitro findings that these receptors are located on sensory neurons, and release ACh when activated (Foxx-Orenstein et al., 1996; Grider et al., 1996; Kadowaki et al., 1993, 1994). Studies in intact dogs indicate that cisapride and prucalopride stimulate GMCs in the proximal colon, which may be the basis of accelerated transit (Rajendran et al., 1992; Sarna and Otterson, 1992). However, the locus of action of 5-HT$_4$ agonists, and the molecular mechanisms by which they stimulate GMCs, are not completely known.

7.4. Emesis

5-HT$_3$ receptors located on vagal afferent neurons, as well as in area postrema, seem to mediate chemotherapy-induced emesis. 5-HT levels in the intestinal mucosa and chemoreceptor trigger zone are increased after cisplatinum treatment (Chbeddu, 1996; Minami et al., 1996). Presumably, the mucosal increase comes from the enterochromaffin cells. 5-HT$_3$ receptor antagonists block the acute phase of cisplatinum-induced emesis; the delayed phase is independent of 5-HT, and is not affected by these receptor antagonists (Jantunen et al., 1997; Marty et al., 1990). A part of the antiemetic effect of 5-HT$_3$ receptor antagonists may also be mediated by the central receptors (Higgins et al., 1989). It is not known, however, whether 5-HT$_3$ receptor antagonists also block the RGCs that precede vomiting. 5-HT$_3$ antagonists also suppress emesis with some efficacy in postoperative and radiation-induced emesis, as well as in that associated with acquired immunodeficiency syndrome (Currow et al., 1997; Roberts and Priestman, 1993; Tramer et al., 1997). 5-HT$_4$ receptors do not seem to directly mediate nausea and vomiting. However, if these symptoms are a result of delayed gastric emptying, they may be effective.

8. SUMMARY

5-HT$_4$ receptor agonists exhibit promise in accelerating gastric emptying and colonic transit. The precise mechanisms of accelerating colonic transit are not known, but the ability of these agonists to stimulate GMCs is likely to play a primary role. The acceleration of gastric emptying is probably caused by the stimulation of a number of factors that regulate this function, such as antro-pyloro-duodenal coordination and spatial and temporal coordination of duodenal contractions. 5-HT$_4$ agonists may act on sensory neurons, motor neurons, or interganglionic neurons to achieve these effects. 5-HT$_3$ antagonists may retard colonic transit in health by altering spatial and temporal organization of phasic contractions. 5-HT$_3$ receptors, however, do not seem to be involved in the stimulation of GMCs in the colon or the small intestine. 5-HT$_3$ receptor antagonists may, therefore, be ineffective in retarding transit, if diarrhea is caused by an increase in the frequency of GMCs.

Drug development in the treatment of GI motility disorders can be facilitated by an understanding of which type(s) of contractions (phasic contractions, ultrapropulsive contractions, tone) should be targeted, what are molecular mechanisms of initiation of different types of contractions, which receptors mediate these contractions, and what is their locus of action. If rhythmic phasic contractions are the target, it is also important to understand that propulsion occurs by the propagation of contractions that are controlled by slow waves. Therefore, the effect of potential drugs on neurotransmitter release, as well as the spatial and temporal organization of slow waves, should be considered. The stimulation of contractions alone does not necessarily accelerate transit. Finally, it is likely that a combination of prokinetic drugs may be required to normalize some motility disorders.

ACKNOWLEDGMENT

Supported in part by NIDDK grant DK 32346 (SKS) and Veterans Medical Research Service (SKS).

REFERENCES

Abell T, Camilleri M, DiMagno E, et al. Long term efficacy of oral cisapride in symptomatic upper gut dysmotility. *Dig Dis Sci* 1991; 36: 616.

Bassotti G, Gaburri M, Imbimbo BP, Rossi L, Farroni F, Pelli MA, Morelli A. Colonic mass movements in idiopathic chronic constipation. *Gut* 1988; 29: 1172–1179.

Bayliss WM, Starling EH. Movements and innervation of the small intestine. J Physiol (London), 1899; 24,100–24,143.

Björnsson ES, Chey WD, Ladabaum U, Woods ML, Hooper FG, Owyang C, Hasler WL. Differential 5-HT$_3$ mediation of human gastrocolonic response and colonic peristaltic reflex. *Am J Physiol* 1998; 275 (*Gastrointest Liver Physiol* 38): G498–G505.

Bockaert J, Sebben M, Dumuis A. Pharmacological characterization of 5-hydroxytryptamine$_4$ (5-HT$_4$) receptors positively coupled to adenylate cyclase in adult guinea pig hippocampal membrane: effect of substituted benzamide derivatives. *Mol Pharmacol* 1989; 340: 403.

Bornstein JC, Furness JB, Kunze WAA. Electrophysiological characterization of myenteric neurons: how do classification schemes relate? *J Autonom Nerv Syst* 1994; 48: 1.

Bornstein JC. Local neural control of intestinal motility: nerve circuits deduced for the guinea pig small intestine. *Clin Exper Pharmacol Physiol* 1994; 21: 441.

Briejer MR, Schuurkes JAJ. 5-HT$_3$ and 5-HT$_4$ receptors and cholinergic and tachykininergic neurotransmission in the guinea-pig proximal colon. *Eur J Pharmacol* 1996; 308: 173–180.

Briejer MR, Van Daele P, Bosmans JP, Ghoos E, Eelen J, Schuurkes JA. Dose-dependent effects after oral and intravenous administration of RO–93877 on colonic motility in conscious dogs. *Gastroenterology* 1997; 112: A704 (Abstract).

Brown NJ, French SJ, Rumsey RDE, Read NW. The effect of a 5-HT$_3$-antagonist on the ileal brake mechanism in the rat. *J Pharm Pharmacol* 1991; 43: 517.

Brown NJ, Horton A, Rumsey RDE, Read NW. Granisetron and ondansetron: Effects on the ileal brake mechanism in the rat. *J Pharm Pharmacol* 1993; 45: 521.

Buchheit KH, Costall B, Engel G, Gunning SJ, Naylor RJ, Richardson BP. 5-Hydroxytryptamine receptor antagonism by metoclopramide and ICS 205–930 in the guinea pig leads to enhancement of contractions of stomach muscle strips induced by electrical field stimulation and facilitation of gastric emptying. *J Pharm Pharmacol* 1985; 37: 664.

Buchheit KH, Buhl T. 5-HT receptor subtypes involved in the stimulatory effect of 5-HT on the peristaltic reflex in vitro. *J Gastrointest Mot* 1993; 5: 49.

Buchheit K-H, Buhl T. Prokinetic benzamides stimulate peristaltic activity in the isolated guinea pig ileum by activation of 5-HT$_4$ receptors. *Eur J of Pharmacol* 1991; 205: 203–208.

Buchheit K-H, Gamse R, Pfannkuche HJ. SDZ 205–557, a selective, surmountable antagonist for 5-HT$_4$ receptors in the isolated guinea pig ileum. *Naunyn Schmiedeberg's Arch Pharmacol* 1992; 345: 387.

Bueno L, Ruckebusch Y. Migrating myoelectrical complexes: disruption, enhancement and disorganization, in *Gastrointestinal Motility in Health and Disease* (Duthie HR, ed.), MTP, Lancaster, UK 1978, pp. 83–91.

Butler A, Elswood CJ, Burridge J, Ireland SJ, Bunce KT, Kilpatrick GJ, Tyers MB. Pharmacological characterization of 5-HT$_3$ receptors in three isolated preparations derived from guinea pig tissues. *Br J Pharmacol* 1990; 101: 591.

Butler A, Hill JM, Ireland SJ, Jordan CC, Tyers MB. Pharmacological properties of GR38032F, a novel antagonist at 5-HT$_3$ receptors. *Br J Pharmacol* 1988; 94: 397.

Camilleri M, Brown ML, Malagelada JR. Impaired transit of chyme in chronic intestinal pseudoobstruction. Correction by cisapride. *Gastroenterology* 1986; 91: 619.

Camilleri M, et al. Effect of six weeks of treatment with cisapride on gastroparesis and intestinal pseudoobstruction. *Gastroenterology* 1989; 96: 704.

Chbeddu LX. Serotonin mechanisms in chemotherapy-induced emesis in cancer patients. *Oncology* 1996; 54(Suppl 1): 18–25.

Clayton NM, Gale JD. 5-HT$_4$ receptors are not involved in the control of small intestinal transit in the fasted conscious rat. *Neurogastroenterol Motility* 1996; 8: 1–8.

Cohen ML, Bloomquist W, Gidda JS, Lacefield W. LY277359 maleate: a potent and selective 5-HT$_3$ receptor antagonist without gastroprokinetic activity. *J Pharmacol Exp Ther* 1990; 254: 350.

Corinaldesi R, Stanghelllini V, Raiti C, et al. Effect of chronic administration of cisapride on gastric emptying of a solid meal and on dyspeptic symptoms in patients with idiopathic gastroparesis. *Gut* 1987; 28: 300.

Costall B, Gunning SJ, Naylor RJ, Tyers MB. Effect of GR38032F, novel 5-HT$_3$-receptor antagonist on gastric emptying in the guinea pig. *Br J Pharmacol* 1987; 91: 263.

Costell B, Naylor RJ, Tuladhar BR. 5-HT$_4$ receptor mediated facilitation of the emptying phase of the peristaltic reflex in the guinea-pig isolated ileum. *Br J Pharmacol* 1993; 110: 1572.

Cowles VE, Sarna SK. Relation between small intestinal motor activity and transit in secretory diarrhea. *Am J Physiol* 1990; 259 (*Gastrointest Liver Physiol* 22): G420–G429.

Craig DA, Clarke DE. Peristalsis evoked by 5-HT and renzapride: evidence for putative 5-HT$_4$ receptor activation. *Br J Pharmacol* 1991; 102: 563–564.

Currow DC, Coughlan M, Fardell B, Cooney NJ. Use of ondansetron in palliative medicine. *J Pain Symptom Manage* 1997; 13: 302–307.

Costa M, Furness JB. Sites of action of 5-hydroxytryptamine in nerve–muscle preparations from the guinea-pig small intestine and colon. *Br J Pharmacol* 1979; 65: 237–248.

Derkach V, Surprenant A, North RA. 5-HT$_3$ receptors are membrane ion channels. *Nature* 1989; 339: 706.

Dumuis A, Stebben E, Monferini M, Nicola M, Turconi M, Ladinsky H, Bochaert J. Azabicycloalkyl benzimidazolone derivatives as a novel class of potent agonists at the 5-HT$_4$ receptor positively coupled to adenylate cyclase in brain. *Naunyn Schmeideberg's Arch Pharmacol* 1991; 343: 245.

Eglen RM, Swank SR, Walsh LKM, Whiting RL. Characterization of 5-HT$_3$ and 'atypical' 5-HT receptors mediating guinea-pig ileal contractions *in vitro*. *Br J Pharmacol* 1990; 101: 513–520.

Eglen RM, Lee C, Smith WL, Johnson LG, Whiting RL, Hedge SS. RS 42358–197, a novel and potent 5-HT$_3$ receptor antagonist, *in vitro* and *in vivo*. *J Pharmacol Exp Ther* 1993; 266: 535.

Emmanuel AV, Kamm MA, Roy AJ, Antonelli K. Effect of a novel prokinetic drug, R093877, on gastrointestinal transit in healthy volunteers. *Gut* 1998; 42: 511–516.

Erspamer V. Occurrence of indolealkylamines in nature, in *Handbook of Experimental Pharmacology: 5-Hydroxytryptamine and Related Indolealkylamines*, vol 19 (Erspamer V, ed.), Springer-Verlag, New York, 1966.

Flynn DL, Zabrowski DL, Becker DP, Nosal R, Villamil CI, Gullikson GW, Moummi C, Yang D-C. SC-53116: the first selective agonist at the newly identified serotonin 5-HT$_4$ receptor subtype. *J Med Chem* 1992; 35: 1486.

Foxx-Orenstein AE, Kuemmerle JF, Grider JR. Distinct 5-HT receptors mediate the peristaltic reflex induced by mucosal stimuli in human and guinea pig intestine. *Gastroenterology* 1996; 111: 1281–1290.

Fortune DH, Ireland SJ, Tyers MB. Phenylbiguanide mimics the effect of 5-hydroxytryptamine on the rat isolated vagus nerve and superior cervical ganglion. *Br J Pharmacol* 1983; 81: 298P.

Fraser R, Horowitz M, Maddox A, et al. Dual effects of cisapride on gastric emptying and antropyloroduodenal motility. *Amer J Phys* 1993; 264 (*Gastrointest Liver Physiol*): G195.

Furness JB, Costa M. Neurons with 5-hydroxytryptamine-like immunoreactivity in the enteric nervous system: their projections in the guinea-pig small intestine. *Neuroscience* 1982; 7: 341.

Gale JD, Grossman CJ, Darton J, Bunce KT, Whitehead JWF, Knight J, et al. GR125487: a selective and high affinity 5-HT$_4$ receptor antagonist. *Br J Pharmacol* 1994a; 113: 120P.

Gale JD, Grossman CJ, Whitehead JWF, Oxford AW, Bunce KT, Humphrey PPA. GR113808: a novel, selective antagonist with high affinity at the 5-HT$_4$ receptor. *Br J Pharmacol* 1994b; 111: 332.

Gershon MD, Ross LL. Location of sites of 5-hydroxytryptamine storage and metabolism by radioautography. *J Physiol* 1966; 186: 477.

Gershon MD, Dreyfus CF, Pickel VM, John TH, Reis, DJ. Serotonergic neurons in the peripheral nervous system: identification in gut by immunohistochemical localization of tryptophan hydroxylase. *Proc Natl Acad Sci USA*, 1977; 74: 3086.

Gershon, MD. Localization and neurochemical aspects of serotonin in the gut, in *Serotonin and Gastrointestinal Function* (Gaginella TS, Galligan JJ, eds.) CRC, New York, 1995.

Gomme L, Verlinden M. Therapeutic efficacy of cisapride in elderly patients with atonic constipation. *Digestion* 1986; 34: 159.

Graf S, Sarna SK. 5-HT induced jejunal motor activity: enteric locus of action and receptor sub-types. *Am J Physiol* 1996; 270 (*Gastrointest Liver Physiol* 33): G992–G1000.

Graf S, Sarna SK. 5-HT-induced colonic contractions: enteric locus of action and receptor subtypes. *Am J Physiol* 1997; 273 (*Gastrointest Liver Physiol* 36): G68–G74.

Grider JR, Kuemmerle JF, Jin J-G. 5-HT released by mucosal stimuli initiates peristalsis by activating 5-HT$_4$/5-HT$_{1p}$ receptors on sensory CGRP neurons. *Am J Physiol* 1996; 270 (*Gastrointest Liver Physiol* 33): G778–G782.

Gullikson GW, Loeffler RF, Viriña MA. Relationship of serotonin–3 receptor antagonist activity to gastric emptying and motor-stimulating actions of prokinetic drugs in dogs. *J Pharmacol Exp Ther* 1991; 258: 103.

Haba T, Sarna SK. Regulation of gastroduodenal emptying of solids by gastropyloroduodenal contractions. *Am J Physiol* 1993; 264 (*Gastrointest Liver Physiol* 27): G261–G271.

Haga N, Mizumoto A, Satoh M, Mochiki E, Mizusawa F, Ohshima H, Itoh Z. Role of endogenous 5-hydroxytryptamine in the regulation of gastric contractions by motilin in dogs. *Am J Physiol* 1996; 270 (*Gastrointest Liver Physiol* 33): G20–G28.

Hasler WL, Heldsinger A, Owyang C. Cisapride acts on muscarinic (glandular

M2) receptors to induce contractions if isolated gastric myocytes: mediation via a calcium-phosphoinositide pathway. *J Pharmacol Exp Ther* 1991; 259: 1294.

Higgins GA, Kilpatrick GJ, Bunce KT, Jones BJ, Tyers MB. 5-HT$_3$ receptor antagonists injected into the area postrema inhibit cisplatin-induced emesis in the ferret. *Br J Pharmacol* 1989; 97: 247–255.

Hirst GDS, Holman ME, Spence I. Two types of neurons in the myenteric plexus of duodenum in guinea pig. *J Physiol* 1974; 236: 303.

Hirst GDS, Silinsky EM. Some effects of 5-hydroxytryptamine, dopamine and noradrenaline on neurones in the submucous plexus of guinea pig small intestine. *J Physiol* 1975; 251: 817.

Horowitz M, Maddern GJ, Maddox A, et al. Effect of cisapride on gastric and esophageal emptying in progressive systemic sclerosis. *Gastroenterology* 1987; 93: 311.

Hoyer D, Clarke DE, Fozard JR, Hartig PR, Martin GR, Mylecharane EJ, Saxena PR, Humphrey PPA. VII. International Union of Pharmacology classification of receptors for 5-hydroxytryptamine (serotonin). *Pharmacol Rev* 1994; 46: 157–203.

Jantunen IT, Kataja VV, Muhonen TT. An overview of randomised studies comparing 5-HT$_3$ receptor antagonists to conventional anti-emetics in the prophylaxis of acute chemotherapy-induced vomiting. *Eur J Cancer* 1997; 33: 66–74.

Jian R, Ducrot F, Piedeloup C, et al. Measurement of gastric emptying in dyspeptic patients: Effect of a new gastrointestinal agent. *Gut* 1985; 26: 352.

Jouët P, Sarna SK, Singaram C, Ryan RP, Hillard CJ, Telford GL, Fink J, Henderson JD. Immunocytes and abnormal gastrointestinal motor activity during experimental ileitis in dogs. *Am J Physiol* 1995; 269 (*Gastrointest Liver Physiol* 32): G913–G924.

Kadowaki M, Wade PR, Gershon MD. Interactions of 5-HT and nicotinic receptors in the peristaltic reflex of the guinea pig distal colon. *Gastroenterology* 1994; 106: A520.

Kadowaki M, Nagakura Y, Tomoi M, Mori J, Kohsaka M. Effect of FK1052, a potent 5-hydroxytryptamine, and 5-hydroxytryptamine$_4$ receptor dual antagonist, on colonic function *in vivo*. *J Pharmacol Exp Ther* 1993; 266: 74.

Karaus M, Sarna SK. Giant migrating contractions during defecation in the dog colon. *Gastroenterology* 1987; 92: 925–933.

Karaus M, Prasad KR, Sarna SK, Lang IM. Differential effects of [Gln^4] neurotensin on circular and longitudinal muscle of dog ileum in vitro. *Am J Physiol* 1987; (*Gastrointest Liver Physiol*): 253: G566–G572.

Kellow JE, Borody TJ, Phillips SF, Tucker RL, Haddad AC. Human interdigestive motility: variations in patterns from esophagus to colon. *Gastroenterology* 1986; 91: 386–395.

Kellow JE, Phillips SF. Altered small bowel motility in irritable bowel syndrome is correlated with symptoms. *Gastroenterology* 1987; 92: 1885–1893.

Kilbinger H, Wolf D. Effects of 5-HT$_4$ receptor stimulation on basal and electrically evoked release of acetylcholine from guinea-pig myenteric plexus. *Naunyn Schmiedeberg's Arch Pharmacol* 1992; 345: 270–275.

Kilpatrick GJ, Butler A, Burridge J, Oxford AW. 1-(*m*-chlorophenyl)-biguanide, a potent high affinity 5-HT$_3$ receptor agonist. *Eur J Pharmacol* 1990; 182: 193.

Krevsky B, Maurer AH, Malmud LS, et al. Cisapride accelerates colonic transit in constipated patients with colonic inertia. *Am J Gastroenterol* 1989; 84: 882.

Kuemmerle JF, Murthy KS, Makhlouf GM. Agonist-activated, ryanodine-sensitive, IP$_3$-insensitive Ca^{2+} release channels in longitudinal muscle of intestine. *Am J Physiol* (*Cell Physiol*) 1994; 266: C1421–C1431.

Kuemmerle JF, Murthy KS, Grider JR, Martin DC, Makhlouf GM. Coexpression of 5-HT$_{2A}$ and 5-HT$_4$ receptors coupled to distinct signaling pathways in human intestinal muscle cells. *Gastroenterology* 1995; 109: 1791–1800.

Lang IM, Sarna SK. Gastrointestinal motor correlates of vomiting in the dog: quantification and characterization as an independent phenomenon. *Gastroenterology* 1986; 90: 4–47.

Lang IM, Marvig J, Sarna SK, Condon RE. The gastrointestinal myoelectric correlates of vomiting in the dog. *Am J Physiol* 1986; 251 (*Gastrointest Liver Physiol* 14): G830–G838.

Linnik MD, Butler BT, Gaddis RR, Ahmed NK. Analysis of serotonergic mechanisms underlying benzamide-induced gastroprokinesis. *J Pharmacol Exp Ther* 1991; 259: 501.

Marty M, Pouillart P, Scholl S, Droz JP, Azab M, Brion N, et al. Comparison of the 5-hydroxytryptamine$_3$ (serotonin) antagonist ondansetron (GR 38032F) with high-dose metoclopramide in the control of cisplatin-induced emesis. *N Engl J Med* 1990; 322: 846–848.

McCallum RW, Prakash C, Campoli-Richardson DM, Goa KL. Cisapride: a preliminary review of its pharmacodynamic and pharmacokinetic properties, and therapeutic use as a prokinetic agent in gastrointestinal motility disorders. *Drugs* 1988; 36: 652–681.

Middlefell VC, Price TL. 5-HT$_3$ receptor agonism may be responsible for the emetic effects of zacropride in the ferret. *Br J Pharmacol* 1991; 103: 1011.

Minami M, Endo T, Hirafuji M. Role of serotonin in emesis. *Nippon Yakurigaka Zasshi Fol Pharmacol Jpn* 1996; 108: 233–242.

Müller-Lissner SA, et al. Treatment of chronic constipation with cisapride and placebo. *Gut* 1987; 28: 1033.

Murthy KS, Grider JR, Makhlouf GM. InsP$_3$-dependent Ca^{2+} mobilization in circular but not longitudinal muscle cells of intestine. *Am J Physiol* 1991; (*Gastrointest Liver Physiol*); 261: G937–G944.

Neild TO. Action of 5-hydroxytryptamine and possible 5-hydroxytryptamine antagonists on neurones of the guinea pig submucous plexus. *Gen Pharmacol* 1980; 12: 284.

Nielsen OH, Hvid-Jacobsen K, Lund P, Langholz E. Gastric emptying and subjective symptoms of nausea: lack of effect of a 5-hydroxytryptamine–3 antagonist ondansetron on gastric emptying in patients with gastric stasis syndrome. *Digestion* 1990; 46: 89.

Nishi S, North RA. Intracellular recordings from the myenteric plexus of guinea pig ileum. *J Physiol* 1973; 231: 471.

Orihata M, Sarna SK. Contractile mechanisms of action of gastroprokinetic agents: cisapride, metoclopramide, and domperidone. *Am J Physiol* 1994; 266 (*Gastrointest. Liver Physiol* 29): G665–G676.

Orihata M, Sarna SK. Nitric oxide mediates mechano- and chemo-receptor activated intestinal feedback control of gastric emptying. *Dig Dis Sci* 1996; 41: 1303–1309.

Ormsbee HS III, Silber DA, Hardy FE Jr. Serotonin regulation of the canine migrating motor complex. *J Pharmacol Exp Ther* 1984; 231: 436–440.

Otterson MF, Sarna SK. Neural control of small intestinal giant migrating contractions. *Am J Physiol* 1994; 266 (*Gastrointest Liver Physiol* 29): G576–G584.

Pan H, Galligan JJ. 5-HT$_{1A}$ and 5-HT$_4$ receptors mediate inhibition and facilitation of fast synaptic transmission in enteric neurons. *Am J Physiol* 1994; 266 (*Gastrointest. Liver Physiol* 29): G230–G238.

Pan H, Galligan JJ. Effects of 5-HT1A and 5-HT4 receptor agonists on slow synaptic potentials in enteric neurons. *Eur J Pharmacol* 1995; 278: 67–74.

Quigley EMM, Phillips SF, Dent J. Distinctive patterns of interdigestive motility of the canine ileocolonic junction. *Gastroenterology* 1984; 87: 836–844.

Rajendran SK, Reiser JR, Bauman W, et al. Gastrointestinal transit after spinal cord injury: effect of cisapride. *Am J Gastroenterol* 1992; 87: 1614.

Richards R, Valenzuela G, McCallum R, et al. Objective and subjective results of a randomized double blind placebo controlled trial using cisapride to treat gastroparesis. *Dig Dis Sci* 1993; 38: 811.

Richardson BP, Engel G, Donatsch P, Stadler PA. Identification of serotonin M-receptor subtypes and their specific blockade by a new class of drugs. *Nature* 1985; 316: 126.

Rizzi CA, Sagrada A, Schiavone A, Schiantarelli P, Cesana R, Schiavi GB, Ladinski H, Donetti A. Gastroprokinetic properties of the benzimidazolone derivative BIMU 1, an agonist at 5-hydroxytryptamine$_4$ and antagonist at 5-hydroxytryptamine$_3$ receptors. *Naunyn Schmiedeberg's Arch Pharmacol* 1994; 349: 338.

Roberts JT, Priestman TJ. A review of ondansetron in the management of radiotherapy-induced emesis. *Oncology* 1993; 50: 173–179.

Sarna SK, Stoddard C, Belbeck L, McWade D. Intrinsic neural control of migrating myoelectric complexes. *Am J Physiol* 1981; 241 (*Gastrointest Liver Physiol* 4): G16–G23.

Sarna SK. Cyclic motor activity; migrating motor complex: 1985. *Gastroenterology* 1985; 89: 894–913.

Sarna SK. Giant migrating contractions and their myoelectric correlates in the small intestine. *Am J Physiol* 1987; 253: G697–G705.

Sarna SK. In vivo myoelectric activity: methods, analysis and interpretation, in *Handbook of Physiology, Gastrointestinal Motility and Circulation*, (Wood JD, ed.) American Physiology Society, Bethesda, MD, 1989, pp. 817–863.

Sarna SK, Otterson MF. Prokinetic effects of cisapride on the colon and the small intestine. *Gastroenterology* 1992; 102: A508.

Sarna SK, Otterson MF. Myoelectric and contractile activities in *Atlas of Gastrointestinal Motility in Health and Disease*, (Schuster MM, ed.) Williams & Wilkins, Baltimore, MD, 1993, pp. 3–42.

Schiavone A, Volonté M, Micheletti R. Gastrointestinal motor effect of benzamide derivatives is unrelated to 5-HT₃ receptor blockade. *Eur J Pharmacol* 1990; 197: 323.

Sethi AK, Sarna SK. Colonic motor activity in acute colitis in conscious dogs. *Gastroenterology* 1991; 100: 954–963.

Sethi AK, Sarna SK. Colonic motor response to a meal in acute colitis. *Gastroenterology* 1991; 101: 1537–1546.

Shi X-Z, Sarna SK. Inflammatory modulation of muscarinic receptor activation in canine ileal circular muscle cells. *Gastroenterology* 1997; 112: 864–874.

Stacher G, Bergmann H, Wiesnargrotzki S, et al. Intravenous cisapride accelerates delayed gastric emptying and increases antral contraction amplitude in patients with primary anorexia nervosa. *Gastroenterology* 1987; 92: 1000.

Steadman CJ, Talley NJ, Phillips SF, Zinsmeister AR. Selective 5-hydroxytryptamine Type 3 receptor antagonism with ondansetron as treatment for diarrhea-predominant irritable bowel syndrome: a pilot study. *Mayo Clin Proc* 1992; 67: 732–738.

Summers RW, Anuras S, Green J. Jejunal manometry patterns in health, partial intestinal obstruction and pseudo-obstruction. *Gastroenterology* 1983; 85: 1290–1300.

Szurszewski JH. Migrating electric complex of the canine small intestine. *Am J Physiol* 1969; 217: 1757–1763.

Talley NJ, Phillips SF, Haddad A, Miller LJ, Twomey C, Zinsmeister AR, Ciociola A. Effect of selective 5-HT₃ antagonist (GR 38032F) on small intestinal transit and release of gastrointestinal peptides. *Dig Dis Sci* 1989; 34: 1511.

Talley NJ, Phillips SF, Haddad A, Miiller LJ, Twomey C, Zinsmeister AR, MacCarty RL, Ciociola A. GR 38032F (ondansetron), a selective 5-HT$_3$ receptor antagonist, slows colonic transit in healthy man. *Dig Dis Sci* 1990; 35: 477–480.

Tonini M, Galligan JJ, North RA. Effects of cisapride on cholinergic neurotransmission and propulsive motility in the guinea pig ileum. *Gastroenterology* 1989; 96: 1257.

Tonini M, Candura SM, Onori L, Coccini T, Manzo L, Rizzi CA. 5-hydroxytryptamine4 receptor agonists facilitate cholinergic transmission in the circular muscle of guinea pig ileum: antagonism by tropisetron and DAU 6285. *Life Sci* 1992; 50: PL173–PL178.

Tramer MR, Reynolds DJ, Moore RA, McQuay HJ. Efficacy, dose-response, and safety of ondansetron in prevention of postoperative nausea and vomiting: a quantitative systematic review of randomized placebo-controlled trials. *Anesthesiology* 1997; 87: 1271–1273.

Tsukamoto M, Sarna SK, Condon RE. Novel motility effect of tachykinins in normal and inflamed colon. *Am J Physiol* 1997; 272 (*Gastrointest Liver Physiol* 35): G1607–G1614.

Van Daele L, DeCupeyere A, Van Kerckhove M. Routine radiologic follow through examination shows effect of cisapride on gastrointestinal transit: a controlled study. *Curr Ther Res* 1984; 36: 1038.

Verheyen K, Vervaeke M, Demyttenaere P, et al. Double blind comparison of two cisapride dosage regimens with placebo in the treatment of functional constipation. *Curr Ther Res* 1987; 41: 978.

Von der Ohe MR, Hanson RB, Camilleri M. Serotonergic mediation of postprandial colonic tonic and phasic responses in humans. *Gut* 1994; 35: 536–541.

Wardle KA, Ellis ES, Baxter GS, Kennett GA, Gastor LM, Sanger GJ. Effects of SB204070, a highly potent and selective 5-HT$_4$ receptor antagonist on guinea pig distal colon. *Br J Pharmacol* 1994; 112: 789.

Wattchow DA, Brookes SJH, Costa M. Morphology and projections of retrogradely labeled myenteric neurons in the human intestine. *Gastroenterology* 1995; 109: 866–875.

Wilmer A, Tack J, Coremans G, Janssens J, Peeters T, Vantrappen G. 5-hydroxytryptamine–3 receptors are involved in the initiation of gastric phase–3 motor activity in humans. *Gastroenterology* 1993; 105: 773–780.

Wood JD. Excitation of intestinal muscle by atropine, tetrodotoxin, and xylocaine. *Am J Physiol* 1972; 222: 118–125.

Yoshida N, Mizumoto A, Iwanaga Y, Itoh Z. Effects of 5-hydroxytryptamine 3 receptor antagonists on gastrointestinal motor activity in conscious dogs. *J Pharmacol Exp Ther* 1991; 256: 272–278.

8 Opioid Receptors

Targets for New Gastrointestinal Drug Development

Pierre J. M. Rivière and Jean-Louis Junien

CONTENTS

1. INTRODUCTION

For centuries, opium and its derivatives have been used for both therapeutic and recreational purposes. One such derivative, morphine, is still one of the most used analgesics. Besides a predominant role in pain control (both somatic and visceral pain), opioids and opioid receptors have a broad spectrum of actions, including modulations of reinforcement and reward pathways, neurotransmitter release, neuroendocrine functions, as well as gastrointestinal (GI) motility, transit, and secretion. The opioid drugs made available, or clinically tested as analgesics, have essentially targeted μ- and κ-receptors in the central nervous system (CNS). The development and use of such compounds have been limited or even discontinued because of their side effects

From: *Drug Development: Molecular Targets for GI Diseases*
Edited by: T. S. Gaginella and A. Guglietta © Humana Press Inc., Totowa, NJ

(constipation, respiratory depression, addiction potential, and/or aversion). Only peripherally acting μ-agonists have been approved for therapeutic use in gastroenterology.

The therapeutic potential of opioids, as well as their side effect properties, have stimulated large scientific, medical, and pharmaceutical research efforts, which have resulted in a significant improvement in the understanding of the opioid field. This chapter reviews current knowledge in molecular biology, distribution, and pharmacology of the opioid receptor subtypes, their putative interest as targets for development of GI drugs, and current status of drug development in this field. New applications could arise for treatment of diarrheic syndromes, motility disorders (postoperative ileus, constipation), and visceral pain (postoperative pain, irritable bowel syndrome [IBS], inflammatory bowel disease [IBD]).

2. OPIOID RECEPTORS

The existence of specific membrane-bound receptors mediating the effects of opioid drugs emerged in the 1970s (Goldstein et al., 1971; Pert and Snyder, 1973; Simon et al., 1973; Terenius, 1973). The opioid receptors were further defined and classified into pharmacological subtypes (Lord et al., 1977; Martin et al., 1976). Martin et al. (1976) showed that a selection of opioids had heterogenous and distinct pharmacological profiles in dogs, and postulated the existence of three opioid receptors subtypes, μ for morphine, κ for ketocyclazocine, and σ for norallylmetazocine (SKF-10,047). Further pharmacological (Musacchio, 1990) and molecular biology (Hanner et al., 1996) studies have suggested that the σ-receptor cannot be classified as an opioid receptor subtype. Contemporaneous with Martin's work, Lord et al. (1977) discovered the existence of another opioid receptor called "delta" (δ), identified in the mouse vas deferens, leading to the commonly accepted division of the opioid receptor family into μ-, δ-, and κ-receptor subtypes. The rodent and human forms of these three receptor subtypes were cloned at the beginning of the 1990s. Further pharmacological subdivisions of each major opioid receptor subtype have been proposed, and are reviewed below.

2.1. Cloned Opioid and Opioid-like Receptors

The mouse δ-opioid receptor (mDOR1) was the first opioid receptor to be cloned (Evans et al., 1992; Kieffer et al., 1992). This opened the way for the cloning of μ- (MOR1) and κ- (KOR1) opioid receptors (Table 1). The pharmacological properties of the cloned MOR1s, DOR1s, and KOR1s were found to closely fit the profile of the postulated μ-, δ-, and κ-receptor subtypes (Knapp et al., 1995; Raynor et al., 1994a, 1994b). In addition to the above three predicted opioid receptor subtypes, an orphan opioid receptor-like 1 receptor (ORL1) was cloned (Mollereau et al., 1994). Whether or not the ORL1 should be considered as an opioid receptor is still debated, on the basis of structural homologies and pharmacological property differences. The ORL1 (Mollereau et al., 1994) and its endogenous ligand (Meunier et al., 1995) are structurally related to the other opioid receptors and opioid ligands, but, unlike the conventional opioid receptors (MOR1, DOR1, and KOR1), ORL1 is not sensitive to naloxone, the nonselective opioid antagonist (Nicholson et al., 1998). The ORL1 is identical to an orphan receptor cloned by others, and referred to as "Kappa 3-related opioid receptor" (KOR1-3) (Pan et al., 1995, 1996, 1998). The mouse-, rat- and human MOR1, DOR1, KOR1, as well as ORL1, have all been cloned (Table 1).

The structural and functional characteristics of the MOR1, DOR1, KOR1, and ORL1 are summarized in Table 2. These receptors share many common features. They have about the same amino acid length (367–400). They all belong to the G-protein-coupled receptor family. These receptors contain hydrophobic α-helices, which correspond to seven putative transmembrane domains, and have short intra- and extracellular loops. The MOR1, DOR1, KOR1, and ORL1 display inhibitory coupling to adenylyl cyclase (Knapp et al., 1995). Each of these receptors can couple to either G_i or G_o proteins. The structure of each opioid receptor subtype is highly preserved among the different species in which they were cloned (about 95% sequence homology between mouse, rat, and human receptors). This is of importance, because it validates the use of rodents to explore opioid systems. Conversely, there is only 50–60% overall sequence homology among the MOR1, DOR1, KOR1, and ORL1. The most divergent regions of these receptors are the N- and C-termini, transmembrane 4, and extracellular loops 2 and 3; the intracellular loops and other transmembrane regions are

Table 1
Cloning of Opioid and Opioid-like Receptors

Cloning of opioid and opioid-like receptors

Species	MOR1	DOR1	KOR1	ORL1
Human	Wang et al., 1994	Knapp et al., 1994; Simonin et al., 1994	Mansson et al., 1994; Simonin et al., 1995; Zhu et al., 1995	Mollereau et al., 1994
Rat	Chen et al., 1993; Thompson et al., 1993; Wang et al., 1993	Abood et al., 1994	Chen et al., 1993; Li et al., 1993; Meng et al., 1993; Minami et al., 1993	Wang et al., 1994
Mouse	Kaufman et al., 1995; Liang et al., 1995	Evans et al., 1992; Kieffer et al., 1992	Yasuda et al., 1993; Tallent et al., 1994	Mollereau et al., 1994; Pan et al., 1995
Guinea Pig			Xie et al., 1994	

Table 2
Structural and Functional Characteristics of Cloned Opioid and opioid-like Receptors

	Cloned opioid and opioid-like receptors			
	MOR1	DOR1	KOR1	ORL1
Human gene localization	6q24-25	1p34.3-p36.1	8q11-12	
Receptor structure	7TMB	7TMB	7TMB	7TMB
Receptor classification	GPCR	GPCR	GPCR	GPCR
Amino acid length	h400	h372	h380	H370
	r398	r372	r380	r367
	m398	m372	m380	m367
Homology among species	97%	94%	93%	99%
Homology with other opioid receptor subtypes	≈60%	≈60%	≈60%	≈50%
Effector, second messenger	Gi/Go Adenylyl cyclase inhibition ↓ cAMP	Gi/Go Adenylyl cyclase inhibition ↓ cAMP	Gi/Go Adenylyl cyclase inhibition ↓ cAMP	Gi/Go Adenylyl cyclase inhibition ↓ cAMP

MOR1, cloned μ-opioid receptor; DOR1, cloned δ-opioid receptor; KOR1, cloned κ-opioid receptor; GPCR, G-protein-coupled receptor; 7TMB, seven transmembrane domains; h, human; r, rat; m, mouse.

more conserved (Fig. 1). The marked structural differences in the extracellular regions of the opioid receptors may serve as a basis for the design of new opioid ligands, with even higher selectivity for each receptor subtype than those currently available. In addition to the structural differences, the genes for the opioid receptor subtypes are localized on different chromosomes, 6q24-25 for hMOR1 (Wang et al., 1994), 1p34.3-p36.1 for hDOR1 (Befort et al., 1994), and 8q11-12 for hKOR1 (Simonin et al., 1995).

2.2. Pharmacological Characterization
of Subtypes of Opioid Receptors

In addition to the cloned opioid receptors, in vitro and in vivo pharmacological data suggest further subdivisions of each major opioid receptor into multiple subtypes. Most of the evidence comes from studies investigating the receptor binding profile of opioid ligands to brain membrane homogenates, or the central antinociceptive activities of opioids.

Early on, it was shown that the μ-receptor population, labeled by [^{3}H]-dihydromorphine in rodent brain membrane homogenates, contains both high- and low-affinity μ-binding sites, termed μ_1 and μ_2, respectively (Hahn and Pasternak, 1982; Nishimura et al., 1984; Pasternak, 1982). In these preparations, morphine preferentially displaces ligand binding at μ_2 sites, and oxymorphonazine (agonist), naloxonazine (irreversible antagonist), and [D-Ala^2,D-Leu^5]enkephalin are potent and selective inhibitors of the μ_1 binding sites. Although both μ_1 and μ_2 sites were found in the brain, only the μ_2 sites have been described in guinea pig ileum (Gintzler and Pasternak, 1983). It was suggested that the antinociceptive effects of morphine are mediated at naloxonazine-sensitive sites (μ_1), but the antitransit effects of morphine were resistant to naloxonazine antagonism (Heyman et al., 1988), suggesting the involvement of μ_2 sites in the latter case. The binding profiles of the cloned MOR1 and μ_1 sites are similar (Raynor et al., 1994a).

Both binding and functional studies suggest that the population of δ-receptors is heterogenous. In mouse brain membranes, [D-Pen^2,D-Pen^5]enkephalin ([^{3}H]-DPDPE) and [D-Ser^2,Leu^5,Thr^6]enkephalin ([^{3}H]-DSLET), two δ-agonists, label two different populations of δ-receptors

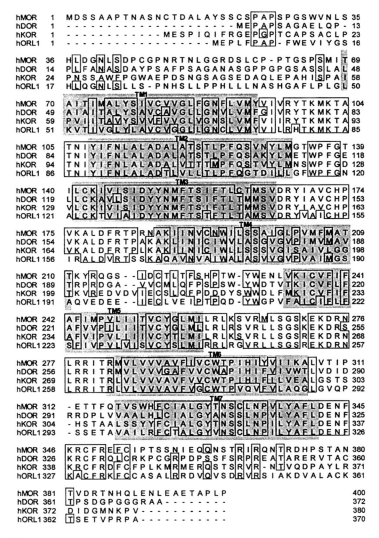

Fig. 1. Compared deduced amino acid sequences of the cloned human µ- (hMOR1), δ- (hDOR1), κ- (hKOR1) opioid receptors and cloned human opioid receptor-like 1 receptor (hORL1), using, respectively, the L25119 (Wang *et al.*, 1994), U10504 (Simonin *et al.*, 1994), U17298 (Mansson *et al.*, 1994), and X77130 (Mollereau *et al.*, 1994) Genbank accession codes. The sequences were aligned and displayed using ClustalX and SeqVu programs. The approximate locations of the putative transmembrane regions are shaded in gray. Identical residues are boxed.

(Sofuoglu et al., 1992). These two binding sites are differently displaced by the δ-antagonists 7-benzylidenenaltrexone (BNTX) and naltrindole-5'-isothiocyanate (5'-NTII): BNTX is selective for the DPDPE-binding site (Portoghese et al., 1992), 5'-NTII is selective for the DSLET-binding site (Chakrabarti et al., 1993). The DPDPE and DSLET sites have been referred as δ_1 and δ_2 sites, respectively.

Functional studies support the idea that opioid δ-receptors may be distinguished on the basis of their involvement in the modulation (i.e., increase or decrease in potency) of μ-mediated antinociception (Mattia et al., 1991). On this basis, it was hypothesized that some opioid δ-receptors exist within a functional complex with μ-receptors ($\delta_{complexed}$ [δ_{cx}] receptors), but other δ sites do not ($\delta_{noncomplexed}$ [δ_{ncx}] receptors). Binding studies have shown that δ_{ncx} can be further subdivided into high- and low-affinity sites, both in rat (Xu et al., 1991) and in mouse (Xu et al., 1998), termed δ_{ncx1} and δ_{ncx2}, respectively. [D-Ala^2]deltorphin II and DPDPE, two δ-receptor agonists, are preferential ligands for the δ_{ncx1} and δ_{ncx2} sites, respectively (Xu et al., 1992). The binding profile of the mouse DOR1 matches the binding profile of δ_{ncx1} sites (Xu et al., 1998) and δ_2 sites (Raynor et al., 1994a). In mice, both DPDPE and [D-Ala^2]deltorphin II have central antinociceptive properties (Qi et al., 1990), but their analgesic responses are differentially blocked by [D-Ala^2,Leu^5,Cys^6]enkephalin (DALCE) and 5'-NTII, two δ-receptor antagonists. DALCE inhibits DPDPE, but not [D-Ala^2]deltorphin II responses; 5'-NTII antagonizes [D-Ala^2]deltorphin II, but not DPDPE analgesia (Jiang et al., 1991). Finally, although it is possible to separately establish tolerance to both [D-Ala^2]deltorphin II and DPDPE, there is no development of antinociceptive cross-tolerance between [D-Ala^2]deltorphin II and DPDPE (Mattia et al., 1991).

Binding studies in guinea pig brain have evidenced two distinct populations of κ-receptors, termed κ_1 (U69,593-sensitive) and κ_2 (U69,593-resistant and bremazocine-sensitive), each one being further subdivided into high- and low-affinity binding sites, leading to the hypothesis of the existence of a total of four κ-receptor subtypes (κ_{1a}, κ_{1b}, κ_{2a}, κ_{2b}) (Rothman et al., 1990). Initial characterizations concluded that the cloned KOR1 has pharmacological characteristics similar to those of the endogenously expressed κ_1-receptor (Raynor et al., 1994a) (Meng et al., 1993). Further studies suggest that the cloned KOR1 displays a binding profile similar to the mouse κ_{1b}-binding site (Lai et al., 1994). According to this classification, fedotozine is listed as a

Table 3
Proposed Correspondence Between Pharmacologically Characterized Opioid Receptor Subtypes and Cloned Receptors

	Cloned opioid and opioid-like receptors			
	MOR1	DOR1	KOR1	hORL1
Pharmacological subtypes	μ_1	δ_2 (δ_{ncx1}, δ_{ncx2})	κ_1 (κ_{1b}?)	κ_3

high-affinity κ_{1a} ligand (Lai et al., 1994). U69,593 and bremazocine, the proposed κ_1- and κ_2-preferred agonists, have both central antinociceptive activity in mice, and their effects are blocked by naloxone, the nonselective opioid antagonist (Horan et al., 1991, 1993). However, their analgesic responses are differentially blocked by (−)UPHIT[*] and quadazocine, two κ-receptor antagonists. The effects of U69,593 are blocked by (−)UPHIT, but not quadazocine; conversely, the effects of bremazocine are blocked by quadazocine, but not by (−)UPHIT (Horan et al., 1991, 1993). Finally, although it is possible to separately induce tolerance to both U69,593 and bremazocine, there is no development of cross-tolerance between the two compounds (Horan and Porreca, 1993).

The pharmacological properties of naloxone benzoylhydrazone (NalBzoH), have suggested the existence of another κ-receptor subtype called κ_3 (Paul et al., 1990). NalBzoH acts as an antagonist to block μ_1-, μ_2- and κ-agonist mediated analgesia, but is also able to induce antinociception, an effect that is blocked by the opiate antagonist WIN44,441. Nalorphine was found to have the same atypical pharmacological profile (Paul et al., 1991). No cross-tolerance could be established between the κ_1-agonist U50,488H and nalorphine. Antisense oligodeoxynucleotides targeted at a newly cloned orphan and opioid related receptor were found to block κ_3-agonist-induced analgesia (Pan et al., 1995). Based on this observation, the orphan receptor was named KOR1-3. Its sequence is identical to that of ORL1 (Mollereau et al., 1994; Pan et al., 1995, 1996).

A correspondence between the cloned opioid receptors and pharmacological subtypes is proposed in Table 3.

[*]1S,ES-trans-2-isothiocyanate-4,5-dichloro-N-methyl-N-[2-(1-pyrrolidinyl) cyclobexyl] benzeneacetamide

All the above observations suggest the existence of functionally differentiated subtypes of μ-, δ-, and κ-opioid receptors. These subtypes were identified by investigating the spinal- and supraspinal opioid control of somatic pain. Whether or not these putative opioid receptor subtypes may be relevant to the control of GI functions, and visceral pain in particular, is still unknown. Should such putative pharmacological subtypes represent true receptor isoforms, minimal progress can be expected in this area until they are actually cloned.

2.3. Localization of Opioid Receptors

The existence of opioid receptors in the intestine and CNS has been known for many years. The recent cloning of the opioid receptors has given new tools for further exploring the anatomical distribution of each receptor subtype. *In situ* hybridization techniques can be used to visualize the receptor mRNAs, and therefore the cells that synthesize the receptors; immunohistochemistry techniques, using receptor-selective antibodies, can be used to visualize the receptor protein. Both methods are highly complementary and useful for exploring receptor trafficking. Only a few studies have explored the anatomical distribution of the cloned opioid receptors in the GI tract.

The presence of MOR1 and KOR1 has been confirmed in the GI tract by immunohistochemistry (Bagnol et al., 1997) and *in situ* hybridization (Fickel et al., 1997). The mRNAs and receptor protein maps overlap very well, confirming the local synthesis of opioid receptors within the GI tract, although receptor trafficking, in particular, from dorsal root ganglia (DRG) via primary sensory afferents cannot be excluded. These findings are in agreement with previous autoradiography data (Dashwood et al., 1985; Nishimura et al., 1986). MOR1 and KOR1 are widely distributed across the wall of the rat GI tract, with the highest level of expression in the stomach and proximal colon (Bagnol et al., 1997; Fickel et al., 1997). MOR1 and KOR1 are present in the myenteric and submucosal plexus, although differences exist: MOR1 is preferentially expressed in submucosal plexus; KOR1 is preferentially expressed in myenteric plexus. The MOR1 and KOR1 are localized on neurons and nerve fibers in myenteric plexus, as well as in the longitudinal and circular muscle layers. MOR1 and KOR1 immunoreactive fibers are very dense in the circular muscle layer, especially in the stomach and the colon. MOR1 and KOR1 immunoreactivity is also present in interstitial cells of Cajal. Neither KOR1 nor MOR1 immunoreactivity is present on smooth muscle cells. This last finding, however, contrasts with previous receptor binding and functional studies (Bitar and Makhlouf, 1985, 1982; Daniel et al., 1987; Grider and Makhlouf, 1991; Kuemmerle and Makhlouf, 1992), and may result from technique limitations. DOR1 mRNA was detected in porcine intestine, and DOR1-like immunoreactivity was localized in neurons within the myenteric and submucous ganglia, longitudinal and circular smooth muscle, and villous lamina propria (Brown et al., 1998). ORL1 receptors have been reported to be widely distributed in peripheral organs, including the intestine, spleen, and vas deferens (Wang et al., 1994).

Outside the intestine, MOR1, DOR1, and KOR1 are widely distributed in the CNS (for review, see Mansour et al., 1995). The distribution on the ascending and descending pain pathways is relevant to the spinal and supraspinal control of visceral pain by opioids. In the ascending pain pathway, MOR1, DOR1, and KOR1 are expressed in the DRG, spinal cord, spinal trigeminal nucleus. However, at the level of the thalamus, MOR1 and KOR1 expression is predominantly observed. In the descending inhibitory pain pathway, all three receptors are expressed in the central gray area, pontine, and gigantocellular and intermediate reticular nuclei, with predominant MOR1 and KOR1 expression in the periaqueductal gray, median raphe, and raphe magnus nuclei. MOR1, DOR1, and KOR1 are expressed in the DRG1, but the three receptor mRNAs are found in different cell populations. MOR1s are localized on large- and medium diameter cells; DOR1s are predominantly on large cells, and KOR1s are on medium and small cells. The functional consequence of this differential distribution is still unknown. Several studies have suggested that, after synthesis in the DRG cell bodies, MOR1, DOR1, and KOR1 migrate by axoplasmic transport to nerve terminals in the spinal cord and the periphery. μ-, δ-, and κ-binding is detected in the superficial lamina of the spinal cord (lamina I and II), in the absence of corresponding receptor mRNAs, suggesting that these binding sites are on presynaptic terminals, and are originating from DRG. Furthermore, a bidirectional transport of opioid receptors has been evidenced in the vagus (Laduron, 1984) and sciatic (Hassan et al., 1993) nerves. The transport occurs in capsaicin-sensitive fibers (Laduron, 1984). The trafficking of opioid receptors toward the periphery is markedly increased in the situation of tissue inflammation, leading to accumulation of opioid binding sites within the damaged tissue

(Hassan et al., 1993), especially μ- and κ-binding sites (Jeanjean et al., 1994, 1995). Transport of opioid receptors through GI primary sensory afferents and its enhancement under inflammation has not yet been described.

The presence of transcripts of the cloned MOR1, DOR1, and KOR1 have been confirmed in rodent and human immune cells (Chuang et al., 1995; Gaveriaux et al., 1995; Sedqi et al., 1995, 1996). δ- and κ-agonists were also shown to inhibit cell proliferation in the T47D human breast cancer cell line (Hatzoglou et al., 1996, 1996; Kampa et al., 1996). These effects were consistent with the presence of opioid-binding sites on the T47D cell line. There has been no confirmation of the expression of the already cloned opioid receptors in this cancer line.

3. ROLE OF OPIOID RECEPTORS IN GI FUNCTIONS AND THERAPEUTIC IMPLICATIONS

3.1. μ-Opioid Receptors

The main GI responses to the activation of μ-opioid receptors by selective agonists include a modulation of intestinal motility, a marked inhibition of intestinal transit (Bueno and Fioramonti, 1988; Burks et al., 1987; Kromer, 1988), and a potent antidiarrheal activity (Ruppin, 1987; Table 4). More recent data have shown that selective μ-opioid receptor agonists exhibit a potent antinociceptive activity in various visceral pain models (Burton and Gebhart, 1998; Danzebrink et al., 1995; Diop et al., 1994; Friese et al., 1997; Langlois et al., 1994; Maves and Gebhart, 1992). Apart from the above major GI responses to opioids, moderate actions on intestinal ion transport and gastric secretion have also been reported. The μ-opioid receptors involved in GI responses to opioids are located in the periphery, spinal cord, and brain (Bueno and Fioramonti, 1988; Burks et al., 1988; Diop et al., 1994).

Loperamide, loperamide-oxide, and trimebutine are the only μ-preferred agonists specifically developed and marketed for GI therapeutic indications. These opioids are peripherally acting compounds. Loperamide is used for the treatment of acute and chronic diarrhea; its mechanism of action has been extensively reviewed (Awouters et al., 1993; De Luca and Coupar, 1996; Ooms et al., 1984; Ruppin, 1987; Schiller

Table 4
Responses to Activation of μ-Opioid Receptors
in Function of Their Localization

	Effect	Receptor localization		
		Periphery	Spinal cord	Brain
Therapeutic targets				
Intestinal motility	↑	•		
	↓↓	•	•	•
Intestinal transit	↓↓↓	•	•	•
Diarrhea	↓↓↓	•	•	•
Intestinal ion transport	↑ (?)	•		•
Visceral pain	↓↓↓		•	•
Somatic pain	↓↓↓	•	•	•
Side effects				
Constipation	↑↑↑	•	•	•
Respiratory depression	↑↑↑			•
Euphoria, addiction	↑↑↑			•

et al., 1984). Loperamide reduces stool weight, frequency of bowel movements, urgency, and fecal incontinence in acute and chronic diarrhea, and is thought to primarily inhibit intestinal and colonic transit. This mechanism increases mucosal contact time, allowing more complete absorption of electrolytes and water. Besides its opiate-receptor-binding and stimulating activity, loperamide also behaves as a calcium–calmodulin antagonist, and as a calcium channel blocker (Ruppin, 1987). Unlike loperamide, which is viewed as a symptomatic treatment of diarrhea, future antidiarrheal drugs are expected to have a selective antisecretory mechanism of action (Aikawa and Karasawa, 1998; Rivière et al., 1990). Among the opioid receptor subtypes, peripheral δ-receptors are the target of choice to achieve such a profile (*see* subheading 3.2.).

Trimebutine is used for the treatment of both acute and chronic abdominal pain in patients with functional bowel disorders, especially IBS (Delvaux and Wingate, 1997). Trimebutine is a preferential, although not selective, μ-agonist; it binds to μ-opioid receptors with an approx 10-fold lower affinity than morphine (Kaneto et al., 1990;

Roman et al., 1987). Trimebutine also binds to δ- and κ-opioid receptors in dog myenteric plexus (Allescher et al., 1991), although no affinity was detected for κ-receptors in brain membrane preparations (Kaneto et al., 1990). In dogs, trimebutine stimulates small intestine motility, by inducing a propagated phase of regular spike activity (phase III), and inhibits colonic motility (Fioramonti et al., 1984). Similar effects are observed in humans: Trimebutine induces phase III-like activity in man (Chaussade et al., 1987; Grandjouan et al., 1989), as well as in children suffering from severe digestive dysmotility (Boige et al., 1987). In dogs, trimebutine-induced phase III-like activity is associated with a significant rise in plasma motilin which precedes the beginning of the premature phase III (Poitras et al., 1989). In IBS patients, trimebutine selectively inhibits long spike bursts, with a greater magnitude in the transverse than the descending colon. The effect is similar in constipated and diarrheic patients (Frexinos et al., 1985). Trimebutine also stimulates gastric emptying, possibly by shortening the lag time at the start of gastric emptying (Okano et al., 1993).

μ-opioid receptors are responsible of a series of receptor specific side effects, such as constipation, respiratory depression, dependence, tolerance, euphoria, and addiction. These side effects are mediated through either peripherally or centrally located μ-opioid receptors (Table 4). Constipation is, however, likely to be mediated at all levels. Studies in rodents have shown that peripheral, intrathecal, and intracerebroventricular administration of selective μ-opioid agonists results invariably in the inhibition of gastric emptying and intestinal transit (Burks et al., 1988; Porreca and Burks, 1983; Porreca et al., 1982, 1983a, 1983b, 1984). Constipation remains a major side effect that continues to limit the use of μ-opioid receptor agonists for pain treatment (Finley, 1990; Schug et al., 1992; Zenz et al., 1992; Zylicz and Twycross, 1991). Constipation is also viewed as a major obstacle to the development of new μ-opioid receptor agonists, being either peripheral or central, for either GI or central therapeutic indications. Despite early experimental work suggesting that opioid antinociception and antitransit activities could be mediated at two different μ-opioid receptor subtypes (*see* subheading 2.2.), there has been no further confirmation of this hypothesis. Unless the existence of such μ-opioid receptor subtypes can be established, it is unlikely that the μ-opioid receptor will represent a molecular target of choice for the development of new GI drugs, whatever the indication.

However, trying to selectively reduce the magnitude of μ-receptor-mediated side effects could be of interest for drug development. One approach could consist of the co-administration of a peripherally restricted opioid antagonist, together with a centrally acting opioid analgesic, the objective being to block peripheral μ-opioid receptors to reduce constipation, while leaving unaffected the central μ-opioid receptors involved in the analgesic activity of the opioid agonist. In recent trials in human volunteers, it was shown that methylnaltrexone, a quaternary opioid antagonist with limited ability to cross the blood–brain barrier, prevents morphine-induced delay in orocecal transit, without affecting morphine-induced analgesia (Yuan et al., 1996, 1997). However, about 40-fold higher doses of methylnaltrexone are required by oral route, suggesting a poor oral bioavailability (Yuan et al., 1997). Another quaternary narcotic antagonist, levallorphan methyl iodide (SR 58002), was shown to have a good peripheral selectivity (>10-fold selectivity) after parenteral administration in rodents (Dragonetti et al., 1983). More recently, Zimmerman et al. (1994) described a novel peripheral opioid antagonist, LY-246736, which distributes selectively to peripheral receptors (>200-fold selectivity), and which has a potent μ-receptor antagonist activity following parenteral, as well as oral, administration in rodents. There has been no report that either SR 58002 or LY-246736 are being developed. However, it may be objected that, if opioid-induced constipation is not exclusively mediated at peripheral μ-receptors, the above strategy would be of limited therapeutic interest.

A second approach to reduce opioid-mediated GI side effects could aim to block the cholecystokinin (CCK)-mediated inhibition of opioid analgesia. When administered systemically or perispinally, CCK potently and specifically antagonizes opiate-induced analgesia (Faris, 1985a, 1985b; Faris et al., 1983). Conversely, systemic, intrathecal, or intracerebral administration of a CCK receptor antagonist potentiates opioid-mediated analgesia (Watkins et al., 1985; O'Neill et al., 1989; Rattray et al., 1988). This effect was proposed to be mediated at spinal CCK_B receptors (Dourish et al., 1990; Wiesenfeld-Hallin et al., 1990). In addition to enhancing opioid-induced analgesia, the blockade of CCK_B receptors also prevents (Dourish et al., 1990; Xu et al., 1992) and may even reverse (Hoffmann and Wiesenfeld-Hallin, 1994) the development of tolerance to morphine. Conversely, CCK antagonists do not modify the antitransit potency of opioids (Singh et al., 1996).

Table 5
Responses to Activation of δ-Opioid Receptors
in Function of Their Localization

		Receptor localization		
	Effect	Periphery	Spinal Cord	Brain
Therapeutic targets				
Diarrhea	↓↓↓	•	•	•
Intestinal ion transport	↓↓↓	•		
Somatic pain	↓↓↓		•	•
Side effects				
Addiction	↑ (?)			•
Convulsions	↑↑			•

The above findings suggest that co-administration of CCK antagonists with μ-opioids could be of clinical interest. This strategy could improve the therapeutic window of morphine-like compounds by reducing the relative impact of their side effects, including constipation.

3.2. δ-Opioid Receptors

Selective δ-opioid receptor agonists have potent antisecretory and antidiarrhreal activity in rodents (Burks et al., 1988). At variance with μ-opioid receptor agonists, these effects are observed in the absence of antitransit or constipating activity (Table 5). Selective δ-receptor agonists enhance intestinal ion transport in a variety of tissue preparations and species (Kachur and Miller, 1982; Kachur et al., 1980; Quito and Brown, 1991; Sheldon et al., 1990; Vinayek et al., 1983). The δ-receptors involved in this response are thought to be primarily located on nerve terminals of submucosal plexus (Sheldon et al., 1990), although the presence of δ-opioid receptors has also been reported on enterocytes (Lang et al., 1996). In addition, DPDPE, the selective δ-receptor agonist, shows antidiarrheal activity after peripheral, spinal, or supraspinal administration in mice (Burks et al., 1988; Lemcke et al., 1991; Shook et al., 1988, 1989). Furthermore, DPDPE does not inhibit intestinal transit at doses that inhibit diarrhea. More recent data have shown that another selective δ-receptor agonist, [D-Ala^2]deltorphin II, also has antidiarrheal activity in rats (Broccardo and Improta, 1992). However, in this case, the antidiarrheal activity is associated with an inhibition of colonic propulsion (Broccardo and Improta, 1992). Several experimental differences may account for the apparent discrepancy in the effects of DPDPE and [D-Ala^2]deltorphin II on transit. The animal species, the GI tract segment considered to evaluate transit, and the drugs used were different. However, DPDPE and [D-Ala^2]deltorphin II have inverse affinity selectivity for the δ$_1$- and δ$_2$-binding sites (*see* subheading 2.2.). DPDPE and [D-Ala^2]deltorphin II are δ$_1$- and δ$_2$-preferred ligands, respectively. On the other hand, it has been suggested that, unlike δ$_1$ sites, δ$_2$ sites have a positive modulatory action on μ-opioid-receptor-mediated responses. Whether or not δ$_1$- and δ$_2$-receptor subtypes could have different GI motility profiles, through a differential modulation of μ-opioid-receptor-mediated responses, is unknown.

It has also been suggested that peripheral δ-opioid receptors could be involved in the control of visceral pain. In rats, intravesical administration of δ-opioid receptor agonists inhibit the nociceptive response to resineferatoxin injected into the urinary bladder (Craft et al., 1995). It was established that the site of action is local, suggesting that δ-opioid receptors may be present on bladder nociceptive afferents, and may be activated for production of peripheral analgesia. Conversely, δ-opioid receptor agonists failed to inhibit the activation of decentralized pelvic afferents induced by colorectal distention in rat (Sengupta et al., 1996). These two sets of data tend to be discordant, especially if it is considered that the urinary bladder and distal colon share common sensory nerves.

There is no report that selective δ-opioid receptor agonist are specifically being developed for GI therapeutic indications. Active drug discovery programs aiming at the identification of δ-opioid receptor agonist are primarily targeting central antinociception (Table 6). The development of a brain-penetrating δ-opioid receptor agonist, BW373U86, was, however, discontinued (Table 6). BW373U86 was shown to produce antinociception after spinal administration in mice (Wild et al., 1993), but this compound was also reported to induce convulsions both in mice (Comer et al., 1993) and monkeys (Dykstra et al., 1993). Both naltrexone and naltrindole produced a dose-dependent rightward shift

Table 6
Status of Drug Development for Agonists and Antagonists at Opioid Receptor Subtypes

Status	Therapeutic indications	Opioid receptor subtype		
		μ	δ	κ
Launched	GI	Loperamide loperamide oxide Trimebutine		
	Pain	Morphine Codeine Dextro-propoxyphen Fentanyl Sufentanyl Remifentanyl		Butorphanol
Development discontinued	GI	SR 58002[1] [a]	BW373U86[c]	Spiradoline[d] Enadoline[e]
	Pain	LY-246736[1] [b]		Fedotozine (PR)[f]
Preclinical or clinical development[2]	Pain	BCH-3963 (C1)[g] SP-130551 (P)[h] KF-24705 (P)[i] 1 series of compounds (P)[j]	SB-237596 (P)[k] 2 series of compounds (P)[l]	Asimadoline (C2)[m] Apadoline (C2)[n] TRK-820 (C2)[o] DuP-747 (P)[p] One series of compound (P)[q] f-f_D-Nle-r-NH2 (P)[r]

PR, preregistration; C2, phase II clinical trials; C1, phase I clinical trials; P, preclinical development; [1] antagonist; [2] new chemical entities only. Source: (Dooley et al., 1998).
Originators: [a] Sanofi; [b] Lilly; [c] Astra; [d] Upjohn; [e] Warner-Lambert; [g] Astra; [h] Sepracor; [i] Kyowa Hakko; [j] Biochem Pharma; [k] SmithKline Beecham; [l] Astra, Delta Pharmaceuticals; [m] Merck KgaA; [n] Rhone-Poulenc Rorer; [o] Toray; [p] NorthStar; [q] Adolor; [r] TPIMS. (Adapted from Pharmaprojects, January 1999; and Dooley et al., 1998.)

in the potency of BW373U86 to induce convulsions (Comer et al., 1993), supporting the selective involvement of central δ-opioid receptors in the convulsive response to BW373U86. It also suggests that any other brain-penetrating δ-opioid agonist is likely to induce similar side effects. Thus, preventing brain penetration for δ-opioid drugs may be required for safety reasons. The most likely therapeutic targets for peripherally selective δ-opioid agonist would be intestinal hypersecretion and diarrheic disorders, as well as visceral pain, providing that the rationale for this later indication could be further substantiated.

3.3. κ-Opioid Receptors

The GI actions triggered by κ-opioid receptors markedly differ from those elicited by μ- or δ-receptors. Unlike μ-opioid receptors, κ-receptors do not mediate transit inhibition or constipation (Burks et al., 1988). Unlike δ-receptors, κ-receptors have almost no effect on intestinal ion transport (Sheldon et al., 1990). In contrast, κ-opioid receptors are consistently and repeatedly shown to mediate potent analgesic responses in various visceral pain models in rodents (Burton and Gebhart, 1998; Craft et al., 1995; Diop et al., 1994a, 1994b; Friese et al., 1997; Langlois et al., 1997, 1994; Sengupta et al., 1996; Su et al., 1997a, 1997b) (Table 7). Although κ-agonists are found to be active after peripheral and supraspinal administration, the periphery has been proposed as the main site of action for κ-agonists in visceral pain. The most supportive evidence of a predominant peripheral site of action comes from recordings of the electrophysiological activity of decentralized primary sensory afferents during colorectal distention (CRD). In these experiments, the administration of κ-, but not μ- or δ-, agonists inhibits, in a dose-related manner, CRD-induced electrical activity (Sengupta et al., 1996). Most of the κ-agonists used in the above visceral pain experiments, such as enadoline, U50488, U69593, or EMD61753, are classical and selective $κ_1$-ligands. In most cases, the analgesic response to these $κ_1$-agonists is blocked by naloxone, the nonselective opioid antagonist, as well as by nor-BNI, a selective κ-antagonist (Diop et al., 1994a, 1994b; Friese et al., 1997; Langlois et al., 1997, 1994). Together, these data suggest that peripheral $κ_1$-receptors located on primary sensory afferents of the gut may effectively inhibit visceral pain, when they are activated. Peripheral $κ_1$-receptors may therefore constitute an interesting molecular target for the development of GI analgesic drugs.

Table 7
Responses to Activation of κ-Opioid Receptors
in Function of Their Localization

		Receptor localization		
	Effect	*Periphery*	*Spinal cord*	*Brain*
Therapeutic targets				
Visceral pain	↓↓↓	•		•
Postoperative ileus	↓↓↓	•		
Somatic pain	↓↓↓	•	•	•
Side effects				
Diuresis	↑↑	•		•
Sedation	↑↑			•
Aversion, dysphoria	↑↑			•

It was suggested that GI inflammation could enhance the antinociceptive activity of κ-agonists in visceral pain (Langlois et al., 1994). Further studies using different experimental conditions failed to confirm this finding (Burton and Gebhart, 1998). In addition to blocking visceral pain, κ-agonists have also been shown to reverse both intestinal transit impairments (Rivière et al., 1993) and pain (Friese et al., 1997) in experimental ileus induced by peritoneal irritation in rats. Because κ-agonists do not have any prokinetic activity, it was suggested that this effect is specific of experimental ileus, and that κ-agonists may selectively target the extrinsic nervous inhibitory pathway that is activated during ileus. This pathway is thought to involve primary sensory afferents, central corticotropin releasing factor (CRF) receptors, and adrenergic inhibitory nerves. Gastric emptying and intestinal transit inhibition in experimental ileus can be prevented by the central administration of a CRF antagonist, and reproduced by a central administration of CRF (Rivière et al., 1994). However, although κ-agonists can reverse experimental ileus, such compounds cannot block CRF-induced gastric emptying and intestinal transit inhibition (Rivière et al., 1994). This suggests that, in experimental ileus, κ-agonists act prior to the activation of central CRF receptors, possibly on the ascending pain pathway. Such a mechanism of action is consistent with the general antinociceptive activity of κ-agonists in visceral pain. It was shown for a selection of κ-agonists that the potency to reverse transit impairments in experimental ileus is directly correlated to the analgesic potency (Friese et al., 1997). Conversely, although being potent analgesics against pain associated with experimental ileus, selective μ-agonists are unable to reverse transit impairments (Friese et al., 1997), possibly because of their antitransit activity.

Fedotozine is the only compound under development for GI therapeutic indications that has a preferred κ-agonist-like profile. When administered by iv or sc route, fedotozine inhibits visceral pain induced by distention in normal duodenum and colon, as well as in irritated colon in rats (Diop et al., 1994a, 1994b; Friese et al., 1997; Langlois et al., 1997, 1994). Fedotozine also reverses experimental ileus in rats (Riviere et al., 1993). The effects of fedotozine were found to be mediated in the periphery. Although having low selectivity for κ-receptors in binding studies (Allescher et al., 1991), fedotozine repeatedly acted as a preferred κ-agonist in vivo, as shown by the blockage of its responses by nor-BNI, the selective κ-antagonist. Fedotozine was found to relieve postprandial fullness, bloating, abdominal pain, and nausea in patients suffering from nonulcer dyspepsia (Fraitag et al., 1994), and was shown effective and safe in the treatment of the abdominal pain and bloating associated with IBS (Dapoigny et al., 1995).

Spiradoline and enadoline (Table 6) are brain-penetrating selective κ-agonists that were initially developed as centrally acting analgesics. These compounds were found efficacious as analgesics, and devoid of the side effects of μ-selective opioids. However, brain-penetrating κ-agonists were found to induce within the analgesic dose range central side effects (dysphoria), which resulted in the discontinuation of their development. It is now widely accepted that peripheral κ-receptors play a role in the control of both somatic and visceral pain, particularly in inflammation. Therefore, peripherally restricted κ-agonists should achieve peripheral analgesia (visceral and somatic) without inducing central side effects. Furthermore, the lack of antitransit and/or constipating activity is expected to be a major advantage over μ-opioid analgesics.

Asimadoline (Table 6) is the first κ-agonist claimed to be peripheral under clinical evaluation. Asimadoline is a nonpeptidic compound, whose chemical structure is very close to those of previously discontinued brain-penetrating κ-agonists. Whether or not this second generation of κ-agonist will be efficacious and safe enough is not known yet.

A tetrapeptide κ-agonist (f-f-$_D$Nle-r-NH$_2$) was recently identified by combinatorial chemistry (Dooley et al., 1998). This compound, as well as derivatives, show unprecedented affinity and selectivity for hKOR1, potent and long-lasting antinociceptive activity, and excellent peripheral selectivity (up to 167-fold better than asimadoline) in rodent models (Rivière et al., 1999).

3.4. ORL1 Receptors

Using a reverse pharmacology approach, the groups of Meunier et al. (1995) and Civelli simultaneously discovered an endogenous 17-amino-acid neuropeptide (Phe-Gly-Gly-Phe-Thr-Gly-Ala-Arg-Lys-Ser-Ala-Arg-Lys-Leu-Ala-Asn-Gln) called either nociceptin (Meunier et al., 1995) or orphanin FQ (Reinscheid et al., 1995), which resembles dynorphin A, and has high-affinity binding and agonist potency at the ORL1. Nociceptin/orphanin FQ (noc/oFQ) was reported to trigger a broad range of pharmacological responses that differ markedly from the pharmacological profile of traditional endogenous opioids (Meunier, 1997). Immunohistochemical studies, using an antibody against noc/oFQ, showed noc/oFQ-immunopositive cells and fibers in the myenteric and submucosal plexus in GI organs, with the highest concentration in proximal colon (Yadzani et al., 1997). Furthermore, peripheral administration of noc/oFQ stimulates colonic motility and transit in rats (Taniguchi et al., 1998; Yadzani et al., 1997), suggesting that noc/oFQ has a specific prokinetic activity on the colon, and may be useful in treating constipation. In the periphery, noc/oFQ inhibits tachykinin release from nerve endings in vitro (Giuliani and Maggi, 1996), inhibits neurogenic inflammation and the release of SP and CGRP from sensory nerve terminals (Helyes et al., 1997), and reduces plasma extravasation (Nemeth et al., 1998). Peripheral administration of noc/oFQ was also shown to inhibit the micturition reflex in rats (Giuliani et al., 1998). Noc/oFQ decreases acetylcholine release induced by electrical stimulation in guinea pig trachea (Patel et al., 1997). Finally, peripheral administration of noc/oFQ in rats induces hypotension and bradycardia (Giuliani et al., 1997; Champion and Kadowitz, 1997), and decreases heart rate and output (Champion et al., 1997; Czapla et al., 1997). These findings are consistent with the fact that noc/oFQ has potent relaxant activity on vascular smooth muscle (Gumusel et al., 1997), and inhibits CGRP-evoked release from capsaicin-sensitive sensory nerve terminals in guinea pig left atria (Giuliani and Maggi, 1997).

It has also been suggested that the ORL1 receptor could be involved in the control of visceral pain, based on results obtained with NalBzoH, the preferential ligand for the κ_3/ORL1 receptor (*see* subheading 2.1.). Like typical κ_1-agonists, NalBzoH inhibits CRD-induced activation of decentralized primary sensory afferents (Su et al., 1997). The responses to NalBzoH are reduced by naloxone. However, the response to either κ_1-agonists or NalBzoH could not be blocked by nor-BNI, a selective κ-antagonist. Based on these observations, the authors suggested that κ_1-and NalBzoH effects on visceral pain could be mediated at an orphan opioid-ORL1 receptor. The involvement of the κ_3/ORL1 receptor is however unlikely since this receptor is naloxone resistant (Nicholson et al., 1998), and that classical κ_1-receptors have no agonist activity at the cloned hORL1 receptor (Mollereau et al., 1994).

4. CONCLUSION

A functional division has emerged regarding the role of different opioid receptor subtypes in the control of GI functions. μ-opioid receptors preferentially alter GI motility transit, and eventually induce constipation. δ-opioid receptors seem to play a preferential role in intestinal ion transport, and have a good potential as antisecretory and antidiarrheal agents. κ-receptors have minimal, if any, impact on GI motility, transit, or secretion. Conversely, peripheral κ-receptors are viewed as a major target for developing analgesics for visceral pain. The combination of their potent visceral antinociceptive activity with their lack of antitransit activity explains the ability of selective κ-agonists to reverse experimental ileus. Both δ and κ central receptors are responsible for unwanted centrally mediated side effects that impose the design of peripherally restricted compounds. The ORL1 receptor will probably be the focus of much exploratory research in the GI field during coming years. The peripherally ORL1-mediated vasodilatation and hypotension may be an obstacle to development of ORL1 agonists for GI indications.

REFERENCES

Abood ME, Noel MA, Farnsworth JS, Tao Q. Molecular cloning and expression of a delta-opioid receptor from rat brain. *J Neurosci Res* 1994; 37: 714-719.

Aikawa N, Karasawa A. Effects of KW–5617 (zaldaride maleate), a potent and selective calmodulin inhibitor, on secretory diarrhea and on gastrointestinal propulsion in rats. *Jpn J Pharmacol* 1998; 76: 199–206.

Allescher HD, Ahmad S, Classen M, Daniel EE. Interaction of trimebutine and Jo–1196 (fedotozine) with opioid receptors in the canine ileum. *J Pharmacol Exp Ther* 1991; 257: 836–842.

Awouters F, Megens A, Verlinden M, Schuurkes J, Niemegeers C, Janssen PA. Loperamide. Survey of studies on mechanism of its antidiarrheal activity. *Dig Dis Sci* 1993; 38: 977–995.

Bagnol D, Mansour A, Akil H, Watson SJ. Cellular localization and distribution of the cloned mu and kappa opioid receptors in rat gastrointestinal tract. *Neuroscience* 1997; 81: 579–591.

Befort K, Mattei MG, Roeckel N, Kieffer B. Chromosomal localization of the delta opioid receptor gene to human 1p34.3-p36.1 and mouse 4D bands by in situ hybridization. *Genomics* 1994; 20: 143–145.

Bitar KN, Makhlouf GM. Selective presence of opiate receptors on intestinal circular muscle cells. *Life Sci* 1985; 37: 1545–1550.

Bitar KN, Makhlouf GM. Specific opiate receptors on isolated mammalian gastric smooth muscle cells. *Nature* 1982; 297: 72–74.

Boige N, Cargill G, Mashako L, Cezard JP, Navarro J. Trimebutine-induced phase III-like activity in infants with intestinal motility disorders. *J Pediatr Gastroenterol Nutr* 1987; 6: 548–553.

Broccardo M, Improta G. Antidiarrheal and colonic antipropulsive effects of spinal and supraspinal administration of the natural delta opioid receptor agonist, [D-Ala2]deltorphin II, in the rat. *Eur J Pharmacol* 1992; 218: 69–73.

Broccardo M, Improta G. Antidiarrheal effect of deltorphin II, a highly selective delta opioid receptor agonist, in the rat. *Pharmacol Res* 1992; 25(Suppl 1): 5–6.

Brown DR, Poonyachoti S, Osinski MA, Kowalski TR, Pampusch MS, Elde RP, Murtaugh MP. Delta-opioid receptor mRNA expression and immunohistochemical localization in porcine ileum. *Dig Dis Sci* 1998; 43: 1402–1410.

Bueno L, Fioramonti J. Action of opiates on gastrointestinal function. *Baillieres Clin Gastroenterol* 1988; 2: 123–139.

Burks TF, Fox DA, Hirning LD, Shook JE, Porreca F. Regulation of gastrointestinal function by multiple opioid receptors. *Life Sci* 1988; 43: 2177–2181.

Burks TF, Galligan JJ, Hirning LD, Porreca F. Brain, spinal cord and peripheral sites of action of enkephalins and other endogenous opioids on gastrointestinal motility. *Gastroenterol Clin Biol* 1987; 11: 44B–51B.

Burton MB, Gebhart GF. Effects of kappa-opioid receptor agonists on responses to colorectal distension in rats with and without acute colonic inflammation. *J Pharmacol Exp Ther* 1998; 285: 707–715.

Chakrabarti S, Sultana M, Portoghese PS, Takemori AE. Differential antagonism by naltrindole–5′-isothiocyanate on [3H]DSLET and [3H]DPDPE binding to striatal slices of mice. *Life Sci* 1993; 53: 1761–1765.

Champion HC, Czapla MA, Kadowitz PJ. Nociceptin, an endogenous ligand for the ORL1 receptor, decreases cardiac output and total peripheral resistance in the rat. *Peptides* 1997; 18: 729–732.

Champion HC, Kadowitz PJ. Nociceptin, an endogenous ligand for the ORL1 receptor, has novel hypotensive activity in the rat. *Life Sci* 1997; 60: PL 241–245.

Chaussade S, Grandjouan S, Couturier D, Thierman-Duffaud D, Henry JF. Induction of phase 3 of the migrating motor complex in human small intestine by trimebutine. *Eur J Clin Pharmacol* 1987; 32: 615–618.

Chen Y, Mestek A, Liu J, Hurley JA, Yu L. Molecular cloning and functional expression of a mu-opioid receptor from rat brain. *Mol Pharmacol* 1993; 44: 8–12.

Chen Y, Mestek A, Liu J, Yu L. Molecular cloning of a rat kappa opioid receptor reveals sequence similarities to the mu and delta opioid receptors. *Biochem J* 1993; 295: 625–628.

Chuang TK, Killam KF JR, Chuang LF, Kung HF, Sheng WS, Chao CC, Yu L, Chuang RY. Mu opioid receptor gene expression in immune cells. *Biochem Biophys Res Commun* 1995; 216: 922–930.

Comer SD, Hoenicke EM, Sable AI, McNutt RW, Chang KJ, De Costa BR, Mosberg HI, Woods JH. Convulsive effects of systemic administration of the delta opioid agonist BW373U86 in mice. *J Pharmacol Exp Ther* 1993; 267: 888–895.

Craft RM, Henley SR, Haaseth RC, Hruby VJ, Porreca F. Opioid antinociception in a rat model of visceral pain: systemic versus local drug administration. *J Pharmacol Exp Ther* 1995; 275: 1535–1542.

Czapla MA, Champion HC, Kadowitz PJ. Decreases in systemic arterial and hindquarters perfusion pressure in response to nociceptin are not inhibited by naloxone in the rat. *Peptides* 1997; 18: 1197–1200.

Daniel EE, Fox JE, Allescher HD, Ahmad S, Kostolanska F. Peripheral actions of opiates in canine gastrointestinal tract: actions on nerves and muscles. *Gastroenterol Clin Biol* 1987; 11: 35B–43B.

Danzebrink RM, Green SA, Gebhart GF. Spinal mu and delta, but not kappa, opioid-receptor agonists attenuate responses to noxious colorectal distension in the rat. *Pain* 1995; 63: 39–47.

Dapoigny M, Abitbol JL, Fraitag B. Efficacy of peripheral kappa agonist fedotozine versus placebo in treatment of irritable bowel syndrome. A multicenter dose-response study. *Dig Dis Sci* 1995; 40: 2244–2249.

Dashwood MR, Debnam ES, Bagnall J, Thompson CS. Autoradiographic localisation of opiate receptors in rat small intestine. *Eur J Pharmacol* 1985; 107: 267–269.

De Luca A, Coupar IM. Insights into opioid action in the intestinal tract. *Pharmacol Ther* 1996; 69: 103–115.

Delvaux M, Wingate D. Trimebutine: mechanism of action, effects on gastrointestinal function and clinical results. *J Int Med Res* 1997; 25: 225–246.

Diop L, Rivière PJ, Pascaud X, Dassaud M, Junien JL. Role of vagal afferents in the antinociception produced by morphine and U–50,488H in the colonic pain reflex in rats. *Eur J Pharmacol* 1994a; 257: 181–187.

Diop L, Rivière PJ, Pascaud X, Junien JL. Peripheral kappa-opioid receptors mediate the antinociceptive effect of fedotozine (correction of fetodozine) on the duodenal pain reflex inrat. *Eur J Pharmacol* 1994b; 271: 65–71.

Dooley CT, Ny P, Bidlack JM, Houghten RA. Selective ligands for the mu, delta, and kappa opioid receptors identified from a single mixture based tetrapeptide positional scanning combinatorial library. *J Biol Chem* 1998; 273: 18,848–18,856.

Dourish CT, O'Neill MF, Coughlan J, Kitchener SJ, Hawley D, Iversen SD. Selective CCK-B receptor antagonist L–365,260 enhances morphine analgesia and prevents morphine tolerance in the rat. *Eur J Pharmacol* 1990; 176: 35–44.

Dragonetti M, Bianchetti A, Sacilotto R, Giudice A, Ferrarese N, Cattaneo C, Manara L. Levallorphan methyl iodide (SR 58002), a potent narcotic antagonist with peripheral selectivity superior to that of other quaternary compounds. *Life Sci* 1993; 33(Suppl 1): 477–480.

Dykstra LA, Schoenbaum GM, Yarbrough J, McNutt R, Chang KJ. Novel delta opioid agonist, BW373U86, in squirrel monkeys responding under a schedule of shock titration. *J Pharmacol Exp Ther* 1993; 267: 875–882.

Evans CJ, Keith De JR, Morrison H, Magendzo K, Edwards RH. Cloning of a delta opioid receptor by functional expression. *Science* 1992; 258: 1952–1955.

Faris PL. Opiate antagonistic function of cholecystokinin in analgesia and energy balance systems. *Ann NY Acad Sci* 1985a; 448: 437–447.

Faris PL. Role of cholecystokinin in the control of nociception and food intake. *Prog Clin Biol Res* 1985b; 192: 159–166.

Faris PL, Komisaruk BR, Watkins LR, Mayer DJ. Evidence for the neuropeptide cholecystokinin as an antagonist of opiate analgesia. *Science* 1983; 219: 310–312.

Fickel J, Bagnol D, Watson SJ, Akil H. Opioid receptor expression in the rat gastrointestinal tract: a quantitative study with comparison to the brain. *Brain Res Mol Brain Res* 1997; 46: 1–8.

Finley RS. Pain management with spinally administered opioids. *Am J Hosp Pharm* 1990; 47: S14–17.

Fioramonti J, Fargeas MJ, Bueno L. Involvement of opiate receptors in the effects of trimebutine on intestinal motility in the conscious dog. *J Pharm Pharmacol* 1984; 36: 618–621.

Fraitag B, Homerin M, Hecketsweiler P. Double-blind dose-response multicenter comparison of fedotozine and placebo in treatment of nonulcer dyspepsia. *Dig Dis Sci* 1994; 39: 1072–1077.

Frexinos J, Fioramonti J, Bueno L. Effect of trimebutine on colonic myoelectrical activity in IBS patients. *Eur J Clin Pharmacol* 1985; 28: 181–185.

Friese N, Chevalier E, Angel F, Pascaud X, Junien JL, Dahl SG, Riviere PJ. Reversal by kappa-agonists of peritoneal irritation-induced ileus and visceral pain in rats. *Life Sci* 1997; 60: 625–634.

Friese N, Diop L, Lambert C, Rivière PJ, Dahl SG. Antinociceptive effects of morphine and U–50,488H on vaginal distension in the anesthetized rat. *Life Sci* 1997; 61: 1559–1570.

Gaveriaux C, Peluso J, Simonin F, Laforet J, Kieffer B. Identification of kappa- and delta-opioid receptor transcripts in immune cells. *FEBS Lett* 1995; 369: 272–276.

Gintzler AR, Pasternak GW. Multiple mu receptors: evidence for mu2 sites in the guinea pig ileum. *Neurosci Lett* 1983; 39: 51–56.

Giuliani S, Lecci A, Tramontana M, Maggi CA. Inhibitory effect of nociceptin on the micturition reflex in anaesthetized rats. *Bri J Pharmacol* 1998; 124: 1566–1572.

Giuliani S, Maggi CA. Prejunctional modulation by nociceptin of nerve-mediated inotropic responses in guinea-pig left atrium. *Eur J Pharmacol* 1997; 332: 231–236.

Giuliani S, Tramontana M, Lecci A, Maggi CA. Effect of nociceptin on heart rate and blood pressure in anaesthetized rats. *Eur J Pharmacol* 1997; 333: 177–179.

Goldstein A, Lowney LI, Pal BK. Stereospecific and nonspecific interactions of the morphine congener levorphanol in subcellular fractions of mouse brain. *Proc Natl Acad Sci USA* 1971; 68: 1742–1747.

Grandjouan S, Chaussade S, Couturier D, Thierman-Duffaud D, Henry JF. Comparison of metoclopramide and trimebutine on small bowel motility in humans. *Aliment Pharmacol Ther* 1989; 3: 387–393.

Grider JR, Makhlouf GM. Identification of opioid receptors on gastric muscle cells by selective receptor protection. *Am J Physiol* 1991; 260: G103–107.

Gumusel B, Hao Q, Hyman A, Chang JK, Kapusta DR, Lippton H. Nociceptin: an endogenous agonist for central opioid like1 (ORL1) receptors possesses systemic vasorelaxant properties. *Life Sci* 1997; 60: PL141–145.

Hahn EF, Pasternak GW. Naloxonazine, a potent, long-lasting inhibitor of opiate binding sites. *Life Sci* 1982; 31: 1385–1388.

Hanner M, Moebius FF, Flandorfer A, Knaus HG, Striessnig J, Kempner E, Glossmann H. Purification, molecular cloning, and expression of the mammalian sigma1-binding site. *Proc Natl Acad Sci USA* 1996; 93: 8072–8077.

Hassan AH, Ableitner A, Stein C, Herz A. Inflammation of the rat paw enhances axonal transport of opioid receptors in the sciatic nerve and increases their density in the inflamed tissue. *Neuroscience* 1993; 55: 185-195.

Hatzoglou A, Bakogeorgou E, Castanas E. Antiproliferative effect of opioid receptor agonists on the T47D human breast cancer cell line is partially mediated through opioid receptors. *Eur J Pharmacol* 1996; 296: 199–207.

Hatzoglou A, Bakogeorgou E, Hatzoglou C, Martin PM, Castanas E. Antiproliferative and receptor binding properties of alpha- and beta-casomorphins in the T47D human breast cancer cell line. *Eur J Pharmacol* 1996; 310: 217-223.

Helyes Z, Nemeth J, Pinter E, Szolcsanyi J. Inhibition by nociceptin of neurogenic inflammation and the release of SP and CGRP from sensory nerve terminals. *Br J Pharmacol* 1997; 121: 613–615.

Heyman JS, Williams CL, Burks TF, Mosberg HI, Porreca F. Dissociation of opioid antinociception and central gastrointestinal propulsion in the mouse: studies with naloxonazine. *J Pharmacol Exp Ther* 1988; 245: 238–243.

Hoffmann O, Wiesenfeld-Hallin Z. CCK-B receptor antagonist Cl 988 reverses tolerance to morphine in rats. *Neuroreport* 1994; 5: 2565–2568.

Horan P, De Costa BR, Rice KC, Porreca F. Differential antagonism of U69,593- and bremazocine-induced antinociception by (−)-UPHIT: evidence of kappa opioid receptor multiplicity in mice. *J Pharmacol Exp Ther* 1991; 257: 1154–1161.

Horan PJ, De Costa BR, Rice K, Haaseth RC, Hruby VJ, Porreca F. Differential antagonism of bremazocine- and U69,593-induced antinociception by quadazocine: further functional evidence of opioid kappa receptor multiplicity in the mouse. *J Pharmacol Exp Ther* 1993; 266: 926–933.

Horan PJ, Porreca F. Lack of cross-tolerance between U69,593 and bremazocine suggests kappa-opioid receptor multiplicity in mice. *Eur J Pharmacol* 1993; 239: 93–98.

Jeanjean AP, Maloteaux JM, Laduron PM. IL–1 beta-like Freund's adjuvant enhances axonal transport of opiate receptors in sensory neurons. *Neurosci Lett* 1994; 177: 75–78.

Jeanjean AP, Moussaoui SM, Maloteaux JM, Laduron PM. Interleukin–1 beta induces long-term increase of axonally transported opiate receptors and substance P. *Neuroscience* 1995; 68: 151–157.

Jiang Q, Takemori AE, Sultana M, Portoghese PS, Bowen WD, Mosberg HI, Porreca F. Differential antagonism of opioid delta antinociception by [D-Ala2,Leu5,Cys6] enkephalin and naltrindole 5′-isothiocyanate: evidence for delta receptor subtypes. *J Pharmacol Exp Ther* 1991; 257: 1069–1075.

Kachur JF, Miller RJ. Characterization of the opiate receptor in the guinea-pig ileal mucosa. *Eur J Pharmacol* 1982; 81: 177–183.

Kachur JF, Miller RJ, Field M. Control of guinea pig intestinal electrolyte secretion by a delta-opiate receptor. *Proc Natl Acad Sci USA* 1980; 77: 2753–2756.

Kampa M, Loukas S, Hatzoglou A, Martin P, Martin PM, Castanas E. Identification of a novel opioid peptide (Tyr-Val-Pro-Phe-Pro) derived from human alpha S1 casein (alpha S1-casomorphin, and alpha S1-casomorphin amide). *Biochem J* 1996; 319: 903–908.

Kaneto H, Takahashi M, Watanabe J. Opioid receptor selectivity for trimebutine in isolated tissues experiments and receptor binding studies. *J Pharmacobiodyn* 1990; 13: 448–453.

Kaufman DL, Keith De JR, Anton B, Tian J, Magendzo K, Newman D, et al. Characterization of the murine mu opioid receptor gene. *J Biol Chem* 1995; 270: 15,877–15,883.

Kieffer BL, Befort K, Gaveriaux-Ruff C, Hirth CG. The delta-opioid receptor: isolation of a cDNA by expression cloning and pharmacological characterization. *Proc Natl Acad Sci USA* 1992; 89: 12,048–12,052.

Knapp RJ, Malatynska E, Collins N, Fang L, Wang JY, Hruby VJ, Roeske WR, Yamamura HI. Molecular biology and pharmacology of cloned opioid receptors. *FASEB J* 1995; 9: 516–525.

Knapp RJ, Malatynska E, Fang L, Li X, Babin E, Nguyen M, et al. Identification of a human delta opioid receptor: cloning and expression. *Life Sci* 1994; 54: PL463–469.

Kromer W. Endogenous and exogenous opioids in the control of gastrointestinal motility and secretion. *Pharmacol Rev* 1988; 40: 121–162.

Kuemmerle JF, Makhlouf GM. Characterization of opioid receptors in intestinal muscle cells by selective radioligands and receptor protection. *Am J Physiol* 1992; 263: G269–276.

Laduron PM. Axonal transport of opiate receptors in capsaicin-sensitive neurones. *Brain Res* 1984; 294: 157–160.

Lai J, Ma SW, Zhu RH, Rothman RB, Lentes KU, Porreca F. Pharmacological characterization of the cloned kappa opioid receptor as a kappa 1b subtype. *Neuroreport* 1994; 5: 2161–2164.

Lang ME, Davison JS, Bates SL, Meddings JB. Opioid receptors on guinea-pig intestinal crypt epithelial cells. *J Physiol (London)* 1996; 497: 161–174.

Langlois A, Diop L, Friese N, Pascaud X, Junien JL, Dahl SG, Riviere PJ. Fedotozine blocks hypersensitive visceral pain in conscious rats: action at peripheral kappa-opioid receptors. *Eur J Pharmacol* 1997; 324: 211–217.

Langlois A, Diop L, Rivière PJ, Pascaud X, Junien JL. Effect of fedotozine on the cardiovascular pain reflex induced by distension of the irritated colon in the anesthetized rat. *Eur J Pharmacol* 1994; 271: 245–251.

Lemcke PK, Shook JE, Burks TF. Spinally mediated opioid antidiarrheal effects. *Eur J Pharmacol* 1991; 193: 109–115.

Li S, Zhu J, Chen C, Chen YW, Deriel JK, Ashby B, Liu-Chen LY. Molecular cloning and expression of a rat kappa opioid receptor. *Biochem J* 1993; 295: 629–633.

Liang Y, Mestek A, Yu L, Carr LG. Cloning and characterization of the promoter region of the mouse mu opioid receptor gene. *Brain Res* 1995; 679: 82–88.

Lord JA, Waterfield AA, Hughes J, Kosterlitz HW. Endogenous opioid peptides: multiple agonists and receptors. *Nature* 1997; 267: 495–499.

Mansour A, Fox CA, Akil H, Watson SJ. Opioid-receptor mRNA expression in the rat CNS: anatomical and functional implications. *Trends Neurosci* 1995; 18: 22–29.

Mansson E, Bare L, Yang D. Isolation of a human kappa opioid receptor cDNA from placenta. *Biochem Biophys Res Commun* 1994; 202: 1431–1437.

Martin WR, Eades CG, Thompson JA, Huppler RE, Gilbert PE. Effects of morphine- and nalorphine-like drugs in the nondependent and morphine-dependent chronic spinal dog. *J Pharmacol Exp Ther* 1976; 197: 517–532.

Mattia A, Vanderah T, Mosberg HI, Porreca F. Lack of antinociceptive cross-tolerance between [D-Pen2, D-Pen5]enkephalin and [D-Ala2]deltorphin II in mice: evidence for delta receptor subtypes. *J Pharmacol Exp Ther* 1991; 258: 583–587.

Maves TJ, Gebhart GF. Antinociceptive synergy between intrathecal morphine and lidocaine during visceral and somatic nociception in the rat. *Anesthesiology* 1992; 76: 91–99.

Meng F, Xie GX, Thompson RC, Mansour A, Goldstein A, Watson SJ, Akil H. Cloning and pharmacological characterization of a rat kappa opioid receptor. *Proc Natl Acad Sci USA* 1993; 90: 9954–9958.

Meunier JC, Mollereau C, Toll L, Suaudeau C, Moisand C, Alvinerie P, et al. Isolation and structure of the endogenous agonist of opioid receptor-like ORL1 receptor. *Nature* 1995; 377: 532–535.

Minami M, Toya T, Katao Y, Maekawa K, Nakamura S, Onogi T, Kaneko S, Satoh M. Cloning and expression of a cDNA for the rat kappa-opioid receptor. *FEBS Lett* 1993; 329: 291–295.

Mollereau C, Parmentier M, Mailleux P, Butour JL, Moisand C, Chalon P, et al. ORL1, a novel member of the opioid receptor family. Cloning, functional expression and localization. *FEBS Lett* 1994; 341: 33–38.

Musacchio JM. Psychotomimetic effects of opiates and the sigma receptor. *Neuropsychopharmacology* 1990; 3: 191–200.

Nemeth J, Helyes Z, Oroszi G, Than M, Pinter E, Szolcsanyi J. Inhibition of nociceptin on sensory neuropeptide release and mast cell-mediated plasma extravasation in rats. *Eur J Pharmacol* 1998; 347: 101–104.

Nicholson JR, Paterson SJ, Menzies JRW, Corbett AD, McKnight AT. Pharmacological studies on the orphan opioid receptor in central and peripheral sites. *Can J Physiol Pharmacol* 1998; 76: 304–313.

Nishimura E, Buchan AM, Mcintosh CH. Autoradiographic localization of mu- and delta-type opioid receptors in the gastrointestinal tract of the rat and guinea pig. *Gastroenterology* 1986; 91: 1084–1094.

Nishimura SL, Recht LD, Pasternak GW. Biochemical characterization of high-affinity 3H-opioid binding. Further evidence for Mu1 sites. *Mol Pharmacol* 1984; 25: 29–37.

Okano H, Saeki S, Inui A, Kawai Y, Ohno S, Morimoto S, et al. Effect of trimebutine maleate on emptying of stomach and gallbladder and release of gut peptide following a solid meal in man. *Dig Dis Sci* 1993; 38: 817–823.

Ooms LA, Degryse AD, Janssen PA. Mechanisms of action of loperamide. *Scand J Gastroenterol Suppl* 1984; 96: 145–155.

O'Neill MF, Dourish CT, Iversen SD. Morphine-induced analgesia in the rat paw pressure test is blocked by CCK and enhanced by the CCK antagonist MK–329. *Neuropharmacology* 1989; 28: 243–247.

Pan YX, Cheng J, Xu J, Rossi G, Jacobson E, Ryan-Moro J, et al. Cloning and functional characterization through antisense mapping of a kappa 3-related opioid receptor. *Mol Pharmacol* 1995; 47: 1180–1188.

Pan YX, Xu J, Pasternak GW. Structure and characterization of the gene encoding a mouse kappa3-related opioid receptor. *Gene* 1996, 171, 255–60.

Pan YX, Xu J, Wan BL, Zuckerman A, Pasternak GW. Identification and differential regional expression of Kor-3/ORL-1 gene splice variants in mouse brain. FEBS Letters 1998; 435: 65–68.

Pasternak GW. (1982) High and low affinity opioid binding sites: relationship to mu and delta sites. *Life Sci* 1996; 31: 1303–1306.

Patel HJ, Giembycz MA, Spicuzza L, Barnes PJ, Belvisi MG. Naloxone-insensitive inhibition of acetylcholine release from parasympathetic nerves innervating guinea pig trachea by the novel opioid, nociceptin. *Br J Pharmacol* 1997; 120: 735–736.

Paul D, Levison JA, Howard DH, Pick CG, Hahn EF, Pasternak GW. Naloxone benzoylhydrazone (NalBzoH) analgesia. *J Pharmacol Exp Ther* 1990; 255: 769–774.

Paul D, Pick CG, Tive LA, Pasternak GW. Pharmacological characterization of nalorphine, a kappa 3 analgesic. *J Pharmacol Exp Ther* 1991; 257: 1–7.

Pert CB, Snyder SH. Opiate receptor: demonstration in nervous tissue. *Science* 1973; 179: 1011–1014.

Pharmaprojects CD-ROM (1999). PJB Publications Ltd.

Poitras P, Boivin M, Lahaie RG, Trudel L. Regulation of plasma motilin by opioids in the dog. *Am J Physiol* 1989; 257: G41–45.

Porreca F, Burks TF. Spinal cord as a site of opioid effects on gastrointestinal transit in the mouse. *J Pharmacol Exp Ther* 1983; 227: 22–27.

Porreca F, Filla A, Burks TF. Spinal cord-mediated opiate effects on gastrointestinal transit in mice. *Eur J Pharmacol* 1982; 86: 135–136.

Porreca F, Filla A, Burks TF. Studies in vivo with dynorphin-(1–9): analgesia but not gastrointestinal effects following intrathecal administration to mice. *Eur J Pharmacol* 1983a; 91: 291–294.

Porreca F, Mosberg HI, Hurst R, Hruby VJ, Burks TF. A comparison of the analgesic and gastrointestinal transit effects of [D-Pen2, L-Cys5]enkephalin after intracerebroventricular and intrathecal administration to mice. *Life Sci* 1983b; 33(Suppl 1): 457–460.

Porreca F, Mosberg HI, Hurst R, Hruby VJ, Burks TF. Roles of mu, delta and kappa opioid receptors in spinal and supraspinal mediation of gastrointestinal transit effects and hot-plate analgesia in the mouse. *J Pharmacol Exp Ther* 1984; 230: 341–348.

Portoghese PS, Sultana M, Nagase H, Takemori AE. Highly selective delta 1-opioid receptor antagonist: 7-benzylidenenaltrexone. *Eur J Pharmacol* 1992; 218: 195–196.

Qi JA, Mosberg HI, Porreca F. Antinociceptive effects of [D-Ala2]deltorphin II, a highly selective delta agonist in vivo. *Life Sci* 1990; 47: PL43–47.

Quito FL, Brown DR. Neurohormonal regulation of ion transport in the porcine distal jejunum. Enhancement of sodium and chloride absorption by submucosal opiate receptors. *J Pharmacol Exp Ther* 1991; 256: 833–840.

Rattray M, Jordan CC, De Belleroche J. Novel CCK antagonist L364,718 abolished caerulein- but potentiates morphine-induced antinociception. *Eur J Pharmacol* 1988; 152: 163–166.

Raynor K, Kong H, Chen Y, Yasuda K, Yu L, Bell GI, Reisine T. Pharmacological characterization of the cloned kappa-, delta-, and mu-opioid receptors. *Mol Pharmacol* 1994a; 45: 330–334.

Raynor K, Kong H, Hines J, Kong G, Benovic J, Yasuda K, Bell GI, Reisine T. Molecular mechanisms of agonist-induced desensitization of the cloned mouse kappa opioid receptor. *J Pharmacol Exp Ther* 1994b; 270: 1381–1386.

Rivière PJ, Pascaud X, Chevalier E, Junien JL. Fedotozine reversal of peritoneal-irritation-induced ileus in rats: possible peripheral action on sensory afferents. *J Pharmacol Exp Ther* 1994; 270: 846–850.

Rivière PJ, Pascaud X, Chevalier E, Le Gallou B, Junien JL. Fedotozine reverses ileus induced by surgery or peritonitis: action at peripheral kappa-opioid receptors. *Gastroenterology* 1993; 104: 724–731.

Rivière PJ, Pascaud X, Junien JL, Porreca F. Neuropeptide Y and JO 1784, a selective sigma ligand, alter intestinal ion transport through a common, haloperidol-sensitive site. *Eur J Pharmacol* 1990; 187: 557–559.

Rivière PJM, Vanderak TW, Houghten R, Schteingart C, Trojnai J, Lai J, Porreca F, Junien JL. Novel D-amino and tetrapeptides demonstrate unprecedented κ-opioid receptor selectivity and antinociception. International Narcotics Research Conference (INRC) July, 1999, Saratoga, New York.

Roman F, Pascaud X, Taylor JE, Junien JL. Interactions of trimebutine with guinea-pig opioid receptors. *J Pharm Pharmacol* 1987; 39: 404–407.

Rothman RB, Bykov V, De Costa BR, Jacobson AE, Rice KC, Brady LS. Interaction of endogenous opioid peptides and other drugs with four kappa opioid binding sites in guinea pig brain. *Peptides* 1990; 11: 311–331.

Ruppin H. Loperamide—a potent antidiarrhoeal drug with actions along the alimentary tract. *Aliment Pharmacol Ther* 1987; 1: 179–190.

Schiller LR, Santa Ana CA, Morawski SG, Fordtran JS. Mechanism of the antidiarrheal effect of loperamide. *Gastroenterology* 1984; 86: 1475–1480.

Schug SA, Zech D, Grond S, Jung H, Meuser T, Stobbe B. A long-term survey of morphine in cancer pain patients. *J Pain Symptom Manage* 1992; 7: 259–266.

Sedqi M, Roy S, Ramakrishnan S, Elde R, Loh HH. Complementary DNA cloning of a mu-opioid receptor from rat peritoneal macrophages. *Biochem Biophys Res Commun* 1995; 209: 563–574.

Sedqi M, Roy S, Ramakrishnan S, Loh HH. Expression cloning of a full-length cDNA encoding delta opioid receptor from mouse thymocytes. *J Neuroimmunol* 1996; 65: 167–170.

Sengupta JN, Su X, Gebhart GF. Kappa, but not mu or delta, opioids attenuate responses to distention of afferent fibers innervating the rat colon. *Gastroenterology* 1996; 111: 968–980.

Sheldon RJ, Riviere PJ, Malarchik ME, Moseberg HI, Burks TF, Porreca F. Opioid regulation of mucosal ion transport in the mouse isolated jejunum. *J Pharmacol Exp Ther* 1990; 253: 144–151.

Shook J, Kazmierski W, Hruby V, Burks T. Precipitation of spinally mediated withdrawal signs by intrathecal administration of naloxone and the mu-receptor antagonist CTP in morphine-dependent mice. *NIDA Res Monogr* 1988; 81: 143–148.

Shook JE, Lemcke PK, Gehrig CA, Hruby VJ, Burks TF. Antidiarrheal properties of supraspinal mu and delta and peripheral mu, delta and kappa opioid receptors: inhibition of diarrhea without constipation. *J Pharmacol Exp Ther* 1989; 249: 83–90.

Simon EJ, Hiller JM, Edelman I. Stereospecific binding of the potent narcotic analgesic (3H) etorphine to rat-brain homogenate. *Proc Natl Acad Sci USA* 1973; 70: 1947–1049.

Simonin F, Befort K, Gaveriaux-Ruff C, Matthes H, Nappey V, Lannes B, Micheletti G, Kieffer B. Human delta-opioid receptor: genomic organization, cDNA cloning, functional expression, and distribution in human brain. *Mol Pharmacol* 1994; 46: 1015–1021.

Simonin F, Gaveriaux-Ruff C, Befort K, Matthes H, Lannes B, Micheletti G, et al. kappa-Opioid receptor in humans: cDNA and genomic cloning, chromosomal assignment, functional expression, pharmacology, and expression pattern in the central nervous system. *Proc Natl Acad Sci USA* 1995; 92: 7006–7010.

Singh L, Field MJ, Hunter JC, Oles RJ, Woodruff GN. Modulation of the in vivo actions of morphine by the mixed CCKA/B receptor antagonist PD 142898. *Eur J Pharmacol* 1996; 307: 283–289.

Sofuoglu M, Portoghese PS, Takemori AE. delta-Opioid receptor binding in mouse brain: evidence for heterogeneous binding sites. *Eur J Pharmacol* 1992; 216: 273–277.

Su X, Sengupta JN, Gebhart GF. Effects of kappa opioid receptor-selective agonists on responses of pelvic nerve afferents to noxious colorectal distension. *J Neurophysiol* 1997; 78: 1003–1012.

Tallent M, Dichter MA, Bell GI, Reisine T. Cloned kappa opioid receptor couples to an N-type calcium current in undifferentiated PC–12 cells. *Neuroscience* 1994; 63: 1033–1040.

Terenius L. Stereospecific interaction between narcotic analgesics and a synaptic plasma membrane fraction of rat cerebral cortex. *Acta Pharmacol Toxicol (Copenhagen)* 1973; 32: 317–320.

Thompson RC, Mansour A, Akil H, Watson SJ. Cloning and pharmacological characterization of a rat mu opioid receptor. *Neuron* 1993; 11: 903–913.

Vinayek R, Brown DR, Miller RJ. Inhibition of the antisecretory effects of [D-Ala2,D-Leu5]enkephalin in the guinea pig ileum by a selective delta opioid antagonist. *Eur J Pharmacol* 1983; 94: 159–161.

Wang JB, Imai Y, Eppler CM, Gregor P, Spivak CE, Uhl GR. mu opiate receptor: cDNA cloning and expression. *Proc Natl Acad Sci USA* 1993; 90: 10,230–10,234.

Wang JB, Johnson PS, Persico AM, Hawkins AL, Griffin CA, Uhl GR. Human mu opiate receptor. cDNA and genomic clones, pharmacologic characterization and chromosomal assignment. *FEBS Lett* 1994; 338: 217–222.

Watkins LR, Kinscheck IB, Mayer DJ. Potentiation of morphine analgesia by the cholecystokinin antagonist proglumide. *Brain Res* 1985; 327: 169–180.

Wiesenfeld-Hallin Z, Xu XJ, Hughes J, Horwell DC, Hokfelt T. PD134308, a selective antagonist of cholecystokinin type B receptor, enhances the analgesic effect of morphine and synergistically interacts with intrathecal galanin to depress spinal nociceptive reflexes. *Proc Natl Acad Sci USA* 1990; 87: 7105–7109.

Wild KD, McCormick J, Bilsky EJ, Vanderah T, McNutt RW, Chang KJ, Porreca F. Antinociceptive actions of BW373U86 in the mouse. *J Pharmacol Exp Ther* 1993; 267: 858–865.

Xie GX, Meng F, Mansour A, Thompson RC, Hoversten MT, Goldstein A, Watson SJ, Akil H. Primary structure and functional expression of a guinea pig kappa opioid (dynorphin) receptor. *Proc Natl Acad Sci USA* 1994; 91: 3779–3783.

Xu H, Lu YF, Partilla JS, Pinto J, Calderon SN, Matecka D, et al. Opioid peptide receptor studies. 8. One of the mouse brain delta(Ncx) binding sites is similar to the cloned mouse opioid delta receptor—further evidence for heterogeneity of delta opioid receptors. *Peptides* 1998; 19: 343–350.

Xu H, Ni Q, Jacobson AE, Rice KC, Rothman RB. Preliminary ligand binding data for subtypes of the delta opioid receptor in rat brain membranes. *Life Sci* 1991; 49: PL141–146.

Xu H, Partilla JS, De Costa BR, Rice KC, Rothman RB. Interaction of opioid peptides and other drugs with multiple delta ncx binding sites in rat brain: further evidence for heterogeneity. *Peptides* 1992; 13: 1207–1213.

Xu XJ, Wiesenfeld-Hallin Z, Hughes J, Horwell DC, Hokfelt T. CI988, a selective antagonist of cholecystokininB receptors, prevents morphine tolerance in the rat. *Br J Pharmacol* 1992; 105: 591–596.

Yasuda K, Raynor K, Kong H, Breder CD, Takeda J, Reisine T, Bell GI. Cloning and functional comparison of kappa and delta opioid receptors from mouse brain. *Proc Natl Acad Sci USA* 1993; 90: 6736–6740.

Yuan CS, Foss JF, O'Connor M, Toledano A, Roizen MF, Moss J. Methylnaltrexone prevents morphine-induced delay in oral-cecal transit time without affecting analgesia: a double-blind randomized placebo-controlled trial. *Clin Pharmacol Ther* 1996; 59: 469–475.

Yuan CS, Foss JF, Osinski J, Toledano A, Roizen MF, Moss J. Safety and efficacy of oral methylnaltrexone in preventing morphine-induced delay in oral-cecal transit time. *Clin Pharmacol Ther* 1997; 61: 467–475.

Zenz M, Strumpf M, Tryba M. Long-term oral opioid therapy in patients with chronic nonmalignant pain. *J Pain Symptom Manage* 1992; 7: 69–77.

Zhu J, Chen C, Xue JC, Kunapuli S, Deriel JK, Liu-Chen LY. Cloning of a human kappa opioid receptor from the brain. *Life Sci* 1995; 56: PL201–207.

Zimmerman DM, Gidda JS, Cantrell BE, Schoepp DD, Johnson BG, Leander JD. Discovery of a potent, peripherally selective trans–3,4-dimethyl–4-(3-hydroxyphenyl)piperidine opioid antagonist for the treatment of gastrointestinal motility disorders. *J Med Chem* 1994; 37: 2262–2265.

Zylicz Z, Twycross RG. Oral opioids in the treatment of cancer pain. *Neth J Med* 1991; 39: 108–114.

9 The Histamine H₃ Receptor

Pharmacotherapy Targets in Gastrointestinal Disorders

Gabriella Coruzzi, Enzo Poli,
Giuseppina Morini, and Giulio Bertaccini

CONTENTS

1. INTRODUCTION

Histamine is widely distributed in the body, although with marked quantitative differences in the various species and tissues, and it produces a variety of biological effects by interacting with specific receptors on the surface of target cells.

From: *Drug Development: Molecular Targets for GI Diseases*
Edited by: T. S. Gaginella and A. Guglietta © Humana Press Inc., Totowa, NJ

Three types of histamine receptors have so far been identified: H_1 receptors, which mediate smooth muscle contraction in the airway, gastrointestinal (GI), and genitourinary systems, and vascular muscle relaxation, and are involved in allergy and anaphylaxis; H_2 receptors, which mediate cardiac effects and the physiological increase in gastric acid secretion; and H_3 receptors, originally identified as autoreceptors in histaminergic neurons of the brain, and, subsequently, in a variety of peripheral tissues, including cardiovascular, respiratory, and GI system (Arrang et al., 1983; Schwartz et al., 1990; Bertaccini and Coruzzi, 1995). Histamine H_3 receptors differ from the other subclasses in location and function, being mostly prejunctionally located, and exerting predominantly an inhibitory control on neural and humoral mediators, including histamine itself.

Over the past few years, the biochemical and functional characterization of H_3 receptors has been a matter for extensive investigation. The major breakthrough in the histamine H_3 receptor field came with the discovery of highly selective and potent agonists and antagonists (Arrang et al., 1987; Leurs et al., 1995), which unraveled the distribution and function of this receptor subtype in different tissues. As expected from the ubiquitous location of histamine in the body, H_3 receptors have also been identified in virtually every tissue, although they are quantitatively less abundant than H_1 and H_2 receptors (Arrang et al., 1987; Korte et al., 1990). This new receptor subtype seems to have multiple cellular locations, which include neurons, enteric ganglia, paracrine and immune cells, and, in some tissues, also smooth muscle cells; therefore it might be regarded as a general regulatory system, which could be a potential target for novel therapeutic drugs.

This chapter focuses on the localization and functional role of histamine H_3 receptors in digestive functions, with particular attention to gastric acid secretion, gastroprotection, and intestinal motility.

2. GASTRIC ACID SECRETION

2.1. Functional Studies In Vitro and In Vivo

Although the first report concerning the acid secretagogue action of histamine dates back to 1920 (Popielski, 1920), the central role of histamine in the regulation of parietal cell acid secretion is a relatively recent concept, with the discovery of histamine H$_2$ receptors by the pioneering work of Black et al. (1972), which changed the old view that gastrin played the fundamental role. It is widely accepted that the stimulation of enterochromaffin-like (ECL) cells to release histamine in response to gastrin and cholinergic stimuli constitutes, in various animal species and in humans, a major stimulatory pathway for acid secretion via the parietal cell. The discovery of histamine H$_3$ receptors gave new impetus for the research in this field and the effects mediated by H$_3$ receptors on gastric acid secretion have been investigated in a variety of experimental techniques in vitro and in vivo in different animal species. The emerging picture, however, is complex, because H$_3$-mediated effects seem to depend on the species, as well as on the secretory stimulus that acts on parietal cells.

Studies carried out in conscious cats and dogs indicate that the predominant effect observed after H$_3$ receptor activation is inhibition (by approx 50%) of acid production, this effect being more evident against indirect stimuli, acting via histamine release from storing cells; the lack of inhibitory effect on direct stimuli, such as exogenous histamine, tends to rule out a location of H$_3$ receptors on parietal cells. In the dog, the inhibition of pentagastrin-induced acid secretion by the H$_3$ receptor agonist (R)α-methylhistamine was accompanied by a reduction of histamine levels in the gastrosplenic vein (Soldani et al., 1996), suggesting that these receptors are located in histamine-producing cells, and control the action of secretory pathways that involve histamine release (Fig. 1). A tonic autoinhibitory control of histamine release mediated by H$_3$ receptors is suggested by the threefold enhancement of histamine release observed with the H$_3$ antagonist, thioperamide, when low doses of pentagastrin are used (Soldani et al., 1996). Regarding the nature of the histaminocyte involved, it is well known that the location of histamine in the gastric mucosa shows considerable variation among species. Three different cell types have been identified: mast cells, ECL cells, and intramural neurons (Waldum and Sandvik, 1989). However, despite a neuronal histamine release in response to electrical stimulation, no histaminergic nerves have been found close to the secretory glands of the stomach (Håkanson and Sundler, 1991). Because mucosal mast cells have very low levels of histidine decarboxylase, and do not respond to gastrin or carbachol (Soll et al., 1988), ECL cells are the most likely source of histamine involved in the regulation of acid secretion.

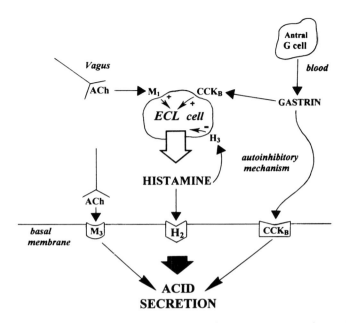

Fig. 1. Schematic model showing the effect of H_3 receptors on the excitatory pathways that control acid secretion by the parietal cell. The model is based on experimental data obtained in the dog (Soldani *et al.*, 1993; 1994; 1996). The activation of H_3 receptors with either histamine or H_3 agonists inhibit histamine release from ECL cells, in response to neural and/or hormonal activation. The inhibitory control does not involve directly parietal cell receptors. ACh, acetylcholine.

A reduction of histamine release from purified ECL cells, together with a physiological inhibitory feedback mechanism mediated by H_3 receptors, have also been detected in the rat stomach (Prinz et al., 1993; Modlin et al., 1995); however, in this species, the picture is rather intriguing. Despite the presence of this receptor subtype on ECL cells, a lack of effects of H_3 ligands on acid production has been reported, both in the isolated stomach (Sandvik et al., 1989) and in intact animals (Coruzzi et al., 1992). Other groups indicated an additional presence of H_3 receptors on fundic D-cells, where they inhibit somatostatin (SS) release (Vuyyuru and Schubert, 1997). The combined reduction in histamine and SS release, which leads to opposite influences on acid secretion, probably explains why peripheral administration of H_3

agonists in intact animals does not have any effect on acid production. The possibility that H_3 receptors regulate acid secretion by central mechanisms has been raised in a recent study (Barocelli et al., 1995).

A role for H_3 receptors in the complex regulation of ECL cell proliferation was suggested by recent findings on isolated rat ECL cells. The selective H_3 receptor agonist, imetit, stimulated gastrin-induced ECL cell proliferation, and the H_3 receptor antagonist, thioperamide, had the opposite effect (Modlin et al., 1995).

In the rabbit, evidence of the location of H_3 receptors in both ECL cells (reduction of histamine synthesis and release) and parietal cells (inhibition of cholinergic stimulation) have been reported (Badò et al., 1992a; Hollande et al., 1993). Furthermore, a negative interaction of H_3 receptors with muscarinic M_3 receptors that occurs through postreceptor mechanisms has also been postulated (Badò et al., 1995).

By contrast, H_3 receptor-mediated effects were not detected in the guinea pig isolated gastric fundus (Bertaccini and Coruzzi, 1995), probably because of the very low amounts (less than 1 fmol/mg of protein) of receptors present in the stomach of this species (Korte et al., 1990). Conversely, in the mouse, it has been reported that histamine, acting via H_3 receptors, actually augments acid secretion by eliminating the inhibitory influence of SS (Vuyyuru et al., 1997).

No functional studies concerning H_3 receptors and acid secretion are available at present in humans; however, the histamine H_3 receptor protein has been purified from the human gastric tumoral cell line HGT-1 and was found to be negatively coupled with phosphatidylinositol turnover (Cherifi et al., 1992).

A summary of the effects mediated by H_3 receptor activation in different species is reported in Tables 1 and 2. It is evident that knowledge of the contribution of H_3 receptors to the regulation of acid secretion is still fragmentary. The multiple location of these receptors on both excitatory and inhibitory pathways makes the picture very complex, at least in some species, and no definite conclusion can be drawn as to the final effect observed in humans.

2.2. H_3 Receptors and Helicobacter Pylori

It is known that *Helicobacter pylori* infection is associated with a wide spectrum of disease conditions, such as duodenal and gastric ulcer and chronic active type B gastritis, which are characterized by

Table 1
Effect of H$_3$ Receptor Activation on Gastric Acid Production

Species	Technique	Effect	Reference
Mouse	Whole stomach in vitro	↑	Vuyyuru and Schubert, 1993
	Gastric glands in vitro	0	Muller et al., 1993
Rat	Pylorus-ligated in vivo	0 (iv) ↓ (icv)	Coruzzi et al., 1992 Barocelli et al., 1995
	Lumen-perfused stomach in vivo	0	Coruzzi et al., 1992
	Vascularly-perfused stomach in vitro	0	Sandvik et al., 1989
	Gastric fundus in vitro	0	Coruzzi et al., 1992
Guinea pig	Gastric fundus in vitro	0	Bertaccini and Coruzzi, 1995
Rabbit	Parietal cells in vitro	0	Beales and Calam, 1997
	Fundic glands in vitro	↓	Badò et al., 1992a
Cat	Gastric fistula in vivo	↓ 2DG and BBS	Coruzzi et al., 1991a
	Gastric fistula and H.P.	↓ Food and PGas	Badò et al., 1991
Dog	Gastric fistula in vivo	↓ 2DG, PGas, BBS	Soldani et al., 1993
Human	Gastric cell line HGT1	↓ IP formation	Cherifi et al., 1992
	Fundic membranes	No effect on AC	Gespach et al., 1988

2DG, 2-deoxy-D-glucose; BBS, bombesin; PGas, pentagastrin. ↓, inhibition; ↑, stimulation; 0, no effect; iv, intravenous; icv, intracerebroventricular; IP, inositol phosphate; AC, adenylyl cyclase; HP, Heidenhain pouch.

completely different acid secretory states (Howden, 1996). In duodenal ulcer patients, the hypergastrinemia and the acid hypersecretion have been related to an impairment of SS-induced inhibitory effects on gastrin and ECL cells. This is supported by a study that showed a lower SS content in *H. pylori*-infected patients (Queiroz et al., 1993). Recently, it has been hypothesized that the reduced SS secretion might be caused by a histamine metabolite, N$^\alpha$-methylhistamine, which is produced by *H. pylori* (Courillon-Mallet et al., 1995). Because this methylated histamine is a potent H$_3$ receptor agonist (Trzeciakowski, 1987; Coruzzi et al., 1991b), it has been proposed that H$_3$ receptors

Table 2
Effect of H$_3$ Receptor Activation on Gastric Endocrine and Paracrine Mediators

Mediator	Effect	Species	Reference
Gastrin	0	Cat	Badò et al., 1990
	0	Dog	Soldani et al., 1993; 1994
Histamine	↑	Mouse	Vuyyuru and Schubert, 1997
	↑	Rat	Vuyyuru et al., 1997
	↓		Sandvik et al., 1989; Prinz et al., 1993 Modlin et al., 1995 Kidd et al., 1996
	↓	Rabbit	Badò et al., 1992a; Hollande et al., 1993;
	↓	Dog	Soldani et al., 1996
Somatostatin	↓	Mouse	Vuyyuru and Schubert, 1997
	↓	Rat	Badò et al., 1992b; Vuyyuru et al., 1995 Konagaya et al., 1998[a]
	↓	Dog	Vuyyuru et al., 1995
	↓	Human	Courillon-Mallet et al., 1995 Vuyyuru et al., 1995
TRH	↓	Rat	Konagaya et al., 1998[a]

0, no effect; ↑, stimulation; ↓, inhibition; [a], also H$_2$ receptors are involved.

are responsible for the reduced SS release from D-cells, and for the consequent hypergastrinemia, increased histamine release, and acid hypersecretion (Courillon-Mallet et al., 1995). This mechanism has been recently confirmed in antral segments of mouse, rat, and human stomach (Vuyyuru et al., 1995; Kaneko et al., 1997), and in conscious cat (Alchepo et al., 1996), but not in rabbit gastric mucosa (Beales and Calam, 1998).

In this respect, it must be considered that N$^\alpha$-methylhistamine could reduce acid secretion by activating H$_3$ receptors on ECL cells, which negatively control histamine synthesis and release; this might counterbalance the acid secretagogue effect caused by reduction of SS release. In keeping with this, a reduced decarboxylase activity was observed in both fundus and antrum of *H. pylori*-infected patients, and this may result from a H$_3$ receptor-mediated downregulation of tissue histamine

operated by Nα-methylhistamine produced by the bacterium (Courillon-Mallet et al., 1995). Finally, the whole picture is complicated by
the potent H_2 receptor agonistic activity of Nα-methylhistamine (Bertaccini et al., 1971), which could perhaps explain an increase in acid
secretion, independent of H_3-mediated mechanisms. Taken together,
these findings suggest that, despite the presence of a histamine-producing bacterium in the gastric mucosa (Velasquez et al., 1996), the
involvement of H_3 receptors in the acid secretory effects of *H. pylori*
needs further investigation.

3. GASTROPROTECTION

Contradictory results, indicating either that histamine protects the
gastric mucosa from an acute insult or induces lesion formation, have
been reported (Aures et al., 1982; Del Soldato, 1984; Galli et al., 1987;
Takeuchi et al., 1987). By contrast, there is ample evidence that the
selective agonist of histamine H_3 receptors, (R)α-methylhistamine, acts
exclusively in a protective manner. (R)α-methylhistamine has been
shown to reduce the severity of acute gastric mucosal damage exerted
by differently acting noxious stimuli, such as cold-restraint stress, nonsteroidal anti-inflammatory drugs (NSAIDs), and absolute or 75% ethanol in the rat (Morini et al., 1995, 1997b; Palitzsch et al., 1995; Belcheva
et al., 1997). In the different experimental models, this compound
appeared to be highly effective, and an almost complete protection has
been observed against lesions induced by the necrotizing agent, ethanol.
Histological studies supported macroscopic findings. Quantitative evaluation of the amount and depth of lesions by light microscopy empha-
sized that the extent of ethanol-induced lesions was reduced by the
H_3 agonist, from 96 to 18% of the total mucosal length examined.
Approximately 80% of the mucosa was found to be preserved in its
integrity throughout the entire thickness (Morini et al., 1997a). Moreover, the severity of gastric lesions was lessened in a similar degree
at 5 min, as well as at 60 min, after the exposure to the damaging
agent, implying that the H_3 agonist allows the mucosa to resist injury
from the time of ethanol exposure (Morini et al., 1998).

The ability of (R)α-methylhistamine to prevent absolute ethanol-
induced lesions was confirmed by light, scanning, and transmission

electron microscopic techniques (Morini et al., 1997a). (R)α-methylhis-tamine has been shown to primarily affect mucus-secreting cells; both surface mucous cells and mucous neck cells were increased in number and in volume, and the secretion of mucus was enhanced (Fig. 2). Although these modifications were just noticeable when (R)α-methyl-histamine was given in absence of noxious stimuli, they were maximized following ethanol exposure. In this latter condition, the thickness of the mucus gel layer adhering to the surface epithelium was almost doubled (Fig. 3). The increase in thickness of adherent mucus layer, a likely consequence of the increased secretory activity, cannot be viewed, however, as entirely responsible for the protective activity of (R)α-methylhistamine. Mucous cells located deep in the low pit and neck region exhibited a disproportionate ratio between the amount of stored and secreted mucus, considering that the intracellular mucus content was increased in the vast majority of mucous cells, and that secretion was observed in a lower percentage. It could be concluded that both extracellular and intracellular mucus account for the protection exerted by (R)α-methylhistamine. Mucosal defense is a complex and dynamic network of factors (Wallace and Granger, 1996), among which mucus is one of the most important. However, the possible influence of (R)α-methylhistamine on other defense levels (microcirculation and mucosal immune system) cannot be excluded, and warrants further investigation; for instance, HCO_3^- secretion was shown to be increased following (R)α-methylhistamine iv bolus in the anaesthetized rat (Coruzzi et al., 1996).

Because the bioavailability of (R)α-methylhistamine is low, espe-cially after oral administration (Garbarg et al., 1989), pharmacokinetic properties of this compound were improved by synthesizing azomethine prodrugs, which are more stable than the parent drug, being resistant to the metabolizing action of N-methyltransferase during the first pass. This leads to higher and slowly decaying plasma levels of the active compound (Krause et al., 1995). Contrary to any expectation, azometh-ine prodrugs and (R)α-methylhistamine reduced gross and histologic damage in the same dose range (Morini et al., 1996). Furthermore, protection by (R)α-methylhistamine was exerted in the same dose range irrespective of the route of administration (intragastric vs intraperitoneal route) (Morini et al., 1995). Yamasaki et al. (1994) demonstrated that the tissue : plasma concentration ratio of (R)α-methylhistamine in rat peripheral tissues is much higher than 1, suggesting the presence of a

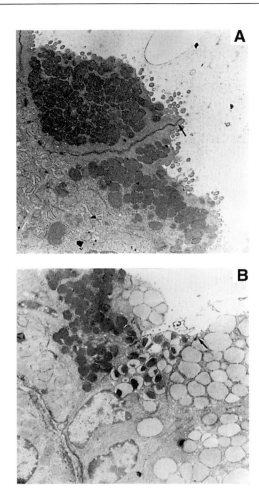

Fig. 2. Electron micrographs of gastric mucosa. (**A**) Rats received (R)α-methylhistamine, 100 mg/kg ig, followed by saline 30 min later. Stomachs were examined 1 h after saline. Surface mucous cells appear to be rich in electron-dark secretory granules in the apical part of the cell. Tight junctions (arrow) are intact (×23,000). (**B**) Rats received (R)α-methylhistamine, 100 mg/kg ig, followed by ethanol 30 min later. Stomachs were examined 1 h after ethanol. Surface mucous cells are shown. Secretory granules appear to be electron-light and enlarged in volume. An increase in the secretory activity of the cells can be derived from the increase in the development of rough endoplasmic reticulum (×10,000).

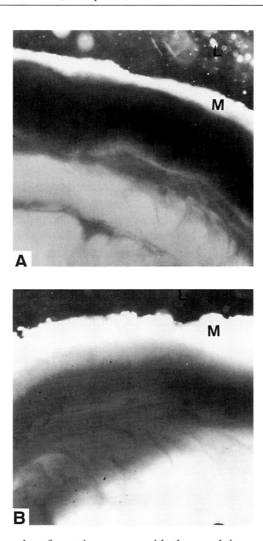

Fig. 3. Photographs of gastric mucosa with the overlying gel mucus layer (M) observed in rats receiving ethanol alone (**A**) or ethanol after a 30-min pretreatment with (R)α-methylhistamine, 100 mg/kg ig (**B**). L, gland lumen. Note the marked variation in the thickness of the surface gel layer between the two sections.

specific transport mechanism for the uptake of (R)α-methylhistamine, or a stronger binding to tissue than to plasma proteins. It is conceivable that the plasma levels of (R)α-methylhistamine are not the major factor in determining its effectiveness in the mucosal defense and that local components could participate.

The question as to whether histamine H_3 receptors mediate gastroprotection by (R)α-methylhistamine remains controversial. (R)α-methylhistamine is a selective agonist of H_3 receptors, and the protective effect exerted in the low-dose range was completely reversed by the selective H_3 receptor antagonist, thioperamide. Furthermore, H_3 receptors have been demonstrated to be stereoselective, the (S)-configured isomer of α-methylhistamine being 100× less potent than the (R)-configured isomer (Arrang et al., 1987). In keeping with this, the (S)-isomer was almost completely devoid of protective activity (G. Morini, unpublished). On the other hand, the H_3 receptor agonists, imetit and immepip, were not effective as gastroprotective agents, and thioperamide was unable to overcome the effect exerted by high doses of (R)α-methylhistamine. These contrasting findings do not allow conclusive statements about the involvement of H_3 receptors in gastroprotection.

4. GI MUCOSAL BLOOD FLOW

Changes in mucosal blood flow may be of importance in the pathophysiology of peptic ulceration, in the pathogenesis of hemorragic gastric mucosal erosions, and in other inflammatory diseases of the intestinal tract. As for other secretagogues, the increase in acid secretion induced by histamine is accompanied by an increase in gastric mucosal blood flow, which is mediated via activation of H_1 and H_2 receptors. No study so far has examined the effect of H_3 ligands on gastric vasculature. Early reports on mesenteric circulation suggest that H_3 receptors exert an inhibitory control of sympathetic nerve activity (Ishikawa and Sperelakis, 1987), which may result in vasodilatation and increase in arteriolar blood flow (Beyak and Vanner, 1995). Such a mechanism could have implications in the complex regulation of mucosal flow by endogenous histamine. This substance, in fact, produces harmful effects in the intestinal mucosa after severe or prolonged intestinal ischemia, but has a beneficial (H_1 receptor-mediated) role in the recovery of mucosal functions after mild ischemia (Fujimoto et al., 1992). More recently, the same group showed that intraperitoneal administration of the H$_3$ antagonist, thioperamide, increased histamine synthesis and release in the rat small intestine (Tsunada et al., 1994). Thus, it might be hypothesized that the blockade of H$_3$ receptors contributes to the restoration of mucosal functions in postischemic intestine, by elevating histamine levels and the degree of activation of H$_1$ receptors.

5. GI MOTILITY

5.1. Functional Studies In Vitro and In Vivo

The histaminergic control of GI motility is very complex and consists of neurally mediated, as well as direct effects on the smooth muscle contractility. Both the classical histamine receptor subtypes, H$_1$ and H$_2$, and the more recently characterized H$_3$, are involved. H$_1$ receptors mediate a direct excitatory response; H$_2$ receptors mediate neurally induced contractions and/or direct muscle relaxation (*see,* for review, Bertaccini and Coruzzi, 1992).

Studies available suggest that the H$_3$ receptor subtype is widely distributed along the GI tract of the guinea pig (Korte et al., 1990), even though marked species-related differences of localization may exist. Histamine H$_3$ receptors are mostly located on nerve terminals of the myenteric plexus, and on pre- and postganglionic cholinergic and nonadrenergic, noncholinergic (NANC) fibers, where they negatively modulate the release of excitatory neurotransmitters, such as acetylcholine and substance P (Table 3, Fig. 4). Therefore, H$_3$ receptor activation causes an attenuation of neurogenic contractions of the smooth muscle, and, possibly, of the propulsive activity of the gut.

The occurrence of histamine H$_3$ receptors in the control of intestinal motility was formerly described in the guinea pig ileum, using N$^\alpha$-methylhistamine and impromidine as agonist and antagonist, respectively (Trzeciakowski, 1987), and was later confirmed in different portions of the guinea pig gut, with the help of more specific agonists, such as (R)α-methylhistamine, imetit, and immepip, and antagonists, such as thioperamide and clobenpropit (Leurs et al., 1995). These

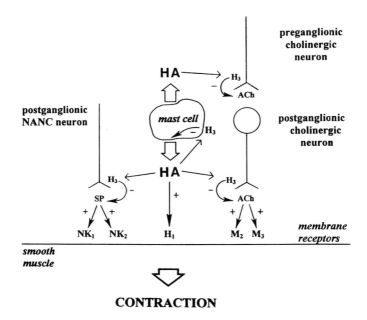

CONTRACTION

Fig. 4. Schematic model showing the role of histamine H_3 receptors in the control of GI motility. The model is based on experimental data from the literature obtained in the guinea pig. The activation of H_3 receptors by exogenous agonists or by endogenous histamine (HA), released from mast cells in response to neurogenic or immunological stimuli, inhibits pre- and postganglionic cholinergic fiber activity, as well as postganglionic nonadrenergic, noncholinergic (NANC) excitatory fibers, thus resulting in a negative modulation of neurogenic contractions of the longitudinal muscle. SP, substance P. Neurokinins other than SP may be involved.

studies were performed in electrically stimulated preparations, in isolated myenteric neurons, and in tissues preincubated with [³H]choline, in which the release of radiolabeled acetylcholine was measured (Table 3).

Several investigations also revealed that the histamine H_3 receptor antagonists, thioperamide, impromidine, and clobenpropit, increased the release of acetylcholine from the myenteric plexus (Poli et al., 1991), and the amplitude of neurogenic contractions in the isolated duodenum (Poli et al., 1997). These findings indicate the possible existence of a negative control exerted by endogenous histamine on cholinergic system activity, which could also be operative in pathophysiological conditions

Table 3
Histamine H_3 Receptor-Mediated Effects on Gastrointestinal Motility

Species	Model	Parameter	Neuron	Effect	Reference
Guinea pig	Isolated ileum	Neurogenic contractions (longitudinal)	Cholinergic	Inhibition	Trzeciakowski, 1987
	Myenteric ganglia	Postsynaptic potentials	Cholinergic	Inhibition	Tamura et al., 1988
	Isolated duodenum	Neurogenic contractions (longitudinal)	Cholinergic	Inhibition	Coruzzi et al., 1991b
	LMMP	^{3}H-Choline release	Cholinergic	Inhibition	Poli et al, 1991
	LMMP	^{3}H-Choline release	Cholinergic	Inhibition	Yau and Youther, 1993
	Isolated ileum	Neurogenic contractions (longitudinal)	Cholinergic	Inhibition	Hew et al., 1990
	Isolated ileum	Neurogenic contractions (longitudinal)	NANC	Inhibition	Taylor and Kilpatrick, 1992
	Isolated ileum	Neurogenic contractions (longitudinal)	Cholinergic, NANC	Inhibition	Leurs et al., 1991
	Isolated ileum	Neurogenic contractions	NANC	Inhibition	Leurs et al., 1991
	Isolated ileum	Neurogenic contraction (circular)	Cholinergic	Inhibition	Poli and Pozzoli, 1997
	Perfused ileum	Distension-evoked emptying waves	Cholinergic	No effect	Poli and Pozzoli, 1997
	Isolated ileum	Distension-evoked excitatory reflexes	Cholinergic, NANC	No effect	Poli and Pozzoli, 1997
	Submucous neurons	EPSP	Cholinergic	Inhibition	Cooke and Wang, 1994
	Isolated oesophagus	Vagally induced contractions	NANC	No effect	Hemedah and Mitchelson, 1997
Rat	Conscious animal	In vivo transit	Not defined (CNS)	Inhibition	Fargeas et al., 1989
Mouse	Conscious animal	In vivo transit		No effect	Oishi et al., 1993
	Conscious animal	In vivo transit		No effect	C. Pozzoli et al., unpublished
Rabbit	Conscious animal	Myoelectrical activity (colon)		No effect	Pozzoli et al., 1997
	Isolated colon	Neurogenic contractions	Cholinergic	No effect	Pozzoli et al., 1997
Man	Isolated colon	Neurogenic contractions	Cholinergic	No effect	G. Bertaccini, unpublished

LMMP, Longitudinal muscle-myenteric plexus of the ileum; NANC, nonadrenergic, noncholinergic; CNS, central nervous system; EPSP, excitatory postsynaptic potential.

253

(inflammatory states, infections, and so on) characterized by an excess of histamine synthesis and/or release from tissue stores.

Histamine H_3 receptors in the intestine undergo desensitization, when maximally stimulated in vitro by agonists like histamine or (R)α-methylhistamine, as described in the guinea pig duodenum (Coruzzi et al., 1991b), and in other areas of the guinea pig intestine, such as ileum (Perez-Garcia et al., 1998) and colon (E. Poli, unpublished). The intimate mechanism of H_3 receptor desensitization has not so far been explored; however, the short-term variation in agonist response is more likely to represent a receptor uncoupling. Phosphorylation phenomena at specific residues of the receptor moiety, typically occurring for G-protein-coupled receptor desensitization, may be involved (Perez-Garcia et al., 1998).

Despite the well-documented inhibitory effects mediated by H_3 receptors in electrically stimulated preparations, the activation of these receptors did not influence reflex-evoked peristaltic motility of the saline-perfused guinea pig ileum (Poli and Pozzoli, 1997), but a well-defined inhibitory effect in response to α$_2$-adrenoceptor and adenosine A$_1$-receptor activation has been observed. Because this model reproduces peristalsis in quasiphysiologic conditions, H_3 receptors apparently play a minor role in the control of the propulsive activity of the gut.

Contrary to what was found in the guinea pig, H_3 receptors were not found in the rabbit colon (Pozzoli et al., 1997), in either in vitro or in vivo experimental models, in which (R)α-methylhistamine, immepip, thioperamide, and clobenpropit were unable to modify spontaneous motility, and neurogenic contractions or electrical activity of the colon. In these respects, the rabbit resembles the rat, another rodent for which H_3 receptors were not detected along the whole GI tract (Bertaccini and Coruzzi, 1995). In this latter species, however, centrally located histamine H_3 receptors may act as an inhibitory control of intestinal activity (Fargeas et al., 1989), even though the exact mechanism has not been identified.

Similar to what is observed in rabbit, the H_3 receptor agonists, (R)α-methylhistamine and N^α-methylhistamine, did not modify the intestinal transit in mice, at doses thought to selectively interact with the H_3 receptor site (Oishi et al., 1993; C. Pozzoli, unpublished). At higher doses (>10–30 mg/kg sc), both drugs caused an inhibition of the intestinal transit. The inhibition induced by N^α-methylhistamine apparently reflects an activation of central inhibitory H_1 receptors (Oishi et al.,

1993), and both H_1 and H_2 receptors are responsible for the inhibitory effect of (R)α-methylhistamine (C. Pozzoli, unpublished).

Preliminary experiments, carried out on human colonic specimens removed during surgery, showed that (R)α-methylhistamine slightly reduced electrically evoked contractions, but this effect seems to be independent of histamine H_3 receptors (Bertaccini and Coruzzi, 1995). Therefore, it is still unclear whether these receptors occur in human intestine, and whether they have a physiological importance in this species.

Intestinal H_3 receptors may also exist outside the myenteric plexus. As in other tissues, such as vessels and bronchi (Oike et al., 1992; Martinez et al., 1997; Cardell and Edvinsson, 1994), postjunctional excitatory histamine H_3 receptors have been found in isolated intestinal cell suspension from longitudinal muscle (Bertaccini et al., 1998), but these receptors do not seem to influence muscular contractility in whole tissues.

Histamine H_3 receptor activation inhibits the release of 5-hydroxy-tryptamine from ECL cells in porcine small intestine (Schwörer et al., 1994), and of histamine from rat peritoneal mast cells (Kohno et al., 1994). These effects, which limit the availability of proinflammatory substances, may represent a protective mechanism known to be involved in the integrated neuroimmune modulation of motility and other visceral functions (Wood, 1992). It has been speculated that histamine released from intestinal mast cells, in response to an antigen challenge, can act on myenteric and submucosal plexus neurons to induce a slow excitatory postsynaptic potential via H_2 receptors (Wood, 1992). By contrast, the suppression of synaptic activity elicited by H_3 receptors may act as a braking mechanism that prevents H_2 receptor-mediated prolonged excitation.

Although mast cells have been implicated in hypersensitivity to rectal distention in rats, studies with H_1, H_2, and H_3 ligands indicated that histamine does not mediate the abdominal response to rectal distention in awake rats (Coelho et al., 1997).

5.2. Signal-Transducing Mechanisms

In the guinea pig duodenum, the inhibitory effect elicited by (R)α-methylhistamine on electrically evoked contractions was partially prevented by pertussis toxin, suggesting that histamine H_3 receptors are coupled to G_i/G_o proteins, as observed in the heart (Endou et al., 1994) and brain cortex (Schlicker et al., 1994b). Furthermore, H_3-receptor-mediated effects seem to be independent of cyclic adenosine monophosphate or guanosine monophosphate (Poli et al., 1993), but markedly reduced in high Ca^{2+} medium or when intracellular Ca^{2+} concentration was increased by the Ca^{2+} agonist, compound Bay K 8644 (Poli et al., 1994). Moreover, H_3 receptor-mediated effects were enhanced in low Ca^{2+} medium and in the presence of the neuronal-type Ca^{2+} channel blocker ω-conotoxin (Poli et al., 1994). Altogether, these experiments suggest that H_3-mediated inhibition of neurogenic contractions is associated with a decrease of Ca^{2+} ion access into the cholinergic axon terminal, with consequent restriction of acetylcholine release. A similar mechanism seems to be operative also in the inhibition of noradrenaline release from sympathetic nerves of the guinea pig heart (Endou et al., 1994) and mouse brain (Schlicker et al., 1994b).

Postreceptor events associated with histamine H_3 receptors closely resemble those of α_2-adrenoceptors, as pointed out in the small intestine (Poli et al., 1994) and in the heart (Endou et al., 1994). Because these receptor systems often coexist on the same nerve terminal, the possibility of presynaptic interaction in mouse brain has been raised (Schlicker et al., 1994b). However, no cooperation (either positive or negative) between H_3 receptors and α_2-adrenoceptors has been demonstrated in the guinea pig duodenum. Here, a negative cooperativity between histamine H_3 receptors and adenosine A_1 receptors has been observed (Poli et al., 1997).

5.3. Histamine H₃ Receptor Heterogeneity

West et al. (1990) proposed for the first time the existence of H_3 receptor subtypes, termed H_{3A} (high-affinity) and H_{3B} (low-affinity), which is based on the biphasic displacement of N^{α}-methylhistamine binding to rat brain homogenates by thioperamide and burimamide. According to this classification, guinea pig ileum, and mouse and rat brain cortex receptors belong to the H_{3A} subtype (Schlicker et al., 1994a; Jansen et al., 1994); those in the guinea pig sympathetic postganglionic nerve terminals belong to the H_{3B} subtype (Hey et al., 1992).

In a subsequent study (Leurs et al., 1996), the new H_3 receptor antagonist, impentamine, was found to discriminate between two functional models, acting as a competitive antagonist in the guinea pig jejunum, but as a partial agonist in the mouse brain. This suggests the existence of H_3 receptor subtypes that seem to be different from those previously proposed. The H_3 receptor mediating inhibition of 5-hydroxytriptamine release from porcine ECL cells has been shown to have a particular pharmacological profile, thus indicating that this receptor does not belong to either H_{3A} or H_{3B} subtype (Schwörer et al., 1994).

6. OTHER FUNCTIONS

There are relatively few studies concerning the role of H_3 receptors in regulating digestive functions other than acid secretion and gut motility. H_3 receptors do not seem to have any role in the regulation of electrolyte intestinal transport in the dog (Rangachari and Prior, 1994). By contrast, in the guinea pig distal colon, H_3 receptors negatively modulate chloride ion secretion by reducing neurotransmission at nicotinic synapses of the submucosal plexus (Cooke and Wang, 1994).

As for the hepatobiliary system, the only study available was carried out in isolated guinea pig and human gallbladder, and does not suggest any role for H_3 receptors in the regulation of gallbladder contractility (Jennings *et al.,* 1995; E. Poli, unpublished). Therefore, the effects induced by histamine are to be ascribed only to the activation of excitatory H_1 and inhibitory H_2 receptors (Waldman et al., 1977).

Finally, very few studies have examined the role of H_3 receptors in the control of pancreatic exocrine secretion. Histamine is distributed in the pancreas of several animal species (Lorenz et al., 1969), and has secretagogue effects mediated by H_1 and H_2 receptors located on pancreatic acinar cells (for review, *see* Bertaccini and Coruzzi, 1992). In the guinea pig pancreas, H_3 receptors are present in amounts comparable to those reported in the GI tract (Korte et al., 1990); their activation was associated with a reduction of nerve-mediated fluid and enzyme secretion (Jennings et al., 1996), and the effect was correlated with the inhibition of [³H]choline from intrinsic cholinergic neurons (Singh et al., 1997). No data are available concerning H_3 receptor-mediated effects on pancreatic blood flow, but the close association of mast cells with blood vessels would suggest a physiological role of histamine in the control of exocrine pancreatic blood flow.

7. THERAPEUTIC IMPLICATIONS

Conversely from drugs acting on histamine H_1 and H_2 receptors, no H_3 ligand has been introduced into therapy. The therapeutic potential of drugs acting on H_3 receptors in the digestive system has not been assessed. Experimental data may indicate future applications of H_3 receptor agonists in diseases characterized by excess acid secretion, or increased exposure of the gastric mucosa to noxious stimuli. However, the availability of efficacious and safe antisecretory agents, such as H_2 receptor antagonists and proton pump inhibitors, offers powerful means in the therapy of peptic ulcer disease, thus minimizing the potential application of H_3 agonists as gastric antisecretory drugs.

By contrast, the recent finding that histamine H_3 receptor agonists may have antinociceptive and anti-inflammatory actions in different experimental models (Ohkubo et al., 1995; Rouleau et al., 1997, Coruzzi and Bertaccini, 1998) may suggest novel therapeutic applications. The major limit to the use of NSAIDs, in fact, is the result of their gastro-lesive potential. H_3 receptor agonists, which combine analgesic and anti-inflammatory actions with antisecretory and gastroprotective effects, may represent the prototype of a novel class of safer NSAIDs that could spare the GI tract. This hypothesis is currently being tested in ongoing clinical trials with prodrugs of $(R)\alpha$-methylhistamine (J.C. Schwartz, personal communication). In this connection, it could be interesting to explore the potential use of H_3 ligands in intestinal inflammatory states. Mast cells have long been suggested to play a role in a variety of chronic inflammatory processes, including inflammatory bowel disease. Some human studies indicate that histamine release is increased in patients with ulcerative colitis (Nolte et al., 1990). Moreover, it has been speculated that mast cells and nerve fibers interact in determining neuronal abnormalities observed in intestinal inflammation (McKay and Bienenstock, 1994). Therefore, the inhibitory control exerted by H_3 agonists on mast cell functions could represent a novel therapeutic approach to limit excess histamine release from tissue stores.

Less encouraging results have been obtained in motility studies, considering that histamine H_3 receptors play a minor role in the regulation of intestinal motility in many species, including man. Because knowledge regarding the occurrence and distribution of these receptors in human GI tract is scanty, further experimental studies are necessary, before hypothesizing future applications of H$_3$ receptor ligands in pathological conditions characterized by deranged motility.

8. CONCLUSIONS

Apart from the primacy of histamine in the regulation of acid secretion, its physiological role in other digestive functions is less clear. There is emerging evidence, however, for a potential role of histamine as a neuro- and immunomodulator in the GI (patho)physiology.

From the available information that has been accumulating, it is clear that histamine H$_3$ receptors are located in different cell types of the GI tract, and constitute a novel inhibitory mechanism that controls the availability of neuromediators and other regulatory substances, in particular, the synthesis and/or release of histamine. This latter aspect could constitute the rationale for a therapeutic intervention, when a modulation of endogenous histamine is required. Regardless of clinical outcome, increased knowledge about the role of histamine H$_3$ receptors will accelerate the understanding of the still enigmatic role of histamine in the GI physiological and pathophysiological processes.

ACKNOWLEDGMENTS

The authors wish to thank colleagues of the Institute of Pharmacology, Maristella Adami and Cristina Pozzoli, and Giulio Soldani from the Laboratory of Veterinary Pharmacology, University of Pisa, who collaborated in the experimental work on H$_3$ receptors. This chapter is dedicated to the memory of Prof. Giulio Bertaccini.

REFERENCES

Alchepo B, Sobhani I, Moizo L, Laigneau JP, Mignon M, Labigne A, Lewin MJM, Badò, A. *Helicobacter* inhibits directly acid secretion by H$_3$ receptor mediator pathway. *Gut* 1996; 39(Suppl 3): A101.

Arrang, JM, Garbarg M, Schwartz JC. Auto-inhibition of brain histamine release mediated by a novel class (H_3) of histamine receptors. *Nature* 1983; 302: 832–837.

Arrang, JM, Garbarg M, Lancelot JC, Lecomte JM, Pollard M, Robba M, Schunack W, Schwartz JC. Highly potent and selective ligands for histamine H_3 receptors. *Nature* 1987; 327: 117–123.

Aures D, Guth PH, Paulsen G, Grossman MI. Effect of increased gastric mucosal histamine on alcohol-induced gastric damage in rats. *Dig Dis Sci* 1982; 27: 347–352.

Badò A, Dubrasquet M, Lewin MJM. Evidence of histamine H_3 receptors in the stomach: physiological role in gastric acid regulation. *Gastroenterology* 1990; 98: A17.

Badò A, Hervatin F, Lewin MJM. Pharmacological evidence for histamine H_3 receptor in the control of gastric acid secretion in cats. *Am J Physiol* 1991; 260: G631–G635.

Badò A, Laigneau JP, Moizo L, Cherifi Y, Lewin MJM. H_3-receptor activation inhibits cholinergic stimulation of acid secretion in isolated rabbit fundic glands. *J Pharmacol Exp Ther* 1995; 275: 1099–1103.

Badò A, Moizo L, Laigneau JP, Lewin MJM. Pharmacological characterization of histamine H_3 receptors in isolated rabbit gastric glands. *Am J Physiol* 1992a; 262: G56–G61.

Badò A, Moizo L, Laigneau JP, Lewin MJM. Gastrin and somatostatin secretion by isolated perfused rat stomach: regulation by the gastric histamine H_3-receptor. *Gastroenterology* 1992b; 102: A916.

Barocelli E, Ballabeni V, Chiavarini M, Impicciatore M. R-α-methylhistamine-induced inhibition of gastric acid secretion in pylorus-ligated rats via central histamine H_3 receptors. *Br J Pharmacol* 1995; 115: 1326–1330.

Beales ILP, Calam J. Effect of N^α-methyl-histamine on acid secretion in isolated cultured rabbit parietal cells: implications for *Helicobacter pylori* associated gastritis and gastric physiology. *Gut* 1997; 40: 14–19.

Beales ILP, Calam J. Histamine H_3 receptor agonist N^α-methylhistamine produced by *Helicobacter pylori* does not alter somatostatin release from cultured fundic D cells. *Gut* 1998; 43: 176–181.

Belcheva A, Marazova K, Lozeva V, Schunack W. Effects of (R)-α-methylhistamine and its prodrug BP 2.94 on gastric mucosal lesions in cold/restraint stressed rats. *Inflamm Res* 1997; 46(Suppl 1): S113–S114.

Bertaccini G, Coruzzi G. Histamine receptors in the digestive system, in *Histamine Receptor* (Schwartz JC, Haas HL, eds.), Wiley Liss, New York, pp. 193–230, 1992.

Bertaccini G, Coruzzi G. An update on histamine H_3 receptors and gastrointestinal functions. *Dig Dis Sci* 1995; 40: 2052–2063.

Bertaccini G, Impicciatore M, Mossini F. Effect of some N-substituted histamine derivatives on gastric secretion. *Naunyn Schmiedeberg's Arch Pharmacol* 1971; 269: 418.

Bertaccini G, Morini G, Coruzzi G, Schunack W. Histamine H₃ receptors in the guinea pig ileum: evidence for a postjunctional location. *J Physiol (Paris)* 1998; in press.

Beyak M, Vanner S. Histamine H₁ and H₃ vasodilator mechanisms in the guinea pig ileum. *Gastroenterology* 1995; 108: 712–718.

Black JW, Duncan W, Durant C, Ganellin CR, Parsons ME. Definition and antagonism of histamine H₂ receptors. *Nature* 1972; 236: 590–593.

Cardell LO, Edvinsson L. Characterization of the histamine receptors in the guinea-pig lung: evidence for relaxant histamine H₃ receptors in the trachea. *Br J Pharmacol* 1994; 111: 445–454.

Cherifi Y, Pigeon C, Le Romancer M, Badò A, Reyl-Desmars, F, Lewin MJM. Purification of a histamine H₃ receptor negatively coupled to phosphoinositide turnover in the human gastric cell line HGT1. *J Biol Chem* 1992; 267: 25,315–25,320.

Coehlo AM, Eeckout K, Fioramonti J, Bueno L. Histamine receptors are not involved in mast cell degranulation-induced delayed rectal allodynia in rats. *Gastroenterology* 1997; 112: A1139.

Cooke HJ, Wang YZ. H₃ receptors: modulation of histamine-stimulated neural pathways influencing electrogenic ion transport in the guinea pig colon. *J Auton Nerv Syst* 1994; 50: 201–207.

Coruzzi G, Adami M, Bertaccini G. Histamine H₃ receptors are not involved in the regulation of rat gastric secretion. *Pharmacology* 1992; 44: 190–195.

Coruzzi G, Bertaccini G. Histamine H₃ receptors mediate both gastroprotective and antiinflammatory effects. *Naunyn Schmiedeberg's Arch Pharmacol* 1998; 358(Suppl 1): R121.

Coruzzi G, Bertaccini G, Schwartz JC. Evidence that histamine H₃ receptors are involved in the control of gastric acid secretion in the conscious cat. *Naunyn Schmiedeberg's Arch Pharmacol* 1991a; 343: 225–227.

Coruzzi G, Gambarelli E, Bertaccini G. Stimulatory effect of (R)α-methylhistamine on duodenal HCO_3^- secretion in anaesthetized rats. *Ital J Gastroenterol* 1996; 28: 520–522.

Coruzzi G, Poli E, Bertaccini G. Histamine receptors in isolated guinea pig duodenal muscle: H₃ receptors inhibit cholinergic neurotransmission. *J Pharmacol Exp Ther* 1991b; 258: 325–331.

Courillon-Mallet A, Launay JM, Roucayrol AM, Callebert J, Emond JP, Tabuteau F, Cattan D. *Helicobacter pylori* infection: physiopathologic implication of Nᵅ-methylhistamine. *Gastroenterology* 1995; 108: 959–966.

Del Soldato P. Studies with specific agonists and antagonists of the role of histamine H₁- and H₂-receptor activation in the pathogenesis of gastric lesions in rats. *Agents Actions* 1984; 14: 139–142.

Endou M, Poli E, Levi R. Histamine H_3-receptor signaling in the heart: possible involvement of G_i/G_0 proteins and N-type Ca^{++} channels. *J Pharmacol Exp Ther* 1994; 269: 221–229.

Fargeas MJ, Fioramonti J, Bueno L. Involvement of different receptors in the central and peripheral effects of histamine on intestinal motility in the rat. *J Pharm Pharmacol* 1989; 41: 534–540.

Fujimoto K, Imamura I, Granger DN, Wada H, Sakata T, Tso P. Histamine and histidine decarboxylase are correlated with mucosal repair in rat small intestine after ischemia-reperfusion. *J Clin Invest* 1992; 89: 126–133.

Galli SJ, Wershil BK, Bose R, Walker PA, Szabo S. Ethanol-induced acute gastric injury in mast cell-deficient and congenic normal mice. *Am J Pathol* 1987; 128: 131–140.

Garbarg M, Trung Tuong MD, Gros C, Schwartz JC. Effects of histamine H_3-receptor ligands on various biochemical indices of histaminergic neuron activity in rat brain. *Eur J Pharmacol* 1989; 164: 1–11.

Gespach C, Fagot D, Emami S. Pharmacological control of the human gastric histamine H_2 receptor by famotidine: comparison with H_1, H_2 and H_3 receptor agonists and antagonists. *Eur J Clin Invest* 1988; 19: 1–10.

Håkanson R, Sundler F. Histamine-producing cells in the stomach and their role in the regulation of acid secretion. *Scand J Gastroenterol* 1991; 26(Suppl 180): 88–93.

Hemedah M, Mitchelson F. Comparison of the effects of histamine and N^{α}-methylhistamine on neural functions in the guinea pig oesophagus and ileum. *J Pharm Pharmacol* 1997; 49: 1217–1221.

Hew RWS, Hodgkinson CR, Hill SJ. Characterization of histamine H_3-receptors in guinea-pig ileum with H_3-selective ligands. *Br J Pharmacol* 1990; 101: 621–624.

Hey YA, Del Prado M, Egan RW, Kreutner W, Chapman RW. Inhibition of sympathetic hypertensive responses in the guinea pig by prejunctional histamine H_3 receptors. *Br J Pharmacol* 1992; 107: 347–351.

Hollande F, Bali JP, Magous R. Autoregulation of histamine synthesis through H_3 receptors in isolated fundic mucosal cells. *Am J Physiol* 1993; 265: G1039–G1044.

Howden CW. Clinical expressions of *Helicobacter pylori* infections. *Am J Med* 1996; 100: S27–S34.

Ishikawa S, Sperelakis N. Novel class (H_3) of histamine receptors on perivascular nerve terminals. *Nature* 1987; 327: 158–160.

Jansen F, Wu TS, Voss HP, Steinbusch HWM, Vollinga RC, Rademaker B, Bast A, Timmerman H. Characterization of the binding of the first selective radiolabelled histamine H_3 receptor antagonist, $[^{125}I]$-iodophenpropit, to rat brain. *Br J Pharmacol* 1994; 113: 355–362.

Jennings LJ, Salido GM, Pariente JA, Davison JS, Singh J, Sharkey KA.

Control of exocrine secretion in the guinea-pig pancreas by histamine H$_3$ receptors. *Can J Physiol Pharmacol* 1996; 74: 744–752.

Jennings LJ, Salido GM, Pozo MJ, Davison JS, Sharkey KA, Lea RW, Singh J. Source and action of histamine in the isolated guinea pig gallbladder. *Inflamm Res* 1995; 44: 447–453.

Kaneko H, Deng W, Yamamoto S, Hayakawa T, Yamashita K, Konagaya T, Kusugami K, Mitsuma T. *Helicobacter pylori*-related urease-ammonia or histamine H$_3$ receptor mediated suppression of rat gastric somatostatin release in vitro. *Gastroenterology* 1997; 112: A166.

Kidd M, Tang LH, Miu K, Lawton GP, Sandor A, Modlin IM. Autoregulation of enterochromaffin-like cell histamine secretion via the histamine 3 receptor subtype. *Yale J Biol Med* 1996; 69: 9–19.

Kohno S, Nakao S, Ogawa K, Yamamura H, Nabe T, Ohata K. Possible participation of histamine H$_3$-receptors in the regulation of anaphylactic histamine release from isolated rat peritoneal mast cells. *Jpn J Pharmacol* 1994; 66: 173–180.

Konagaya T, Kusugami K, Yamamoto H, Kaneko H, Nagai H, Mitsuma T. Effect of histamine on thyrotropin-releasing hormone and somatostatin secretion in rat stomach. *Hepato-Gastroenterology* 1998; 45: 567–572.

Korte A, Myers J, Shih NY, Egan RW, Clark MA. Characterization and tissue distribution of H$_3$ histamine receptors in guinea pigs by N$^\alpha$-methylhistamine. *Biochem Biophys Res Comm* 1990; 168: 979–986.

Krause M, Rouleau A, Stark H, Luger P, Lipp R, Garbarg M, Schwartz JC, Schunack W. Synthesis, X-ray cristallography, and pharmacokinetics of novel azomethine prodrugs of (R)-α-methylhistamine: highly potent and selective histamine H$_3$ receptor agonists. *J Med Chem* 1995; 38: 4070–4079.

Leurs R, Brozius MM, Smit MJ, Bast A, Timmerman H. Effects of histamine H$_1$-, H$_2$- and H$_3$-receptor selective drugs on the mechanical activity of guinea pig small and large intestine. *Br J Pharmacol* 1991; 102: 179–185.

Leurs R, Kathmann M, Vollinga RC, Menge WMPB, Schlicker E, Timmerman H. Histamine homologues discriminating between two functional H$_3$ receptor assays. Evidence for H$_3$ receptor heterogeneity? *J Pharmacol Exp Ther* 1996; 276: 1009–1015.

Leurs R, Smit MJ, Timmerman H. Molecular pharmacological aspects of histamine receptors. *Pharmacol Ther* 1995; 66: 413–463.

Lorenz W, Schauer A, Heitland S, Calvoer R, Werle E. Biochemical and histochemical studies on the distribution of histamine in the digestive tract of man, dog and other mammals. *Naunyn Schmiedeberg's Arch Pharmak Exp Pathol* 1969; 265: 81–100.

Martinez AC, Novella S, Raposo R, Recio P, Labadia A, Costa G. Histamine receptors in isolated bovine oviductal arteries. *Eur J Pharmacol* 1997; 326: 163–173.

McKay DM, Bienenstock J. Interaction between mast cells and nerves in the gastrointestinal tract. *Immunol Today* 1994; 15: 533–538.

Modlin IM, Lawton GP, Tang LH, Miu K, Schwartz JC. Histamine–3 receptor modulation of ECL cell histamine secretion and DNA synthesis. *Gastroenterology* 1995; 108: A992.

Morini G, Grandi D, Bertaccini G. (R)-alpha-methylhistamine inhibits ethanol-induced gastric lesions in the rat: involvement of histamine H_3 receptors? *Digestion* 1995; 56, 145–152.

Morini G, Grandi D, Bertaccini G. Comparison of the protective effect of (R)-α-methylhistamine and its prodrugs on gastric mucosal damage induced by ethanol in the rat. *Gen Pharmacol* 1996; 27: 1391–1394.

Morini G, Grandi D, Arcari ML, Galanti G, Bertaccini G. Histological effect of (R)-α-methylhistamine on ethanol damage in rat gastric mucosa. Influence on mucus production. *Dig Dis Sci* 1997a; 42: 1020–1028.

Morini G, Grandi D, Gentili S, Bertaccini G. Rapid onset of (R)-α-methylhistamine protection in response to ethanol-induced histological damage in rat gastric mucosa. *Life Sci* 1998; 62: PL13–18.

Morini G, Grandi D, Krause M, Schunack W. Gastric mucosal injury by nonsteroidal anti-inflammatory drugs is reduced by (R)-α-methylhistamine and its pro-drugs in the rat. *Inflamm Res* 1997b; 46(Suppl 1): S101–S102.

Muller MJ, Padol I, Hunt RH. Acid secretion in isolated murine gastric glands: classification of histaminergic and cholinergic receptors. *Gastroenterology* 1993; 104(Suppl): A151.

Nolte H, Spjeldnaes N, Kruse A, Windelborg B. Histamine release from gut mast cells from patients with inflammatory bowel diseases. *Gut* 1990; 31: 791–794.

Oike M, Kitamura K, Kuriyama H. Histamine H_3 receptor activation augments voltage-dependent Ca^{2+} currents via GTP hydrolysis in rabbit saphenous artery. *J Physiol (London)* 1992; 448: 133–152.

Ohkubo T, Shibata M, Inoue M, Kaya H, Takahashi H. Regulation of substance P release mediated via prejunctional histamine H_3 receptors. *Eur J Pharmacol* 1995; 273: 83–88.

Oishi R, Adachi N, Saeki K. N^α-methylhistamine inhibits intestinal transit in mice by central histamine H_1 receptor activation. *Eur J Pharmacol* 1993; 237: 155–159.

Palitzsch KD, Morales RE, Kronauge JF, Bynum TE, Szabo S. Effect of histamine on hemorrhagic mucosal lesions is related to vascular permeability in rats: studies with histamine, H_1-, H_2- and H_3-agonists and bradykinin. *Eur J Gastroenterol Hepatol* 1995; 7: 447–453.

Perez-Garcia C, Morales L, Alguacil LF. Histamine H_3 receptor desensitization in the guinea pig ileum. *Eur J Pharmacol* 1998; 341: 253–256.

Poli E, Coruzzi G, Bertaccini G. Histamine H_3 receptors regulate acetylcholine release from the guinea pig ileum myenteric plexus. *Life Sci* 1991; 48: PL63–PL68.

Poli E, Pozzoli C. Histamine H$_3$ receptors do not modulate reflex-evoked peristaltic motility in the isolated guinea-pig ileum. *Eur J Pharmacol* 1997; 327: 49–56.

Poli E, Pozzoli C, Bertaccini G. Interaction between histamine H$_3$ receptors and other prejunctional receptor systems in the isolated guinea pig duodenum. *J Pharmacol Exp Ther* 1997; 281: 393–399.

Poli E, Pozzoli C, Coruzzi G, Bertaccini G. Histamine H$_3$ receptor-mediated inhibition of duodenal cholinergic transmission is independent of intracellular cyclic AMP and GMP. *Gen Pharmacol* 1993; 24: 1273–1278.

Poli E, Pozzoli C, Coruzzi G, Bertaccini G. Signal transducing mechanisms coupled to histamine H$_3$ receptors and *alpha*–2 adrenoceptors in the guinea pig duodenum: possible involvement of N-type Ca^{++} channels. *J Pharmacol Exp Ther* 1994; 270: 788–794.

Popielski L. B-Imidazolyläthylamin und die Organextrakte. I. B-Imidazolyläthylamin als mächtiger Erreger der Magendrüsen. *Pflüegers Arch* 1920; 178: 214–236.

Pozzoli C, Poli E, Costa A, De Ponti F. Absence of histamine H$_3$ receptors in the rabbit colon: species difference. *Gen. Pharmacol* 1997; 28: 217–221.

Prinz C, Kajimura M, Scott DR, Mercier F, Helander HF, Sachs G. Histamine secretion from rat enterochromaffinlike cells. *Gastroenterology* 1993; 105: 449–461.

Queiroz DMM, Mendes EM, Rocha GA, Moura SB, Resende LMH, Barbosa AJA, et al. Effect of *Helicobacter pylori* eradication on antral gastrin and somatostatin immunoreactive cell density and gastrin and somatostatin concentrations. *Scand J Gastroenterol* 1993; 28: 858–864.

Rangachari PK, Prior T. Functional subtyping of histamine receptors on the canine proximal colonic mucosa. *J Pharmacol Exp Ther* 1994; 271: 1016–1026.

Rouleau A, Garbarg M, Ligneau X, Mantion C, Lavie P, Advenier C, et al. Bioavailability, antinociceptive and antiinflammatory properties of BP 2–94, a histamine H$_3$ receptor agonist prodrug. *J Pharmacol Exp Ther* 1997; 281: 1085–1094.

Sandvik AK, Lewin MJM, Waldum HL. Histamine release in the isolated vascularly perfused stomach of the rat: regulation by autoreceptors. *Br J Pharmacol* 1989; 96: 557–562.

Schlicker E, Kathmann M, Reidemeister S, Stark H, Schunack W. Novel histamine H$_3$ receptor antagonists: affinities in an H$_3$ receptor binding assay and potencies in two functional H$_3$ receptor models. *Br J Pharmacol* 1994a; 112: 1043–1048.

Schlicker E, Malinowska B, Kathmann M, Gothert M. Modulation of neurotransmitter release *via* histamine H₃ heteroreceptors. *Fundam Clin Pharmacol* 1994b; 8: 128–137.

Schwartz JC, Arrang JM, Garbarg M, Pollard H. Third histamine receptor subtype: characterization, localisation and functions of the H₃ receptor. *Agents Actions* 1990; 30: 13–19.

Schwörer H, Reimann A, Ramadori G, Racké K. Characterization of histamine H₃ receptors inhibiting 5-HT release from porcine enterochromaffin cells: further evidence for H₃ receptor heterogeneity. *Naunyn Schmiedeberg's Arch Pharmacol* 1994; 350: 375–379.

Singh J, Pariente JA, Salido JM. Physiological role of histamine in the exocrine pancreas. *Inflamm Res* 1997; 46: 159–165.

Soldani G, Garbarg M, Intorre L, Bertini S, Rouleau A, Schwartz JC. 1996; Modulation of pentagastrin-induced histamine release by histamine H₃ receptors in the dog. *Scand J Gastroenterol* 1996; 31: 631–638.

Soldani G, Intorre L, Bertini S, Luchetti E, Coruzzi G, Bertaccini G. Regulation of gastric acid secretion by histamine H₃ receptors in the dogs: an investigation into the site of action. *Naunyn Schmiedeberg's Arch Pharmacol* 1994; 350: 218–223.

Soldani G, Mengozzi G, Intorre L, De Giorgi G, Coruzzi G, Bertaccini G. Histamine H₃ receptor-mediated inhibition of gastric acid secretion in conscious dogs. *Naunyn Schmiedeberg's Arch Pharmacol* 1993; 347: 61–65.

Soll AH, Toome M, Culp D, Shanahan F, Beaven MA. Modulation of histamine release from canine gastric parietal cells. *Am J Physiol* 1988; 254: G40–G48.

Tamura K, Palmer JM, Wood JD. Presynaptic inhibition produced by histamine at nicotinic synapses in enteric ganglia. *Neuroscience* 1988; 25: 171–179.

Takeuchi K, Nishiwaki H, Furukawa O, Okabe S. Cytoprotective action of histamine against 0.6 *N* HCl-induced gastric mucosal injury in rats: comparative study with adaptive cytoprotection induced by exogenous acid. *Jpn J Pharmacol* 1987; 44: 335–344.

Taylor SJ, Kilpatrick GJ. Characterization of histamine-H₃ receptors controlling non-adrenergic non-cholinergic contractions of the guinea pig isolated ileum. *Br J Pharmacol* 1992; 105: 667–674.

Trzeciakowski JP. Inhibition of guinea pig ileum contractions mediated by a class of histamine receptors resembling the H₃ subtype. *J Pharmacol Exp Ther* 1987; 243: 874–880.

Tsunada S, Fujimoto K, Gotoh Y, Sakai T, Kang M, Sakata T, Granger DN, Tso P. Role of histamine receptors in intestinal repair after ischemia-reperfusion in rats. *Gastroenterology* 1994; 107: 1297–1304.

Velasquez RD, Brunner G, Varrentrapp M, Tsikas D, Frolich JC. Helicobacter pylori produces histamine and spermidine. *Z Gastroenterol* 1996; 34: 116–122.

Vuyyuru L, Harrington L, Arimura A, Schubert ML. Reciprocal inhibitory paracrine pathways link histamine and somatostatin secretion in the fundus of the stomach. *Am J Physiol* 1997; 273: G106–G111.

Vuyyuru L, Schubert ML. Participation of H$_3$-receptors of the fundus in the regulation of gastric acid secretion. *Gastroenterology* 1993; 104: A220.

Vuyyuru L, Schubert ML. Histamine, acting via H$_3$ receptors, inhibits somatostatin and stimulates acid secretion in isolated mouse stomach. *Gastroenterology* 1997; 113: 1545–1552.

Vuyyuru L, Schubert ML, Harrington L, Arimura A, Makhlouf GM. Dual inhibitory pathways link antral somatostatin and histamine secretion in human, dog, and rat stomach. *Gastroenterology* 1995; 109: 1566–1574.

Waldman DB, Zfass AM, Makhlouf GM. Stimulatory (H$_1$) and inhibitory (H$_2$) histamine receptors in gall-bladder muscle. *Gastroenterology* 1977; 72: 932–936.

Waldum HL, Sandvik AK. Histamine and the stomach. *Scand J Gastroenterol* 1989; 24: 130–139.

Wallace JL, Granger DN. Cellular and molecular basis of gastric mucosal defense. *FASEB J* 1996; 10: 731–740.

West RE, Zweig A, Shih NY, Siegel MI, Egan RW, Clark MA. Identification of two H$_3$ histamine receptor subtypes. *Mol Pharmacol* 1990; 38: 610–613.

Wood JD. Histamine signals in enteric neuroimmune interactions. *Ann NY Acad Sci* 1992; 664: 275–283.

Yau WM, Youther ML. Selective inhibition of acetylcholine release from myenteric plexus by histamine$_3$ receptor activation. *Gastroenterology* 1993; 104: A605.

Yamasaki S, Sakurai E, Hikichi N, Sakai N, Maeyama K, Watanabe T. Disposition of (R)-α-methylhistamine, a histamine H$_3$-receptor agonist, in rats. *J Pharm Pharmacol* 1994; 46: 371–374.

INDEX